Computed Tomography Imaging in 2012

Guest Editors

STEPHAN ACHENBACH, MD
TAKESHI KONDO, MD, PhD
JAGAT NARULA, MD, PhD

CARDIOLOGY CLINICS

www.cardiology.theclinics.com

Consulting Editor
MICHAEL H. CRAWFORD, MD

February 2012 • Volume 30 • Number 1

SAUNDERS an imprint of ELSEVIER, Inc.

W.B. SAUNDERS COMPANY
A Division of Elsevier Inc.

1600 John F. Kennedy Blvd. • Suite 1800 • Philadelphia, PA 19103-2899

http://www.theclinics.com

CARDIOLOGY CLINICS Volume 30, Number 1
February 2012 ISSN 0733-8651, ISBN-13: 978-1-4557-3837-3

Editor: Barbara Cohen-Kligerman
Developmental Editor: Teia Stone

Cardiology Clinics (ISSN 0733-8651) is published quarterly by Elsevier Inc., 360 Park Avenue South, New York, NY 10010-1710. Months of issue are February, May, August, and November. Business and Editorial Offices: 1600 John F. Kennedy Blvd., Ste. 1800, Philadelphia, PA 19103-2899. Customer Service Office: 3251 Riverport Lane, Maryland Heights, MO 63043. Periodicals postage paid at New York, NY and additional mailing offices. Subscription prices are $305.00 per year for US individuals, $488.00 per year for US institutions, $150.00 per year for US students and residents, $373.00 per year for Canadian individuals, $606.00 per year for Canadian institutions, $432.00 per year for international individuals, $606.00 per year for international in-stitutions and $212.00 per year for Canadian and international students/residents. To receive student/resident rate, orders must be accompanied by name of affiliated institution, data of term, and the *signature* of program/residency coordinator on institu-tion letterhead. Orders will be billed at individual rate until proof of status is received. Foreign air speed delivery is included in all *Clinics* subscription prices. All prices are subject to change without notice. **POSTMASTER:** Send address changes to *Cardiology Clinics*, Elsevier Health Sciences Division, Subscription Customer Service, 3251 Riverport Lane, Maryland Heights, MO 63043. **Customer Service: 1-800-654-2452 (U.S. and Canada); 314-447-8871 (outside U.S. and Canada). Fax: 314-447-8029. E-mail: journalscustomerservice-usa@elsevier.com (for print support); journalsonlinesupport-usa@ elsevier.com (for online support).**

Reprints. For copies of 100 or more, of articles in this publication, please contact the Commercial Reprints Department, Elsevier Inc., 360 Park Avenue South, New York, NY 10010-1710. Tel.: 212-633-3812; Fax: 212-462-1935; E-mail: reprints@elsevier.com.

Cardiology Clinics is also published in Spanish by McGraw-Hill Interamericana Editores S. A., P.O. Box 5-237, 06500, Mexico D. F., Mexico; in Portuguese by Reichmann and Alfonso Editores Rio de Janeiro, Brazil; and in Greek by Dimitrios P. Lagos, 8 Pondon Street, GR115-28 Ilissia, Greece.

Cardiology Clinics is covered in *MEDLINE/PubMed (Index Medicus)*, *Excerpta Medica*, *The Cumulative Index to Nursing and Allied Health Literature* (CINAHL).

Printed and bound by CPI Group (UK) Ltd, Croydon, CR0 4YY

Transferred to Digital Print 2012

Contributors

CONSULTING EDITOR

MICHAEL H. CRAWFORD, MD
Professor of Medicine, University of California;
Lucie Stern Chair in Cardiology and Chief of
Clinical Cardiology, University of California,
San Francisco Medical Center, San Francisco,
California

GUEST EDITORS

STEPHAN ACHENBACH, MD
Professor of Cardiology, Department
of Cardiology, University of Giessen,
Giessen, Germany

TAKESHI KONDO, MD, PhD
Department of Cardiology, Takase Clinic,
Takasaki, Japan

**JAGAT NARULA, MD, PhD, FACC,
FAHA, FRCP**
Philip J. and Harriet L. Goodhart Chair in
Cardiology, Professor of Medicine, Associate
Dean for Global Health, Mount Sinai School
of Medicine; Director, Cardiovascular Imaging
Program, Zena and Michael A. Wiener
Cardiovascular Institute and Marie-Josée and
Henry R. Kravis Center for Cardiovascular
Health, Mount Sinai School of Medicine,
New York, New York

AUTHORS

STEPHAN ACHENBACH, MD
Professor of Cardiology, Department
of Cardiology, University of Giessen,
Giessen, Germany

AMR M. AJLAN, MD, FRCPC
Department of Radiology, St Paul's Hospital,
University of British Columbia, Vancouver,
British Columbia, Canada

PAUL APFALTRER, MD
Department of Radiology and Radiological
Science, Medical University of South Carolina,
Charleston, South Carolina; Institute of Clinical
Radiology and Nuclear Medicine, University
Medical Center Mannheim, Medical Faculty
Mannheim - Heidelberg University,
Mannheim, Germany

REZA ARSANJANI, MD
Department of Imaging, Cedars-Sinai Medical
Center, Los Angeles, California

DANIEL S. BERMAN, MD
Department of Imaging, Cedars-Sinai Medical
Center; Cedars-Sinai Heart Institute,
Los Angeles, California

PHILIPP BLANKE, MD
Department of Radiology and Radiological
Science, Medical University of South Carolina,
Charleston, South Carolina; Department of
Diagnostic Radiology, University Hospital
Freiburg, Freiburg, Germany

MICHAEL K. CHEEZUM, MD
Cardiology Service, Walter Reed National
Military Medical Center, Bethesda, Maryland

ULLRICH EBERSBERGER, MD
Department of Radiology and Radiological
Science, Medical University of South Carolina,
Charleston, South Carolina; Department of
Cardiology and Intensive Care Medicine, Heart
Center Munich-Bogenhausen, Munich,
Germany

COLLIN FISCHER, MD
Cardiology Service, Walter Reed National
Military Medical Center, Bethesda, Maryland

SHINICHIRO FUJIMOTO, MD, PhD
Department of Cardiology, Takase Clinic,
Takasaki, Japan

PANKAJ GARG, MD
University of California, Irvine, California

RICHARD T. GEORGE, MD
Assistant Professor of Medicine, Director of
Outreach Cardiovascular Imaging, Division of
Cardiology, Department of Medicine, Johns
Hopkins University School of Medicine,
Baltimore, Maryland

RAMIL GOEL, MD
Mayo Clinic, Scottsdale, Arizona

ABHA GUPTA, MD
Mayo Clinic, Scottsdale, Arizona

RONEN GURVITCH, MD
Division of Cardiology, St Paul's Hospital,
University of British Columbia, Vancouver,
British Columbia, Canada

CAMERON J. HAGUE, MD
Department of Radiology, St Paul's Hospital,
University of British Columbia, Vancouver,
British Columbia, Canada

UDO HOFFMANN, MD, MPH
Cardiac MR PET CT Program, Harvard Medical
School, Massachusetts General Hospital,
Boston, Massachusetts

EDWARD A. HULTEN, MD, MPH
Non-invasive Cardiovascular Imaging
Program; Departments of Medicine and
Radiology, Brigham and Women's Hospital,
Harvard Medical School, Boston,
Massachusetts

JUHANI KNUUTI, MD
Professor; Director, Turku PET Centre,
Turku University Hospital, University of Turku,
Turku, Finland

MINISHA KOCHAR, MD
Department of Cardiology, Kaiser Permanente,
Panorama City, California

TAKESHI KONDO, MD, PhD
Department of Cardiology, Takase Clinic,
Takasaki, Japan

TROY M. LABOUNTY, MD, FSCCT
Departments of Medicine, Imaging, and
Biomedical Sciences, Cedars-Sinai Heart
Institute, Cedars-Sinai Medical Center,
Los Angeles, California

MATHIAS LANGER, MD
Department of Diagnostic Radiology,
University Hospital Freiburg, Freiburg,
Germany

JONATHON LEIPSIC, MD, FRCPC, FSCCT
Vice Chairman, Department of Radiology,
Division of Cardiology, St Paul's Hospital,
University of British Columbia, Vancouver,
British Columbia, Canada

DONALD M. LLOYD-JONES, MD, ScM
Associate Professor, Department of Preventive
Medicine, Northwestern University Feinberg
School of Medicine, Chicago, Illinois

VISHAL C. MEHRA, MD, PhD
Cardiovascular Fellow, Division of Cardiology,
Department of Medicine, Johns Hopkins
University School of Medicine, Baltimore,
Maryland

JAMES K. MIN, MD, FSCCT
Departments of Medicine, Imaging, and
Biomedical Sciences, Cedars-Sinai Heart
Institute, Cedars-Sinai Medical Center,
Los Angeles, California

KENTA MURANAKA, RT
Chief Radiological Technologist, Center for
Radiological Science, Iwate Medical University
Hospital, Morioka, Japan

JAGAT NARULA, MD, PhD, FACC, FAHA, FRCP
Philip J. and Harriet L. Goodhart Chair in Cardiology, Professor of Medicine, Associate Dean for Global Health, Mount Sinai School of Medicine; Director, Cardiovascular Imaging Program, Zena and Michael A. Wiener Cardiovascular Institute and Marie-Josée and Henry R. Kravis Center for Cardiovascular Health, Mount Sinai School of Medicine, New York, New York

TAMAR S. POLONSKY, MD, MSCI
Assistant Professor of Medicine, Section of Cardiology, Department of Medicine, University of Chicago Medical Center, Chicago, Illinois

SUBHA V. RAMAN, MD
Division of Cardiology, Department of Medicine, The Ohio State University School of Medicine, Columbus, Ohio

ANTTI SARASTE, MD
Associate Professor, Department of Medicine; Turku PET Centre, Turku University Hospital, University of Turku, Turku, Finland

ANDREAS SCHINDLER, BS
Department of Radiology and Radiological Science, Medical University of South Carolina, Charleston, South Carolina

CHRISTOPHER L. SCHLETT, MD, MPH
Cardiac MR PET CT Program, Harvard Medical School, Massachusetts General Hospital, Boston, Massachusetts

U. JOSEPH SCHOEPF, MD
Department of Radiology and Radiological Science, Medical University of South Carolina, Charleston, South Carolina

HARALD SEIFARTH, MD
Cardiac MR PET CT Program, Harvard Medical School, Massachusetts General Hospital, Boston, Massachusetts; Department of Clinical Radiology, University of Münster, Germany

LESLEE J. SHAW, PhD
Division of Cardiology, Department of Medicine, Emory University School of Medicine, Atlanta, Georgia

AHMAD M. SLIM, MD, FACC, FACP
Director, Cardiovascular Research and Assistant Professor of Medicine, Cardiology Service, San Antonio Military Medical Center, Fort Sam Houston, Texas

RYAN M. SMITH, DO
Cardiology Service, Walter Reed National Military Medical Center, Bethesda, Maryland

JEREMY J. SONG, BS
University of California, Irvine, California

RYOICHI TANAKA, MD, PhD
Assistant Professor, Division of Cardiovascular Radiology, Department of Radiology, Iwate Medical University Hospital, Morioka, Japan

QUYNH A. TRUONG, MD, MPH
Cardiac MR PET CT Program, Harvard Medical School, Massachusetts General Hospital, Boston, Massachusetts

TODD C. VILLINES, MD, FACC, FSCCT
Associate Professor of Medicine; Co-Director, Cardiac CT Program; Director of Cardiovascular Research, Walter Reed National Military Medical Center, Uniformed Services University, Bethesda, Maryland

GABRIEL VOROBIOF, MD
Memorial Heart & Vascular Institute, Long Beach Memorial Medical Center, Long Beach, California; Assistant Professor of Medicine (Cardiology), Division of Cardiology, Department of Medicine, University of California Irvine, Irvine, California

NATHAN D. WONG, PhD
University of California, Irvine, California

KUNIHIRO YOSHIOKA, MD, PhD
Associate Professor, Division of Cardiovascular Radiology, Department of Radiology, Iwate Medical University Hospital, Morioka, Japan

Contents

Cardiac computed tomography (CT) and its main clinical application, coronary CT angiography, have made major progress during the past years. Advances were driven by progress in CT hardware technology and CT image reconstruction and processing software. Technical innovations have successfully been used to lower the radiation exposure of coronary CT angiography and to improve image quality, especially in challenging situations, such as individuals with high heart rates or severe calcification. Some of the most important recent contributions have been the development of area detectors, dual-source CT, and the introduction of iterative reconstruction algorithms.

Coronary CT angiography is a rapidly growing technique that offers distinct advantages over traditional imaging techniques. However, because of rapid growth of this technique, radiation dose safety has been placed under the spotlight. There are several main determinants of total radiation dose, and these are outlined in this review. Integration of these dose-saving techniques will go a long way in maintaining diagnostic image quality and improving patient safety.

The presence of coronary artery calcium is closely associated with the presence of atherosclerotic lesions in the coronary vasculature. Detection of coronary calcium by imaging techniques has evolved over the last few decades and has become especially more sophisticated with advanced imaging technology. Whereas the status of coronary artery calcium as a marker of increased cardiovascular risk is well established, the indication for testing continues to be a topic of debate.

Measurement of traditional risk factors remains the foundation of current clinical practice guidelines when screening for coronary heart disease (CHD) risk. However, many adults who experience CHD events are not identified as higher risk based on their traditional risk factors. Observational data show that the coronary artery calcium (CAC) score improves risk prediction, even after taking into account traditional risk factors. The authors have outlined several principles of CAC testing into a list of dos and don'ts to help maximize its potential benefit while minimizing potential harm.

Coronary computed tomographic angiography (CCTA) has emerged as a novel non-invasive method for the evaluation of not only coronary artery stenosis but also arterial wall and plaque features. Recent developments in CCTA technology enable the simultaneous assessment of coronary stenosis, atherosclerotic plaque characteristics, physiologic significance of lesion-specific ischemia, and cardiac function. Through these studies, the prognostic significance of individual coronary lesions and ventricular function can be determined and used to direct therapy. Future studies are needed to establish the totality of coronary artery plaque measures that improve clinical utility.

Coronary computed tomographic angiography (CTA) is a promising noninvasive tool that allows the visualization of plaque morphology. Plaques characterized by positive remodeling, low attenuation, and napkin ring circular enhancement on contrast-enhanced coronary CTA have been regarded as rupture-prone vulnerable plaques, which account for about 60% of all vulnerable lesions and may be precursors of plaque rupture. In this article, the authors discuss the various features related to plaque morphology that are essential to detect vulnerable plaques while performing coronary CTA.

Coronary computed tomography angiography (CTA) is a highly accurate noninvasive test that is increasingly used in symptomatic patients primarily for the diagnosis of coronary artery disease (CAD). Beyond its proven accuracy, data have now clearly demonstrated the incremental prognostic information available from coronary CTA related to the presence, extent, and severity of obstructive and nonobstructive CAD across a variety of clinical settings and patient populations. Current evidence supports the use of coronary CTA not only for the diagnosis of CAD in appropriately selected symptomatic patients but also to further refine their cardiovascular risk assessment following testing.

One of the main problems in coronary angiography using 64-row computed tomography (CT) is that the presence of severe calcification interferes with the assessment of lesions, which reduces diagnostic accuracy and may even make assessment of some coronary artery segments impossible. With 320-row CT, it is possible to avoid this problem by performing subtraction coronary CT, which fully exploits the performance capabilities of the CT system. However, subtraction coronary CT has several limitations. When these limitations have been overcome, this technique is expected to become a useful method for assessing patients with severe calcification and evaluating coronary artery stents.

CT Detection of Pulmonary Embolism and Aortic Dissection   103

Philipp Blanke, Paul Apfaltrer, Ullrich Ebersberger, Andreas Schindler, Mathias Langer, and U. Joseph Schoepf

Triage of patients with acute, potentially life-threatening chest pain is one of the most daunting challenges currently facing emergency department physicians. Acute aortic syndrome and pulmonary embolism are two potentially underlying causes. For both, computed tomography has become the de facto clinical reference standard for diagnosis. This article discusses state-of-the-art computed tomography for the detection of these disorders, including recent advances and future perspectives.

Cardiac CT in the Emergency Department   117

Harald Seifarth, Christopher L. Schlett, Quynh A. Truong, and Udo Hoffmann

Current triage strategies are not effective in correctly identifying patients suffering from acute coronary syndrome (ACS). The diagnostic workup of patients presenting with acute chest pain continues to represent a major challenge for emergency department (ED) personnel. This statement holds especially true for patients with a low to intermediate likelihood for ACS. Taking current concepts for the diagnosis and management of patients presenting with acute chest pain to the ED into account, this article discusses the evidence and potential role of coronary computed tomography angiography to improve management of patients with possible ACS.

Myocardial Perfusion by CT Versus Hybrid Imaging   135

Richard T. George, Vishal C. Mehra, Antti Saraste, and Juhani Knuuti

Coronary computed tomography angiography (CTA) is a reliable diagnostic test for the anatomic diagnosis of obstructive coronary artery disease (CAD). Although coronary CTA shows high sensitivity and negative predictive value for detecting stenosis greater than or equal to 50% diameter, it is limited in its ability to diagnose myocardial ischemia. Advances in computed tomography (CT) technology alone and technology that hybridizes CT with single-photon emission CT and positron emission tomography allow for the combined anatomic and physiologic diagnosis of CAD. This article summarizes these combined technologies, emphasizing the merits and limitations of each technology and their clinical implications.

MDCT to Guide Transcatheter Aortic Valve Replacement and Mitral Valve Repair   147

Jonathon Leipsic, Cameron J. Hague, Ronen Gurvitch, Amr M. Ajlan, Troy M. Labounty, and James K. Min

Percutaneous management of valvular heart disease is becoming a reality, with multicenter trials supporting minimally invasive procedures for both aortic and mitral valve disease. Historically, the treatment of choice has been aortic valve replacement with conventional surgery for patients with severe aortic stenosis, as the prognosis of untreated patients is poor, particularly if the patient is symptomatic. Transcatheter aortic valve replacement is now available as a minimally invasive option to treat select high-risk patients with severe aortic stenosis. At present more than 30,000 procedures have been performed worldwide, mostly confined to patients at high surgical risk. The short- and medium-term outcomes have been promising.

Cardiology Clinics

READ THE CLINICS ONLINE!
Access your subscription at:
www.theclinics.com

Foreword
Update on Cardiac CT

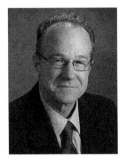

Michael H. Crawford, MD
Consulting Editor

The February 2012 issue of *Cardiology Clinics* is our latest update on cardiac CT. The first was in November of 2003 and the second in November of 2009. Thus, the time between publications has shortened by 50%, which reflects the rapid developments in this field. It is also noteworthy that this issue is truly international, with one guest editor from Europe and one from Asia. Cardiology advances now come from all over the developed world. Being American-centric no longer serves the interests of our readers or those who discover a *Clinics* article on an Internet search.

This issue covers basic technical aspects of CT technology, including radiation exposure, but most of the articles are on clinical uses for this technique. Diagnostic and prognostic uses are discussed. CT can now analyze myocardial perfusion and left ventricular performance, heretofore reserved for radionuclide imaging and MRI. Perhaps more remarkable is that CT is now being used to guide procedures such as coronary and valve interventions. As any clinician knows, CT angiography is used routinely now in emergency departments to diagnose various vascular events with great success. Perhaps we are approaching the triple cardiovascular event rule out test with CT angiography: pulmonary embolus, coronary occlusion, and aortic dissection, excluded with one contrast injection. We can certainly use CT to diagnose each individually with great accuracy. All these topics are ably discussed by the experts selected by our international guest editors.

The final article is a discussion of how to and how not to use CT imaging in coronary disease. Although it sounds like it is good for everything, there are competing technologies, some less expensive, some without radiation exposure, and some better developed for certain applications. Dr Robert Bonow takes us through the appropriate use of this technology today. This is very important in an era of cost containment in health care.

Finally, I would like to thank Drs Achenbach, Kondo, and Narula for assembling an outstanding and timely update on CT in cardiology practice.

Michael H. Crawford, MD
Division of Cardiology, Department of Medicine
University of California San Francisco Medical Center
505 Parnassus Avenue, Box 0124
San Francisco, CA 94143-0124, USA

E-mail address:
crawfordm@medicine.ucsf.edu

doi:10.1016/j.ccl.2012.01.001
0733-8651/12/$ – see front matter

Cardiac CT Imaging: Precocious Maturity?

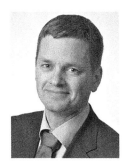 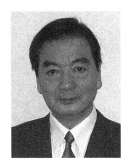 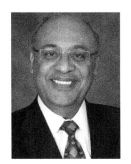

Stephan Achenbach, MD   Takeshi Kondo, MD, PhD   Jagat Narula, MD, PhD, FRCP

Guest Editors

It is not very frequently that an entirely new diagnostic modality is created to offer new possibilities and opportunities to clinicians in a short span of time. Computed tomography (CT) made its way into the cardiovascular arena approximately 10 years ago, when the first multidetector CT systems were introduced. Engineers then devised methods for synchronizing data acquisition and data reconstruction with the electrocardiograms. Much effort has focused on using CT imaging to visualize the coronary vessels, and coronary CT angiography has matured rapidly to find its way into clinical practice and a few official guidelines for selected patients. Although the emergence of coronary angiography has been the most noticeable development in the field of CT, many other innovations deserve our attention. Potential applications of CT imaging now range from left ventricular function to delayed myocardial contrast enhancement, from coronary plaque analysis to fractional flow reserve by luminal contrast gradient, and from risk stratification in primary prevention to the guidance of coronary or cardiac interventions.

To this issue of *Cardiology Clinics*, outstanding investigators have contributed state-of-the-art review articles, which on one hand illustrate the great breadth of applications of cardiac CT and on the other discuss some of the most striking recent developments. We thank the authors for their tremendous effort which has made it possible to provide you with the most current and comprehensive compendium of cardiac applications of CT imaging. We hope that you will find this issue interesting to read, useful for your practice, and as fascinating as we do, considering the rapid growth of knowledge and the swift pace at which new applications of cardiac CT are becoming available.

Stephan Achenbach, MD
University of Erlangen
Erlangen, Germany

Takeshi Kondo, MD, PhD
Takase Clinic
Takasaki, Japan

Jagat Narula, MD, PhD, FRCP
Mount Sinai School of Medicine
New York, NY, USA

E-mail addresses:
Stephan.Achenbach@uk-erlangen.de
(S. Achenbach)
tkondo@fujita-hu.ac.jp (T. Kondo)
narula@mountsinai.org (J. Narula)

Cardiol Clin 30 (2012) xiii
doi:10.1016/j.ccl.2011.12.002
0733-8651/12/$ – see front matter © 2012 Elsevier Inc. All rights reserved.

Technical Advances in Cardiac CT

Stephan Achenbach, MD[a],*, Takeshi Kondo, MD, PhD[b]

KEYWORDS

- Cardiac • Computed tomography
- Coronary CT angiography • Technological advances

Cardiac computed tomography (CT) and its main clinical application, coronary CT angiography (CTA), have made major progress during the past years. The advances were driven by 2 main factors. On one hand, clinical evaluation was performed in comparative validation studies and, more recently, numerous prospective trials and cohort studies. On the other hand, however, progress in CT technology has continuously contributed to increasing image quality and the robustness of cardiac CT. Improvements in CT imaging technology are not limited to hardware, but also include new software solutions, such as refined image reconstruction methods. Next to the progress regarding image quality, achieved through increased temporal and spatial resolution, new technologies can be used, and have been used successfully, to lower radiation exposure of cardiac CT, which is of critical importance, especially for coronary CTA. The following article outlines some of the major recent advances in cardiac CT technology and the potential clinical implications.

COMPUTED TOMOGRAPHY HARDWARE
Historical Development

The first coronary CTA procedures were performed using the electron beam computed tomography (EBCT) system, in the mid-1990s.[1,2] This system was able to acquire cross-sectional CT images without mechanical motion. Instead, X rays were created by an electron beam that could be electronically deflected and swept across stationary targets that were arranged around the patient. This system permitted a temporal resolution of 100 milliseconds per image. Image acquisition was prospectively triggered by the electrocardiogram (ECG). The system, however, was limited to single-slice acquisition, with a slice thicknesses of 1.5 to 3.0 mm and, hence, did not provide sufficient spatial resolution for reliable and detailed imaging of the coronary arteries. However, because EBCT had demonstrated the feasibility of CT-based noninvasive coronary, CTA motivated CT manufacturers to design mechanical spiral or helical CT systems that would also permit cardiac and coronary imaging. Consequently, multidetector row CT (MDCT) and retrospectively ECG-gated image reconstruction were introduced. The simultaneous acquisition of several cross-sections was the prerequisite to cover the volume of the heart with thin collimation but in a sufficiently short time to allow the completion of the image-acquisition process within a single breath hold. The first generation of MDCT systems with the ability to visualize the coronary arteries was a 4-slice CT, introduced around the year 2000. The image-acquisition process would require approximately 30 to 35 seconds, with a slice collimation of 4.0 × 1.0 mm, at gantry rotation times of 500 milliseconds (with an ensuing temporal resolution of 250 milliseconds).[3,4] In the following years, manufacturers were able to increase the number of simultaneously acquired slices and did so simultaneously, going from 4 to 16 and 64 simultaneously acquired slices (some manufacturers had iterations in between,

Conflict of interest: Stephan Achenbach has received research support and speaker honoraria from Siemens Healthcare; Takeshi Kondo has received research support from Toshiba Medical Systems.

[a] Department of Cardiology, University of Giessen, Klinikstrasse 33, 35392 Giessen, Germany
[b] Department of Cardiology, Takase Clinic, 885-2, Minami-Orui, Takasaki 370-0036, Japan
* Corresponding author.
E-mail address: stephan.achenbach@uk-erlangen.de

Cardiol Clin 30 (2012) 1–8
doi:10.1016/j.ccl.2011.11.002

such as 40-slice systems). This increase was accompanied by slight reductions in slice collimation (to 0.5–0.75 mm) and increased gantry rotation time. Overall, the effect was improved spatial resolution (thinner slice collimation), improved temporal resolution (increased gantry rotation speed), and shorter overall image-acquisition time (going from approximately 30 heartbeats for 4-slice CT to approximately 4 to 8 heartbeats for 64-slice CT). The shorter acquisition time helped to improve substantially image quality because of the shorter required breath hold (diminishing the risk of breathing artifacts) and the ability of using higher contrast-injection rates (providing better contrast between vessel lumen and surrounding tissues) without having to use unreasonably high volumes of injected contrast agent. Image quality was further enhanced by stronger tubes, which lead to reduced image noise, a parameter of major importance when imaging the coronary vessels.

Currently, 64-slice CT is regarded as the minimum required technical standard for robust clinical applications of coronary CTA.[5] Several multicenter trials have documented the diagnostic accuracy of 64-slice CT for the detection of coronary artery stenoses using retrospectively ECG-gated spiral or helical acquisition.[6–8] However, some limitations do remain. One factor is the limited temporal resolution as compared with the rapid motion of the heart and coronary arteries, especially in patients with a heart rate of more than 60 beats per minute. Another potential problem is caused by the fact that image acquisition requires several heart beats, even though the number of cardiac cycles that are required for one data set are substantially less than for 4- or 16-slice CT. Still, the image-acquisition period of 4 to 8 heartbeats incorporates some vulnerability to breathing artifacts in patients who are not fully cooperative and to the occurrence of arrhythmias or ectopic beats, which may render retrospectively ECG-gates image reconstruction inaccurate.[9]

Manufacturers have chosen different strategies to improve their products beyond the 64-slice CT. Most manufacturers increased the number of simultaneously acquired slices, which will shorten the number of heartbeats that are required to complete the acquisition of a cardiac CT data set (wide-detector CT). One manufacturer, on the other hand, designed a system that incorporates 2 x-ray tubes and detectors arranged in a 90° angulation, (dual-source CT [DSCT]). This arrangement improves the temporal resolution of the acquired images by a factor of 2.

Wide-Detector CT

Artifacts of the 64-slice multi-detector-row CT include helical artifacts, misalignment artifacts, banding artifacts, breath-hold duration, high radiation exposure caused by overlapping image acquisition, and severe impact of arrhythmias on image quality. CT systems with 256 or 320 detector rows have become available (sometimes referred to as area detectors). The width of a single detector row (collimation) is 0.5 to 0.6 mm. Hence, the systems can cover up to 160 mm in a single rotation (0.5 mm x 320.0 = 160 mm), which permits prospectively triggered axial acquisition with a stationary table and ideally covers the volume of the heart within a single cardiac cycle. The lack of slice overlap leads to low radiation exposure, and misalignment artifacts do not occur (**Fig. 1**).[10,11] Rotation time is 350 milliseconds for the 320-slice system and 275 milliseconds for the 256-slice system. Single-beat acquisition with a consequent temporal resolution of 140 to 175 milliseconds is used for patients with low heart rates. For patients with higher heart rates (typically more than 60 beats/min), image acquisition is

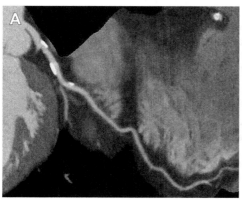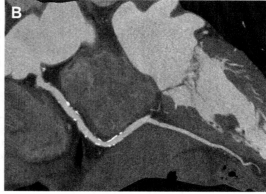

Fig. 1. Coronary CTA images acquired with the most recent CT hardware. (*A*) A 320-slice CT, (*B*) high-pitch spiral acquisition with dual-source CT.

repeated during several consecutive heartbeats to allow for multi-segment reconstruction, which leads to improved temporal resolution, which can be achieved by averaging x-ray data obtained during consecutive cardiac cycles. The resulting temporal resolution varies with the heart rate in a nonlinear fashion. Because of the ability to cover the volume of the heart, ideally in a single beat (for low heart rates) or in 2 to 3 consecutive beats (for higher heart rates), the amount of required contrast agent can be kept low.[10–13] A 1-beat acquisition would be desirable for any application of cardiac CT. It yields a data set free of step artifacts and free of artifacts caused by the averaging of several cardiac cycles. Furthermore, contrast enhancement is uniform throughout the data set, so for applications that depend on homogenous contrast enhancement, such as studies of myocardial perfusion, the conditions are ideal. Similarly, a data set recorded coherently during a single time point of the cardiac cycle may be particularly useful to flow or, as a substitute, contrast-enhancement gradients within the coronary arteries, going from proximal to distal,[14–16] but this concept has not been fully explored.

Dual-Source CT

X-ray data acquired in approximately 180° of projections are required to reconstruct one cross-sectional CT image. In conventional CT systems with 1 tube and detector (single-source CT), it is consequently necessary to collect x-ray data during a one-half rotation of the gantry for image reconstruction, and the temporal resolution per image is roughly equal to one-half of the gantry rotation time (this holds true for the center of the scan field and, in reality, it is a little more to compensate for the fan angle of the x-ray beam).

In dual-source CT (DSCT), the gantry contains not 1 but 2 x-ray tubes and 2 detectors.[17] The tubes are arranged in a 90° angle. This arrangement permits the collection of x-ray data in 180° of projections during only a quarter rotation of the gantry. Hence, temporal resolution is equal to one-quarter of the gantry rotation time and 2 times faster than that for single-source CT imaging. DSCT became available around the year 2005, with 2 × 64 simultaneously acquired slices and a rotation time of 33 milliseconds and, more recently, with 2 × 128 simultaneously acquired slices and a gantry rotation time of 0.28 seconds. This system provides for a temporal resolution of 75 milliseconds per image, independent from heart rate. Next to improved image quality for low heart rates, the higher temporal resolution as compared with single-source CT makes this technology less vulnerable to high heart rates[18,19] and some investigators suggest that heart-rate control is no longer required. One publication compared the 64-slice single-source CT coronary angiography to 2 × 64-slice DSCT and was able to demonstrate that diagnostic accuracy for stenosis detection was significantly reduced if no heart-rate control (ie, beta blocker premedication for patients with a heart rate >65/min) was used for single-source CT but not for DSCT.[20]

Recently, a new image-acquisition protocol has been described for DSCT, prospectively ECG triggered high-pitch spiral acquisition.[21–23] With a pitch of 3.4, this scan mode allows a complete image acquisition for coronary CT angiography with a time interval of approximately 250 milliseconds in a single cardiac cycle. Under the prerequisite of a low (<60 beats/min) and stable heart rate, high image quality can be achieved at very low doses (see **Fig. 1**).[24–26]

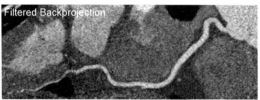

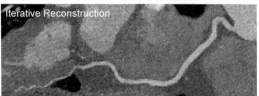

Fig. 2. Reduction of image noise through iterative reconstruction. A coronary CT angiogram was acquired using 80 kV tube voltage (effective dose, 0.32 mSv) in a patient with a body weight of 93 kg. Conventional filtered back projection (*top*) shows considerable image noise. Through iterative reconstruction (*below*), image noise can be reduced substantially.

Dual-Energy CT

Simultaneous yet separate acquisition of CT data at different energy (kilovolt) levels may have potential advantages because the x-ray absorption of elements, such as iodine, but also of physiologic material, such as kidney stones, change in a nonlinear way for varying x-ray tube voltages. The subtraction of x-ray data obtained at different energy levels may, therefore, substantially increase contrast between these materials and all surrounding structures. Dual-energy CT can be achieved by simultaneous acquisition with 2 tubes and 2 detectors (DSCT) by extremely rapid

Table 1
Comparison of the technical details of the most recent CT scanner generations

Name		Toshiba Aquilion ONE	GE Discovery CT 750HD	Siemens Definition Flash	Philips Brilliance iCT
Basic Performance	No. of detectors	320	64	64 × 2	128
	Thickness of detectors	0.5 mm	0.625 mm	0.6 mm	0.625 mm
	No. of channels	896	912	736 + 480	672
	No. of slices acquirable	640 using double-slice technology	128 using 2 energies	128 using Flying Focal	256 using Smart Focal
	Dual energy	High-speed energy switching using 1 source	High-speed energy switching using 1 source	Simultaneous exposure using dual sources	Sequential dual energy scan (dual spin)
	Gantry rotation speed	0.35 s	0.35 s	0.28 s	0.27 s
	Drive mechanism	Direct drive	Belt drive	Direct drive	Air bearing drive
	Opening size	720 mm	700 mm	780 mm	700 mm
	Tilt angle	±22°	±30°	—	—
Tube and Generator	Anode heat capacity	7.5 MHU	8.0 MHU	0.53 MHU (effective 30 MHU)	8.0 MHU (effective 30 MHU)
	Anode cooling efficiency	1.386 kHU/min	2.100 kHU/min	7.300 kHU/min	1.608 kHU/min
	Capacity	70 kW	100 kW	100 kW × 2	120 kW
	Tube voltage	80/100/120/135 kV	80/100/120/140 kV	80/100/120/140 kV	80/120/140 kV
	Tube current	10–580 mA	10–835 mA (570 mA using small focus)	20–800 mA	10–1000 mA
Computer System	Hard-disk capacity	3.8 TB	2 × 147 GB (15,000 rpm)	596 GB	1.17 TB
	Memory capacity	8 G	8 G	8 G	4 G
	Image-storage capacity	500G (800,000 images)	250,000 images	146 GB (260,000 images)	292 GB (514,000 images)
	Reconstruction	ConeXact, ConeXact+, VolumExact, VolumExact+	ASiR + 3D reconstruction	2D AMPR	3D COBRA

Image Quality				
Spatial resolution	18.0 lp/cm (MTF 0%)	21.5 lp/cm (MTF 0%)	30.0 lp/cm (MTF 0%)	24.0 lp/cm (MTF 0%)
Density resolution	2 mm/0.3%	2 mm/0.3% (90 mGy: standard, 54 mGy: ASiR)	5 mm/0.3%	4 mm/0.3%
Dose Reduction				
Software	Volume EC (SureExposure3D), Boost3D, QDS, Scan Simulator, Dose Summary, Real-time Helical recon, Flash Helical (SureCardio prospective), AIDR	Auto mA (Z-axis), Smart mA (X-Y axis), AAR Advanced Artifact Reduction, Cardiac Image Filters, Volara HD, ASiR	CARE Dose, CARE Dose4D, AAR, Adaptive Filter, Simulation of Dose, SAFIRE	DoseRight ACS, DoseRight D-DOM, DoseRight Z-DOM, iDose4
Prospective ECG gating scan	Nonhelical 1-beat volume scan	SnapShot Pulse	Adaptive Cardio Sequence, Flash Spiral	Step & Shoot Cardiac
Maximum View Rate	2572 view/s	7131 view/s	4608 view/s	3200 view/s
Pitch Factor	0.555–1.5	—	0.4–2.0 (option: 0.17)	0.04–1.5
Temporal Resolution				
Nonsector half recon	175 ms	175 ms	83 ms	135 ms
Sector (segment) reconstruction	35 ms	—	42 ms	34 ms
Phase Setting	Relative or absolute of RR	Relative of RR	Relative or absolute of RR	Beat-to-beat variable delay algorism
Bed				
Lowest position	330 mm	430 mm	480 mm	520 mm
Width	470 mm	420 mm	430 mm	410 mm
Capacity	300 kg	227 kg	220 kg	204 kg (295 kg: option)
Maximum acquisition length	1500 or 2000 mm	1700 or 2000 mm	2000 mm	1750 mm

Abbreviations: 2D, 2 dimensional; 3D, 3 dimensional; AIDR, adaptive iterative dose reduction; AMPR, axial multiplanar reconstruction; ASiR, adaptive statistical iterative reconstruction; COBRA, a commercial software package; iDose4, Philips iterative reconstruction technique; MTF, modulation transfer function; RR, R-R interval; SAFIRE: sinogram affirmed Iterative reconstruction.

switching of the emitted x-rays between different energy levels or by the design of detectors, which combine different elements with varying sensitivity to discrete kilovolt levels. Potential clinical applications in cardiovascular imaging include, for example, the improved delineation of vascular calcium (and its separation from the contrast-enhanced lumen)[27] and improved visualization of differences in myocardial contrast enhancement when myocardial perfusion is studied during exercise or at rest.[28] The full spectrum of potential clinical applications remains to be explored and validated.

SOFTWARE
Iterative Reconstruction

CT imaging is a 2-step process. First, x-ray data are acquired, and in a second step, images are reconstructed from the collected x-ray information. Both steps critically influence image quality. Image reconstruction from the numerical x-ray data has conventionally been performed by a process called filtered back projection, which does not make full use of the information contained in the x-ray data that were acquired. However, it is computationally rapid and, with currently available computer processors, allows image generation at a rate of several images per second. Iterative reconstruction is computationally more elaborate but makes more effective use of the acquired x-ray information. Improvements in computer processing power now permit the use of such algorithms for image reconstruction with reasonable computing times and they have become commercially available. Currently, these methods are applied not so much to improve the image quality of existing protocols but to reduce the noise level of low-dose acquisitions and, hence, permit coronary CTA with very low radiation exposure (**Fig. 2**). Clinical trials have demonstrated the ability to lower the dose with this method,[29,30] but applications are not yet widespread. It can be expected that substantial improvements in image-reconstruction methodology will occur in the near future, both as a consequence of further software development and as a consequence of increasing computing power.

Image Interpretation and Analysis

Next to image generation, powerful software can also be used to aid image interpretation. Software-based approaches can be used to perform morphologic image analysis, much like a physician would, or software-based algorithms can be used to extract additional information from the data set that is beyond the ability of a human reader. For morphologic image analysis, software

algorithms have become available and could theoretically act as a 24/7 expert interpreter of coronary CTA data sets for a first read, with the ability to clear rule-out cases quickly. Alternatively, they could serve as an over-read even for experienced operators, minimizing errors caused by oversight. Little data are currently available regarding the accuracy or added value of such computer programs.[31] For the identification and quantification of coronary atherosclerotic plaque, a laborious task it attempted manually, software is also available and has been validated against reference methods, such as intravascular ultrasound.[32]

An interesting aspect is the use of software-based image interpretation algorithms, which extract information from the data set that is not visible to the human reader. One example is the calculation of the gradient of contrast attenuation within a coronary artery, from the proximal segments toward the distal segments, with the underlying concept that reduced flow caused by a proximal stenosis should lead to a faster drop in contrast attenuation.[14–16] This calculation may help differentiate flow-relevant from nonrelevant lesions (even though it needs to be kept in mind that CTA data sets are acquired at rest, not under stress conditions). Another interesting approach is the use of computational flow dynamics to calculate blood flow in the coronary arteries based on the 3-dimensional anatomy provided by CT.[33] Initial data indicate that such an approach may derive the CT-based fractional flow reserve (FFR), which correlates closely to the invasively measured FFR. Although the comparison of resting CT data with invasive FFR obtained during maximum vasodilation remains a limitation, initial data show an impressive ability of CT-based FFR to improve the accuracy of coronary CTA when compared with invasively measured FFR. More than sensitivity, specificity was improved. It is reasonable to expect that software-based interpretation will become a major area of research and development in future years.

FUTURE DEVELOPMENTS

Undoubtedly, both hardware and software for cardiac CT will continue to be improved. However, it is pure speculation that improvements can be expected to become available and in what time frame this will be the case. It is important to note that many aspects are interleaved; higher temporal resolution will require stronger x-ray tubes (or more sensitive detectors) because less time is available to collect the photons for image reconstruction. Higher spatial resolution requires a substantially higher radiation dose to avoid excessive image noise.

More sensitive detectors, routine use of iterative reconstruction, or a combination of both will, hence, be the prerequisite before further improved spatial resolution can be considered (**Table 1**). Close collaboration between clinicians, imaging researchers, hardware engineers, and software developers will, hence, be necessary to guide the further development of this promising method and to make full use of its potential.

REFERENCES

1. Moshage W, Achenbach S, Seese B, et al. Coronary artery stenoses: three-dimensional imaging with electrocardiographically triggered, contrast agent-enhanced, electron beam CT. Radiology 1995;196: 707–14.

2. Schmermund A, Rensing BJ, Sheedy PF, et al. Intravenous electron-beam computed tomographic coronary angiography for segmental analysis of coronary artery stenoses. J Am Coll Cardiol 1998;31:1547–54.

3. Achenbach S, Ulzheimer S, Baum U, et al. Non-invasive coronary angiography by retrospectively ECG-gated multi-slice spiral CT. Circulation 2000;102: 2823–8.

4. Achenbach S, Giesler T, Ropers D, et al. Detection of coronary artery stenoses by contrast-enhanced, retrospectively ECG-gated, multi-slice spiral CT. Circulation 2001;103:2535–8.

5. Abbara S, Arbab-Zadeh A, Callister TQ, et al. SCCT guidelines for performance of coronary computed tomographic angiography: a report of the Society of Cardiovascular Computed Tomography Guidelines Committee. J Cardiovasc Comput Tomogr 2009;3:190–204.

6. Budoff MJ, Dowe D, Jollis JG, et al. Diagnostic performance of 64-multidetector-row coronary computed tomographic angiography for evaluation of coronary artery stenosis in individuals without known coronary artery disease. J Am Coll Cardiol 2008;52:1724–32.

7. Meijboom WB, Meijs MF, Schuijf JD, et al. Diagnostic accuracy of 64-slice computed tomography coronary angiography: a prospective, multicenter, multivendor study. J Am Coll Cardiol 2008;52: 2135–44.

8. Miller JM, Rochitte CE, Dewey M, et al. Diagnostic performance of coronary angiography by 64-row CT. N Engl J Med 2008;359:2324–36.

9. Achenbach S. Cardiac CT: state of the art for the detection of coronary arterial stenosis. J Cardiovasc Comput Tomogr 2007;1:3–20.

10. Matsutani H, Sano T, Kondo T, et al. Comparison of radiation dose reduction of prospective ECG-gated one beat scan using 320 area detector CT coronary angiography and prospective ECG-gated helical scan with high helical pitch (FlashScan) using 64

11. Weigold W, Olszewski M, Walker M. Low-dose prospectively gated 256-slice coronary computed tomographic angiography. Int J Cardiovasc Imaging 2009;25:217–30.

12. Dewey M, Zimmermann E, Deissenrieder F, et al. Noninvasive coronary angiography by 320-row computed tomography with lower radiation exposure and maintained diagnostic accuracy: comparison of results with cardiac catheterization in a head-to-head pilot investigation. Circulation 2009;120:867–75.

13. de Graaf FR, Schuijf JD, van Velzen JE, et al. Diagnostic accuracy of 320-row multidetector computed tomography coronary angiography in the non-invasive evaluation of significant coronary artery disease. Eur Heart J 2010;31:1908–15.

14. Steigner ML, Mitsouras D, Whitmore AG, et al. Iodinated contrast opacification gradients in normal coronary arteries imaged with prospectively ECG-gated single heart beat 320-detector row computed tomography. Circ Cardiovasc Imaging 2010;3:179–86.

15. Chow BJ, Kass M, Gagné O, et al. Can differences in corrected coronary opacification measured with computed tomography predict resting coronary artery flow? J Am Coll Cardiol 2011;57:1280–8.

16. Choi JH, Min JK, Labounty TM, et al. Intracoronary transluminal attenuation gradient in coronary CT angiography for determining coronary artery stenosis. JACC Cardiovasc Imaging 2011;4: 1149–57.

17. Flohr TG, McCollough CH, Bruder H, et al. First performance evaluation of a dual-source CT (DSCT) system. Eur Radiol 2006;16:256–68.

18. Ropers U, Ropers D, Pflederer T, et al. Influence of heart rate on the diagnostic accuracy of dual-source computed tomography coronary angiography. J Am Coll Cardiol 2007;50:2393–8.

19. Scheffel H, Alkadhi H, Plass A, et al. Accuracy of dual-source CT coronary angiography: first experience in a high pre-test probability population without heart rate control. Eur Radiol 2006;16:2739–47.

20. Achenbach S, Ropers U, Kuettner A, et al. Randomized comparison of 64-slice single- and dual-source computed tomography for the detection of coronary artery disease. J Am Coll Cardiol Img 2008;1:177–86.

21. Achenbach S, Marwan M, Schepis T, et al. High-pitch spiral acquisition: a new scan mode for coronary CT angiography. J Cardiovasc Comput Tomogr 2009;3:117–21.

22. Hausleiter J, Bischoff B, Hein F, et al. Feasibility of dual-source cardiac CT angiography with high-pitch scan protocols. J Cardiovasc Comput Tomogr 2009;3:236–42.

multidetector-row CT coronary angiography. Nihon Hoshasen Gijutsu Gakkai Zasshi 2010;66:1548–54 [in Japanese].

23. Lell M, Hinkmann F, Anders K, et al. High-pitch electrocardiogram-triggered computed tomography of the chest: initial results. Invest Radiol 2009;44:728–33.

24. Achenbach S, Marwan M, Ropers D, et al. Coronary computed tomography angiography with a consistent dose below 1 mSv using prospectively ECG-triggered high-pitch spiral acquisition. Eur Heart J 2010;31:340–6.

25. Alkadhi H, Stolzmann P, Desbiolles L, et al. Low-dose, 128-slice, dual-source CT coronary angiography: accuracy and radiation dose of the high-pitch and the step-and-shoot mode. Heart 2010;96:933–8.

26. Achenbach S, Goroll T, Seltmann M, et al. Detection of coronary artery stenoses by low-dose, prospectively ECG-triggered high-pitch spiral coronary CT angiography. JACC Cardiovasc Imaging 2011;4:328–37.

27. Stolzmann P, Leschka S, Scheffel H, et al. Characterization of urinary stones with dual-energy CT: improved differentiation using a tin filter. Invest Radiol 2010;45:1–6.

28. Schwarz F, Ruzsics B, Schoepf UJ, et al. Dual-energy CT of the heart–principles and protocols. Eur J Radiol 2008;68:423–33.

29. Leipsic J, Labounty TM, Heilbron B, et al. Estimated radiation dose reduction using adaptive statistical iterative reconstruction in coronary CT angiography: the ERASIR study. AJR Am J Roentgenol 2010;195:655–60.

30. Bittencourt MS, Schmidt B, Seltmann M, et al. Iterative reconstruction in image space (IRIS) in cardiac computed tomography: initial experience. Int J Cardiovasc Imaging 2011;27:1081–7.

31. Boogers MJ, Schuijf JD, Kitslaar PH, et al. Automated quantification of stenosis severity on 64-slice CT: a comparison with quantitative coronary angiography. JACC Cardiovasc Imaging 2010;3:699–709.

32. Dey D, Schepis T, Marwan M, et al. Automated three-dimensional quantification of noncalcified coronary plaque from coronary CT angiography: comparison with intravascular US. Radiology 2010;257:516–22.

33. Koo BK, Erglis A, Doh JH, et al. Diagnosis of ischemia-causing coronary stenoses by noninvasive fractional flow reserve computed from coronary computed tomographic angiograms results from the prospective multicenter DISCOVER-FLOW (Diagnosis of Ischemia-Causing Stenoses Obtained Via Noninvasive Fractional Flow Reserve) study. J Am Coll Cardiol 2011;58:1989–97.

Minimizing Radiation Dose for Coronary CT Angiography

Gabriel Vorobiof, MD[a,b,*], Stephan Achenbach, MD[c],
Jagat Narula, MD, PhD, FRCP[a,b,d]

KEYWORDS

- Coronary artery disease • Coronary CT
- Computed tomography • Radiation dose

Coronary computed tomographic angiography (CTA) allows noninvasive visualization of the coronary arteries, and, since the advent of 64-slice multidetector computed tomography scanners in 2005, it has become sufficiently robust for clinical applications. The new method is increasingly penetrating clinical practice. At the same time, the overall volume of imaging procedures, especially computed tomography (CT), in the United States has increased substantially.[1] Concerns have been raised that the increasing volume of CT examinations and the associated radiation exposure may lead to an increased incidence of malignancies.[2] Coronary CTA has been under particular scrutiny because the radiation dose of this technique can be relatively high. This is of particular concern because coronary CTA examinations are considered particularly for low-risk and often young individuals and there is even speculation about potential screening applications.[3] However, new image acquisition protocols have recently been developed to specifically reduce radiation exposure while preserving image quality. This review focuses on the available techniques to reduce the radiation exposure of coronary CTA examinations and provides specific information on the imaging protocols that can be integrated into contemporary clinical practice.

IONIZING RADIATION BACKGROUND

The general principle of contemporary CT imaging involves the use of an x-ray source rotating rapidly around a detector plate at opposite ends of a gantry wherein lies the patient. By virtue of x-ray production by the x-ray tube, CT scans are considered sources of ionizing radiation. Ionizing radiation is defined as electromagnetic radiation with sufficient energy to displace electrons from molecules with subsequent creation of ions or charged particles. Federal attention to this issue has resulted in increased oversight and plans for greater regulation of the public's exposure to medical radiation (CT, nuclear medicine, radiotherapy, and fluoroscopies).[4]

The radiation dose of CT examinations is commonly expressed in terms of 2 parameters: CT dose index (CTDI) and dose-length product (DLP) (**Table 1**). CTDI represents the integrated dose from 1 axial CT scan (1 rotation of the x-ray tube) and forms the principal measure from which all other dose estimations are derived. CTDI volume (CTDIvol) is a further measure used to describe the radiation dose. It factors in the pitch (table speed relative to gantry rotation) and represents the average radiation dose in 3 dimensions. It is typically reported in milligrays (mGy). The DLP

[a] Memorial Heart & Vascular Institute, Department of Cardiology, Long Beach Memorial Medical Center, 2801 Atlantic Avenue, Long Beach, CA 90806, USA
[b] Division of Cardiology, Department of Medicine, University of California Irvine, 101 The City Drive South Orange, Irvine, CA 92868, USA
[c] Department of Cardiology, University of Giessen, Klinikstrasse 33, 35392 Giessen, Germany
[d] Division of Cardiology, Mount Sinai School of Medicine, One Gustave L. Levy Place Box 1030, New York, NY 10029, USA
* Corresponding author. Memorial Heart & Vascular Institute, 2801 Atlantic Avenue, Long Beach, CA 90806.
E-mail address: gvorobiof@gmail.com

Cardiol Clin 30 (2012) 9–17
doi:10.1016/j.ccl.2011.11.003

Table 1
Glossary

Abbreviation	Description
Electrocardiographic tube current modulation (ECG TCM)	ECG TCM is a technique that reduces x-ray tube potential during nonessential parts of acquisition, such as systolic phases (eg, 0%–50% of the R-R interval), and optimizes it for the diastolic portions (eg, 60%–80% of the R-R interval)
CTDI	Represents the radiation dose of a single slice from the primary beam and scatter from surrounding slices
CTDIvol	A measure used to describe radiation dose factoring in pitch, which represents the average radiation dose in 3 dimensions, and is typically reported in milligrays
DLP	DLP reflects the total energy absorbed attributable to a complete CT scan acquisition and is determined by multiplying CTDIvol by the scan length in the z direction
Pitch	Pitch is a dimensionless variable and refers to the speed of the table relative to the gantry rotation speed. Pitch is therefore the amount of overlap between contiguous slabs of data
Field of view (FOV)	The predetermined area or space that is being imaged. FOV is measured in centimeters and is a function of the x-ray beam width
Slice thickness (mm)	The thickness of tissue that is being acquired and later averaged to be displayed for interpretation. This is typically analogous to the detector width on multislice CT systems

reflects the total energy absorbed attributable to a complete CT scan acquisition and is determined by multiplying CTDIvol by the scan length in the z-direction. DLP is commonly reported by all CT vendors as part of a CT imaging study. The DLP does not incorporate the type of tissue that is exposed to the radiation. However, the so-called effective dose (E, measured in millisieverts [mSv]), which pays tribute to the fact that different tissue types have different sensitivities to radiation, can be estimated based on the DLP by using anatomy-specific conversion factors (k). A conversion factor of 0.014 is often used for thoracic and cardiac CT imaging.[5] The advantage of the effective dose is that it can be used to compare radiation exposures of different imaging modalities.

The correct conversion factor to use in coronary CT has been disputed, and there are indications that a higher value may be necessary, especially in the female population.

The parameter E describes the effective dose delivered only to the volume of tissue that is being irradiated, with the tissues' radiosensitivities adjusted when incorporating the k factor. However, the radiosensitivity of tissues involved in CT varies between men and women despite a single recommended k factor for thoracic imaging without gender-specific values. Therefore, when patients differ in age, size, and shape from phantom models from which the k factor is derived, E can vary significantly.

Mean effective radiation doses are given in **Table 2** for commonly performed procedures and expressed in millisieverts (mSv).

To understand why coronary CTA may be a potential source for relatively high radiation dose studies, it is worthwhile reviewing how a coronary CTA study is acquired. Visualization of the coronary arteries is possibly the most challenging CT task because it requires both a high temporal resolution to negate the motion of the coronaries as well as high spatial resolution to differentiate small structures such as the coronaries and adjacent tissues.[6] Coronary CTA requires synchronization of both the acquisition and the reconstruction of images to the patient's cardiac cycle (a process known as cardiac gating). This is typically done by monitoring the patient's electrocardiogram via an electrocardiographic gating monitor attached to the CT machine. To obtain image datasets with the least motion artifact and because the coronaries are moving throughout the cardiac cycle, the x-ray tube needs to be turned on throughout the acquisition period (approximately 10 s for 64-slice CT). Acquisition can be achieved either via retrospective gating (acquisition throughout the patient's cardiac cycle) or through prospective triggering (turning the x-ray tube on only during preselected portions of the cardiac cycle). In addition, to obtain high-resolution images of small structures such as the coronary arteries, image noise needs to be kept

**Table 2
Mean effective radiation doses**

	Dose (mSv)
Natural environmental exposure	2–3
Commercial flight	0.005/h
CXR (posteroanterior, lateral)	0.04–0.06
Diagnostic catheterization	2–10
Percutaneous coronary intervention	25
Tl-Tl stress redistribution SPECT	22
Tl-Tc SPECT MPI	23–41
Tc-Tc SPECT MPI	15
Rubidium Rb 82 PET	12–13
Ammonia N 13 PET	2
FDG F 18 PET	7
Head CT	5
Chest CT	12
Pelvis CT	15
Coronary calcium score (EBCT)	0.8–1.3
Coronary calcium score (64-slice MDCT)	2–3
Cardiac MDCT (4 slice)	3–13
Cardiac MDCT (8 slice)	12–24
Cardiac MDCT (64 slice)	9–24
Cardiac MDCT (320 slice)	6
Prospective MDCT (64 slice)	2–3

Abbreviations: CXR, chest radiography; EBCT, electron beam CT; FDG, fludeoxyglucose; MDCT, multidetector CT; MPI, myocardial perfusion imaging; PET, positron emission tomography; SPECT, single photon emission CT; Tc, technetium; Tl, thallium.

Data from Einstein AJ, Moser KW, Thompson RC, et al. Radiation dose to patients from cardiac diagnostic imaging. Circulation 2007;116(11):1290–305. Available at: http://www.ncbi.nlm.nih.gov/pubmed/17846343.

to a minimum. This is accomplished by increases in x-ray tube voltage and tube current.

CURRENT STRATEGIES TO REDUCE RADIATION DOSE

There is a high variability of overall effective radiation doses between sites that perform coronary CTA.[7] Multiple techniques now exist to reduce overall radiation dose drastically on routine coronary CTA studies (**Table 3**). Ideally, standardized protocols for each laboratory need to be established depending on local availability of CT scanner technology and operator comfort for the routine and seamless integration of these recommendations. We recommend using a standard protocol

involving a stepwise series of measures that can be used to lower overall dose substantially.

Cardiac Gating Mode

All coronary CTA studies are done by timing the scan acquisition and subsequent image reconstruction to the patient's intrinsic cardiac rate and rhythm, a process known as cardiac gating. Two methods are currently available for acquisition of coronary CTA: retrospective gating and prospective triggering.

Retrospective acquisition has been the default technique used to date; however, it is associated with higher radiation doses because of continuous incident x-rays being generated throughout the cardiac cycle. Acquisition is achieved using a spiral method as the patient table moves within the system gantry. This affords the possibility of reconstructing data from any of the cardiac phases, thus improving diagnostic performance in situations in which suboptimal image quality is encountered because of coronary motion. Retrospective gating also affords the advantage of creating suitable cine loops for ventricular function and volume.

Prospective acquisition allows for the x-ray beam to be turned on only during predefined phases of the cardiac cycle (typically diastolic phases, eg, 65%–75%) and turns the beam off completely at all other phases.[8] Acquisition is typically accomplished sequentially in an axial orientation with stepwise motion of the table on alternating heartbeats.

An important reason for the dramatic differences in overall radiation doses between the 2 techniques is the pitch factor (pitch refers to the speed of the table relative to the gantry rotation). Retrospectively gated studies have greater slice overlap (higher pitch) with a resultant higher overall dose.

This development has led to substantial dose improvements over retrospective gating. The results of the PROTECTION III (Prospective Multicenter Study on Radiation Dose Estimates of Cardiac CT Angiography III) trial demonstrated that in 400 patients the overall radiation was reduced by 69% (3.5 vs 11.2 mSv) by sequential (prospective triggering) versus spiral acquisition (retrospective gating) modes.[9] Importantly, image quality was not different in the 2 groups. The key to successful use of low-dose strategies is aggressive control of the heart rate, which, in turn, avoids false-positive findings and reduces equivocal examinations that require further testing. A recent meta-analysis of 61 coronary CTA studies found a mean effective dose of 3.4 ± 1.4 mSv for prospectively triggered versus 9.4 ± 4.8 mSv for retrospectively acquired scans.[10] The duration of x-ray exposure during diastole (padding or pulsing

Table 3
Strategies for dose reduction

Strategy	Description	Relative Dose Reduction (%)	Pros	Cons
X-ray Source Related				
Electrocardiographically controlled tube current modulation	Modulation of x-rays during nonessential phases	25 to 48[20]	Automated, simple to set up	Reduced systolic image quality
Automated exposure control	Modulation of radiation dose based on body size and morphology	4 to 50[37]	Automated	Minimal impact on overall dose
Tube voltage	Reduction of tube voltage from 120 to 100 kV	46 to 49[7,20,38]	Robust improvements with minimal change in image noise	Not automated, obesity
Cardiac gating	Retrospective vs prospective	78[7,39]	Robust improvements with no change in image quality	Requires regular slow heart rate <65 beats per minute
Hardware (relative to a Siemens single-source 64 slice)		11 to 97 increase[7]		
Modulation of Patient Exposure				
FOV and filters	Predetermined area or space that is being imaged	Small, medium, or large FOV	Simple to select as part of standardized protocol based on patient weight	If too small, anatomic structures may be partially imaged
z-axis length	The scan length from the superior to inferior borders of the FOV	−5 for each 1-cm decrease in length[7]	Significant reductions in overall dose	Difficult to determine exactly where ideal superior-inferior borders should be in each patient
Pitch	Table speed relative to gantry rotation	Variable	Semiautomated based on chosen protocol	Small changes to pitch create large changes in radiation dose
Miscellaneous				
Bolus method	Timing bolus vs bolus tracking	Unknown	—	—
Noncontrast CT	Can be used to assess for coronary calcium score or intramural hematoma of the aorta	16[7]	A single axial slice can be used instead of bolus tracking/timing	Can provide additional prognostic information. Allows for precise determination of scan length

window) directly influences the radiation dose, such that every 100 milliseconds of additional padding increases overall radiation dose by 45%.[11] Requirements for successful prospective cardiac gating are a slow and regular heart rate (ideally, a rate <60 beats per minute and variability of <5 beats per minute). The practical aspects of narrowing the pulsing window are more challenging than the strategies previously mentioned. Certain CT manufacturers limit the maximal tube current during prospective acquisition mode, making this a suboptimal technique in large patients. An alternative form of prospective gating has been introduced that allows for helical scanning during the diastolic portion of the cardiac cycle without the need to use alternate heart beats for table motion (the patient table moves continuously throughout the study).[12]

Tube Current Modulation

Tube current is a measure of the x-ray quantity or number of photons being generated to travel across the patient. Higher tube current produces higher sampling rate with resultant better image quality and less image noise, however, at the cost of higher radiation dose. Tube current, similar to tube voltage, can be predefined by the operator before the scan is acquired. All these factors need to be assessed when prescribing tube current before acquisition in coronary CTA. Algorithms based on patient size and weight have been proposed to produce reliable and reproducible diagnostic image quality.[13]

Tube current modulation (TCM) refers to the temporal change in tube current during a CT imaging study. This can be in the form of electrocardiographic dose modulation, which is a technique that lowers the x-ray tube output during the noncritical portions of the cardiac cycle, that is, systolic phases, and maximizes tube current during the middiastolic period. The tube current can be reduced by 50% to 96% depending on the manufacturer to allow for lower-resolution nondiastolic images and higher-resolution images during diastole. These adjustments can be made before scan acquisition and tailored to individual patient requirements, including performing optimal image acquisition during systolic phases for patients with elevated heart rates. Although images acquired during lower tube current produce higher noise, these are generally sufficient for the evaluation of cardiac volume and function (ejection fraction). Depending on the chosen phases for dose modulation and degree of tube output reduction, overall radiation doses can be reduced by 50% to 60% using this technique.[14] The overall

efficiency of TCM is significantly dependent on patient heart rate because longer diastolic periods allow for higher potential dose reduction through the application of shorter pulsing intervals. The efficiency of TCM is enhanced by slow regular heart rates, and, as a result, atrioventricular nodal blockers (such as β-blockers) are recommended for enhanced radiation dose reduction.[15]

Depending on the system being used, tube current can be also varied based on patient size and patient morphology in the x, y, and z planes. Image noise is increased during portions where attenuation is highest (lateral projection through the thorax vs anteroposterior) and can vary by up to 3 orders of magnitude between the lowest and highest attenuation structures.[16] Lowering the tube current when imaging through body structures with reduced attenuation results in effective reductions in radiation dose of up to 20%. Most 64-slice CT systems use these dose modulation techniques, which, given 350-millisecond gantry rotation times, include near real-time performance. However, as long as the scan range encompasses only the heart, the overall effect on total radiation dose is expected to have minimal impact.

All conventional CT scanners come equipped with some form of TCM, and all standard coronary CTA protocols should incorporate this feature.

Scan Length

One of the principal determinants of the amount of radiation exposure during CT imaging is the craniocaudal length along the patient's longitudinal axis (z-axis). The relationship between craniocaudal scan length and effective dose is linear. There is evidence to suggest that for every 1-cm increase in z-axis length, an additional 5% effective radiation dose is delivered.[7] Routine use of a noncontrast CT for coronary artery calcium scoring is one technique that has been shown to optimize planning of scan length, which leads to an overall dose reduction of 16% (the difference between the scout-based scan length determination and calcium score–based method was 1.7 ± 0.9 mSv), even when factoring in the additional dose from the calcium score scan itself.[17] For coronary CTA imaging of patients after cardiopulmonary bypass surgery, extension of the scan length is necessary up to the lung apices superiorly to include the origin of the left or right internal mammary artery as it arises proximally from the subclavian artery. In these situations, we advocate the use of prospective triggering[14] or variable pitch techniques (if available), which can increase pitch during the noncardiac portions of the study, thereby minimizing radiation exposure.

Tube Voltage

The default tube voltage that is used in coronary CTA is 120 kV, with the option to modify this to a voltage between 80 and 140 kV. Rather counterintuitive, it is important to realize that a higher tube voltage yields images with reduced image contrast and reduced tube voltage leads to images with higher contrast. A major advantage of a higher tube voltage includes higher -quality images, that is, reduced image noise. However, this comes at the not insignificant expense of substantially higher radiation dose. The change in radiation exposure is proportional to the square root of the change in tube voltage.[18] Substantial evidence now exists that for routine coronary CTA studies performed on patients with a body mass index less than 25 to 30 kg/m^2 or body weight less than 85 to 90 kg, reducing tube voltage from 120 to 100 kV maintains diagnostic image quality while reducing radiation dose by approximately 40%.[7,19–22] Interesting work examining the effects of ionizing radiation from CT on DNA double-stranded breaks in blood lymphocytes has revealed less DNA damage at 100 kV.[23] As a result, these investigators recommend that all patients who are not overweight undergo coronary CTA with a reduced tube voltage, that is, 100 kV. This technique requires no other changes to the acquisition protocol. It is recommended to use a further reduced tube voltage of 80 kV in underweight adults and pediatric patients.[24,25]

Field of View and X-Ray Filters

All efforts should be made to narrow the field of view (FOV) when planning a coronary CTA study. In most coronary CTA studies, a small FOV (<32 cm) should be selected because this will ensure that the entire cardiac anatomy fits comfortably within the acquisition area. Selection of the FOV determines the size of the x-ray filter, known as a bow-tie filter, that is used. Bow-tie filters (named for their shape) are graphite filters effective in minimizing radiation dose by reducing x-ray variation as seen by the detector plate. This is done through a process of reducing x-rays in the center of the tube and increasing x-rays at the periphery. Other CT filters can be selected among some vendors, such as noise reducing and edge preserving filters, which can amount to at least a 25% reduction on effective radiation dose.[26,27]

Iterative reconstruction is a newly developed reconstruction technique that reduces image noise and improves low contrast detectability and image quality. Radiation dosing can be reduced by up to 40% with claims of no loss of image quality.[28] Data on this technique are limited; however, this seems to be a promising new technique to reduce radiation dose further.[29,30]

Pitch

Pitch refers to the speed of the table relative to the gantry rotation such that a pitch of 1.0 reflects contiguously acquired slabs without overlap. The default pitch for retrospectively acquired coronary CTA is 0.2, which reflects 80% overlap between individual slices, although most vendors vary the pitch automatically based on the patient's heart rate (higher pitch for higher heart rates). Varying the pitch significantly affects total radiation exposure such that changes in pitch are inversely proportional to radiation dose.

Newer CT systems have the ability to perform very high pitch (>3) spiral acquisitions in a different manner to conventional helical systems with no gaps in data through the use of dual-source coverage, faster gantry rotation, and table motion times. Acquisition occurs during the diastolic phase, and data cannot be reconstructed like traditional retrospectively gated studies. These newer systems have been shown to maintain excellent quality and reduce estimated radiation doses to submillisievert levels for routine coronary CTA studies (0.83 mSv).[31] This is at least one order of magnitude less radiation dose compared with commonly used procedures in cardiac imaging and represents a major achievement in the attempt to reduce overall patient exposure from medical imaging.

CT Scanner Hardware

CT scanner hardware continues to improve with the use of newer materials and faster gantries. There is tremendous variation in terms of the radiation dose delivered depending on the vendor-specific CT system (97% difference between the highest vs lowest dose system; 95% confidence interval, 88%–106%).[17] This effect is thought to be predominantly as a result of the scan mode and less due to the hardware itself. This argues that independent of institutional experience and protocols, there are significant hardware-related differences that have a substantial role in determining overall radiation dose.

Through the use of dual–x-ray source CT, radiation doses can be reduced compared with single-source CT, particularly at high heart rates as a result of higher pitch acquisition (>70 beats per minute).[7] In addition, dual-source CT offers the ability to perform acquisition at twice the temporal resolution of conventional single-source CT systems and possesses the ability to acquire in dual energy mode. Dual energy acquisition is primarily being investigated for iodine mapping in CT stress myocardial perfusion imaging and the ability to subtract vascular wall calcification.[5] Increasing total slice number is another approach, and the latest generation CT systems have 128-slice, 256-slice, and 320-slice detectors. In the case of 320-slice volume acquisition, the radiation dose has been shown to be 91% lower in phantom scans (when optimizing exposure control and tube current) compared with traditional helical scanning with similar image noise.[32] This improved efficiency in terms of dose savings reflects the fact that newer-generation CT systems are equipped and used in a predominantly prospectively triggered mode instead of the traditional retrospective gating. Compared with conventional coronary angiography, 320-slice CT was found to reduce the radiation dose by about half (median, 4.2 vs 8.5 mSv; $P<.05$).

Newer gemstone detector plates possess a higher efficiency, resulting in higher-quality images with better spatial resolution (0.23 mm), higher signal to noise ratio, and reduced beam-hardening artifacts. We believe that as scanner technology improves, these types of technological enhancements will continue to be used in future systems, resulting in lower patient exposure to radiation.

Other Techniques

Every center interested in performing coronary CTA imaging should work closely with their individual CT vendor to modify existing protocols to optimize and take advantage of vendor-specific dose reduction strategies. Standardized protocols that have been successfully shown to reduce radiation doses across a variety of institutions should be implemented.[7] Technologists need to have a firm understanding of basic CT radiation physics and, specifically, have undergone coronary CTA training for optimal results. Given the renewed focus on radiation safety by the US Food and Drug Administration and closer media attention, the Society of Cardiovascular Computed Tomography recommends inclusion of the radiation dose (as DLP or effective dose in millisieverts) as an optional component of the physician report of coronary CTA studies.[7] Ongoing quality control and laboratory improvement efforts should be an integral part of every active center's workflow to ensure consistency and patient safety.

LIMITATIONS

There are several ways to derive effective dose calculations, and these may vary considerably depending on the method and weighting factor used. Monte Carlo–based techniques determine specific organ doses by simulating the absorption and scattering of x-rays in various tissues using a mathematical model of the human body. Appropriate organ risk weighting factors have been published and recently updated by the International Commission on Radiological Protection (ICRP).[33,34] Therefore, several calculation methods exist for determining the effective radiation dose, and results can vary among studies depending on which method is used. Monte Carlo methods using the same weighting factors are generally in good agreement.[35] However, effective doses based on the new ICRP 103 recommendations vary considerably compared with those based on ICRP 60 because of the change in weighting factors[36]; thus careful interpretation of the results is necessary.

SUMMARY

Coronary CTA imaging is a rapidly growing technique that offers many distinct advantages over traditional cardiac imaging techniques. However, because of the rapid growth of this technique, radiation dose safety has been placed under the spotlight. There are several main determinants of total radiation dose, and these are outlined in this review. Integration of these dose-saving techniques will go a long way in maintaining diagnostic image quality and improving patient safety.

REFERENCES

1. Brenner DJ, Hall EJ. Computed tomography—an increasing source of radiation exposure. N Engl J Med 2009;357(22):2277–84. Available at: http://dx.doi.org/10.1056/NEJMra072149. Accessed October 10, 2011.
2. Einstein AJ, Henzlova MJ, Rajagopalan S. Estimating risk of cancer associated with radiation exposure from 64-slice computed tomography coronary angiography. JAMA 2007;298(3):317–23. Available at: http://jama.ama-assn.org/cgi/content/abstract/298/3/317. Accessed October 10, 2011.
3. Choi EK, Choi SI, Rivera JJ, et al. Coronary computed tomography angiography as a screening tool for the detection of occult coronary artery disease in asymptomatic individuals. J Am Coll Cardiol 2008;52(5):357–65. Available at: http://content.onlinejacc.org/cgi/content/abstract/52/5/357. Accessed October 10, 2011.
4. FDA unveils initiative to reduce unnecessary radiation exposure from medical imaging. Available at: http://www.fda.gov/newsevents/newsroom/press announcements/ucm200085.htm. Accessed October 10, 2011.

5. Einstein AJ, Moser KW, Thompson RC, et al. Radiation dose to patients from cardiac diagnostic imaging. Circulation 2007;116(11):1290–305. Available at: http://www.ncbi.nlm.nih.gov/pubmed/17846343. Accessed October 10, 2011.

6. Alkadhi H. Radiation dose of cardiac CT—what is the evidence? Eur Radiol 2009;19(6):1311–5. Available at: http://www.springerlink.com/content/j31xr42363556161. Accessed October 10, 2011.

7. Hausleiter J, Meyer T, Hermann F, et al. Estimated radiation dose associated with cardiac CT angiography. JAMA 2009;301(5):500–7. Available at: http://www.ncbi.nlm.nih.gov/pubmed/19190314. Accessed October 10, 2011.

8. Husmann L, Valenta I, Gaemperli O, et al. Feasibility of low-dose coronary CT angiography: first experience with prospective ECG-gating. Eur Heart J 2008;29(2):191–7. Available at: http://www.ncbi.nlm.nih.gov/pubmed/18089704. Accessed October 10, 2011.

9. Hausleiter J, Meyer TH, Martuscelli E, et al. Prospective randomized trial on radiation dose estimates Of CT AngIOgraphy In: PatieNts Scanned With A Sequential Scan Protocol — the PROTECTION III study. In: 5th Annual Scientific Meeting of the Society of Cardiovascular Computed Tomography. Las Vegas, NV, July 15–18, 2010.

10. Efstathopoulos EP, Pantos I, Thalassinou S, et al. Patient radiation doses in cardiac computed tomography: comparison of published results with prospective and retrospective acquisition. Radiat Prot Dosimetry 2011;1–9. Available at: http://www.ncbi.nlm.nih.gov/pubmed/21324959. Accessed October 10, 2011.

11. Labounty TM, Leipsic J, Min JK, et al. Effect of padding duration on radiation dose and image interpretation in prospectively ECG-triggered coronary CT angiography. AJR Am J Roentgenol 2010;194(4):933–7. Available at: http://www.ncbi.nlm.nih.gov/pubmed/20308494. Accessed October 10, 2011.

12. DeFrance T, Dubois E, Gebow D, et al. Helical prospective ECG-gating in cardiac computed tomography: radiation dose and image quality. Int J Cardiovasc Imaging 2010;26(1):99–107. Available at: http://www.ncbi.nlm.nih.gov/pubmed/19898955. Accessed October 10, 2011.

13. Hoang JK, Hurwitz LM, Boll DT. Optimization of tube current in coronary multidetector computed tomography angiography: assessment of a standardized method to individualize current selection based on body habitus. J Comput Assist Tomogr 2009;33(4):498–504. Available at: http://www.ncbi.nlm.nih.gov/pubmed/19638839. Accessed October 10, 2011.

14. Blanke P, Bulla S, Baumann T, et al. Thoracic aorta: prospective electrocardiographically triggered CT angiography with dual-source CT—feasibility, image quality, and dose reduction. Radiology 2010;255(1):207–17. Available at: http://radiology.rsna.org/content/255/1/207.full. Accessed October 10, 2011.

15. Jakobs TF, Becker CR, Ohnesorge B, et al. Multislice helical CT of the heart with retrospective ECG gating: reduction of radiation exposure by ECG-controlled tube current modulation. Eur Radiol 2002;12(5):1081–6. Available at: http://www.ncbi.nlm.nih.gov/pubmed/11976849. Accessed October 10, 2011.

16. Mastora I, Remy-Jardin M, Suess C, et al. Dose reduction in spiral CT angiography of thoracic outlet syndrome by anatomically adapted tube current modulation. Eur Radiol 2001;11(4):590–6. Available at: http://www.ncbi.nlm.nih.gov/pubmed/11354753. Accessed October 10, 2011.

17. Leschka S, Kim CH, Baumueller S, et al. Scan length adjustment of CT coronary angiography using the calcium scoring scan: effect on radiation dose. AJR Am J Roentgenol 2010;194(3):W272–7. Available at: http://www.ajronline.org/cgi/content/abstract/194/3/W272. Accessed October 10, 2011.

18. Abbara S, Arbab-Zadeh A, Callister TQ, et al. SCCT guidelines for performance of coronary computed tomographic angiography: a report of the Society of Cardiovascular Computed Tomography Guidelines Committee. J Cardiovasc Comput Tomogr 2009;3(3):190–204. Available at: http://www.ncbi.nlm.nih.gov/pubmed/19409872. Accessed October 10, 2011.

19. Bischoff B, Hein F, Meyer T, et al. Impact of a reduced tube voltage on CT angiography and radiation dose: results of the PROTECTION I study. JACC Cardiovasc Imaging 2009;2(8):940–6. Available at: http://www.ncbi.nlm.nih.gov/pubmed/19679281. Accessed October 10, 2011.

20. Raff GL, Chinnaiyan KM, Share DA, et al. Radiation dose from cardiac computed tomography before and after implementation of radiation dose-reduction techniques. JAMA 2009;301(22):2340–8. Available at: http://www.ncbi.nlm.nih.gov/pubmed/19509381. Accessed October 10, 2011.

21. Pflederer T, Rudofsky L, Ropers D, et al. Image quality in a low radiation exposure protocol for retrospectively ECG-gated coronary CT angiography. AJR Am J Roentgenol 2009;192(4):1045–50. Available at: http://www.ajronline.org/cgi/content/abstract/192/4/1045. Accessed October 10, 2011.

22. Feuchtner GM, Jodocy D, Klauser A, et al. Radiation dose reduction by using 100-kV tube voltage in cardiac 64-slice computed tomography: a comparative study. Eur J Radiol 2010;75(1):e51–6. Available at: http://www.sciencedirect.com/science/article/B6T6F-4WYNCVR-2/2/435251cf9a285976c7fd704f43d93368. Accessed October 10, 2011.

23. Kuefner MA, Anders K, Achenbach S, et al. Effect of CT scan protocols on x-ray induced DNA double-strand

breaks in blood lymphocytes of patients undergoing coronary CT angiography. In: 5th Annual Scientific Meeting of the Society of Cardiovascular Computed Tomography. Las Vegas, NV, July 15–18, 2010.

24. Herzog C, Mulvihill DM, Nguyen SA, et al. Pediatric cardiovascular CT angiography: radiation dose reduction using automatic anatomic tube current modulation. AJR Am J Roentgenol 2008;190(5): 1232–40. Available at: http://www.ajronline.org/cgi/content/abstract/190/5/1232. Accessed October 10, 2011.

25. Suess C, Chen X. Dose optimization in pediatric CT: current technology and future innovations. Pediatr Radiol 2002;32(10):729–34. DOI:10.1007/s00247-002-0800-x. Available at: http://dx.doi.org/10.1007/s00247-002-0800-x. Accessed October 10, 2011.

26. Wessling J, Esseling R, Raupach R, et al. The effect of dose reduction and feasibility of edge-preserving noise reduction on the detection of liver lesions using MSCT. Eur Radiol 2007;17(7):1885–91. Available at: http://www.springerlink.com/content/n03326847hp45378. Accessed October 10, 2011.

27. Kakeda S, Korogi Y, Ogawa M, et al. Reduction of the radiation dose for multidetector row CT angiography of cerebral aneurysms using an edge-preserving adaptive filter: a vascular phantom study. AJNR Am J Neuroradiol 2010;31(5):827–9. Available at: http://www.ajnr.org/cgi/content/abstract/31/5/827. Accessed October 10, 2011.

28. Hara AK, Paden RG, Silva AC, et al. Iterative reconstruction technique for reducing body radiation dose at CT: feasibility study. AJR Am J Roentgenol 2009; 193(3):764–71. Available at: http://www.ncbi.nlm.nih.gov/pubmed/19696291. Accessed October 10, 2011.

29. Heilbron BG, Leipsic J. Submillisievert coronary computed tomography angiography using adaptive statistical iterative reconstruction—a new reality. Can J Cardiol 2010;26(1):35–6. Available at: http://www.pubmedcentral.nih.gov/articlerender.fcgi?artid=2827222&tool=pmcentrez&rendertype=abstract. Accessed October 10, 2011.

30. Leipsic J, LaBounty TM, Heilbron B, et al. Estimated radiation dose reduction using adaptive statistical iterative reconstruction in coronary CT angiography: the ERASIR study. AJR Am J Roentgenol 2010;195(3): 655–60. Available at: http://www.ajronline.org/cgi/content/abstract/195/3/655. Accessed October 10, 2011.

31. Achenbach S, Marwan M, Ropers D, et al. Coronary computed tomography angiography with a consistent dose below 1 mSv using prospectively electrocardiogram-triggered high-pitch spiral acquisition. Eur Heart J 2010;31(3):340–6. Available at: http://eurheartj.oxfordjournals.org/content/31/3/340.abstract. Accessed October 10, 2011.

32. Wang M, Qi HT, Wang XM, et al. Dose performance and image quality: dual source CT versus single source CT in cardiac CT angiography. Eur J Radiol 2009;72(3):396–400. Available at: http://www.sciencedirect.com/science/article/B6T6F-4TKBP57-3/2/5a927cfd40893b539bc3dab90a5d2e90. Accessed October 10, 2011.

33. ICRP. ICRP publication 60: 1990 Recommendations of the International Commission on Radiological Protection. Elsevier; 1991. Available at: http://www.amazon.com/ICRP-Publication-Recommendations-International-Radiological/dp/0080411444. Accessed October 10, 2011.

34. The 2007 Recommendations of the International Commission on Radiological Protection. ICRP publication 103. Ann ICRP 2007;37(2–4):1–332. Available at: http://www.ncbi.nlm.nih.gov/pubmed/18082557. Accessed October 10, 2011.

35. McCollough CH, Schueler BA. Calculation of effective dose. Med Phys 2000;27(5):828–37. Available at: http://www.ncbi.nlm.nih.gov/pubmed/10841384. Accessed October 10, 2011.

36. Matsubara K, Koshida K, Suzuki M, et al. Effective dose evaluation of multidetector CT examinations: influence of the ICRP recommendation in 2007. Eur Radiol 2009;19(12):2855–61. Available at: http://www.ncbi.nlm.nih.gov/pubmed/19585122. Accessed October 10, 2011.

37. Raff GL, Abidov A, Achenbach S, et al. SCCT guidelines for the interpretation and reporting of coronary computed tomographic angiography. J Cardiovasc Comput Tomogr 2009;3(2):122–36. Available at: http://www.ncbi.nlm.nih.gov/pubmed/19272853. Accessed October 10, 2011.

38. Hausleiter J, Meyer T, Hadamitzky M, et al. Radiation dose estimates from cardiac multislice computed tomography in daily practice: impact of different scanning protocols on effective dose estimates. Circulation 2006;113(10):1305–10. Available at: http://www.ncbi.nlm.nih.gov/pubmed/16520411. Accessed October 10, 2011.

39. Greess H, Wolf H, Baum U, et al. Dose reduction in computed tomography by attenuation-based on-line modulation of tube current: evaluation of six anatomical regions. Eur Radiol 2000;10(2):391–4. Available at: http://www.ncbi.nlm.nih.gov/pubmed/10663775. Accessed October 10, 2011.

Coronary Artery Calcification and Coronary Atherosclerotic Disease

Ramil Goel, MD[a,1], Pankaj Garg, MD[b,1],
Stephan Achenbach, MD[c], Abha Gupta, MD[a],
Jeremy J. Song, BS[b], Nathan D. Wong, PhD[b],
Leslee J. Shaw, PhD[d,*], Jagat Narula, MD, PhD, FRCP[e]

KEYWORDS

- Acute coronary syndrome • Hyper lipidemia
- Metabolic syndrome • Diabetes • Smoking
- Coronary angiography • Framingham risk score

As I examin'd the external surface of the heart, the left coronary artery appear'd to have been chang'd into a bony canal, from its very origin to the extent of many fingers breadth, where it embraces the greater part of the basis. And part of that very long branch, also, which it sends down upon the anterior surface of the heart, was already become bony to so, great a space, as could be cover'd by three fingers plac'd transversely.

—John Baptist, 1761

HISTORICAL PERSPECTIVE

This quote about the transformation of normal coronary arteries into "bony canals" seen on necropsy is taken from the 1761 treatise on anatomy by John Baptist, the first professor of Anatomy at the University of Padua.[1] However, it seems the earliest documented discoveries of the presence of calcium deposits in the coronary arterial system were perhaps made even earlier independently by Bellini, a physician and anatomist in the late seventeenth century, and by Thebesius, another anatomist in the early eighteenth century.[2] Until the 1930s, calcium deposition in coronary arteries post mortem was regarded as an "ancillary" degenerative process marking the terminal effects of atherosclerosis.[2,3] It was only in the 1950s that radiologic detection of coronary arterial calcium was made using fluoroscopy.[4] By the 1960s the relationship between coronary calcification as seen on imaging and coronary atherosclerosis was well established, and investigators as far back as then had mooted the idea of using imaging to detect such lesions to identify high-risk patients who may benefit from early aggressive risk factor modification.[5,6] By the 1970s, it was well recognized that "coronary

[a] Mayo Clinic, 13400 East Shea Boulevard, Scottsdale, AZ 85259, USA
[b] University of California, Sprague Hall 112, Irvine, CA 92697-4101, USA
[c] Department of Cardiology, University of Giessen, Klinikstrasse 33, 35392 Giessen, Germany
[d] Division of Cardiology, Department of Medicine, Emory Clinical Cardiovascular Research Institute, Emory University School of Medicine, 1462 Clifton Road NE, Room 530, Atlanta, GA 30306, USA
[e] Mount Sinai School of Medicine, One Gustave L. Levy Place, Box 1030, New York, NY 10029-6574, USA
[1] Contributed equally to the article.
* Corresponding author.
E-mail address: Lshaw3@emory.edu

Cardiol Clin 30 (2012) 19–47
doi:10.1016/j.ccl.2011.10.001
0733-8651/12/$ – see front matter © 2012 Published by Elsevier Inc.

calcification is easily detected, occurs frequently, increases with age, and indicates severe underlying lesions."[7] Coronary calcification was also noted to be a prognostic marker of survival independent of coronary atherosclerosis seen on fluoroscopy.[8] **Table 1** displays some important chronologic landmarks in the development of coronary artery calcification (CAC) as a marker of coronary atherosclerosis.

By the 1980s, there seemed to be enough rationale and pathophysiologic basis for developing the measurement of coronary calcification as a clinically useful marker for coronary artery disease (CAD). This cause was further aided by the development of a tool that would allow for the quantification of calcium deposits in the coronary arterial system, the high-resolution ultrafast computed tomography (CT) or electron-beam CT (EBCT).[9,10] A system of quantification and scoring was also developed for EBCT, the Agatston score, based on number, areas, and peak Hounsfield CT numbers of the calcific lesions detected, which has continued to this day as the standard scoring technique.[11] A new method to improve scoring based on the CT interpolated volume technique was introduced in 1998; because this score correlates nearly perfectly with the Agatston score, its use has been limited mainly to studies of serial changes or progression of coronary calcium, and the Agatston score remains the standard scoring technique.[12] Subsecond multirow detector CT (MDCT) scanning seems to be a rapidly emerging technology and may hold some advantages over EBCT, particularly the newer-generation greater slice and multisource scanners whereby problems of motion artifact are minimized.[13]

PATHOPHYSIOLOGY OF CORONARY ARTERY CALCIUM

The process of vascular calcification is almost exclusively related to atherosclerosis, barring rare cases of hypervitaminosis D, Monckeberg sclerosis, and infantile calcifications. The calcification of the atherosclerotic lesion begins at the stage of fatty streak formation as early as in the second decade of life.[14] The lesions even in younger adults reveal aggregates of crystalline calcium among the lipid particles of the lipid core.[14] The quantity of coronary artery calcium correlates with the burden of atherosclerosis in different individuals, and to some extent also with different segments of the coronary artery tree in the same individual.[15]

Pioneering work by pathologists in the mid twentieth century had established that the primary cause of calcification in coronary arteries was atherosclerosis,[16] and that advanced coronary atheromas may contain as much as 1.4 g of calcium mineral per 100 g of wet weight.[2] Calcification was then thought of as a feature of advanced atherosclerotic plaques and was described as a "terminal process, a monumental deposit in dead and dying tissue."[3]

The process of vascular calcification is not well understood, but may resemble the mineralization

Table1
Historical perspective on the development of coronary artery calcium as a marker of coronary atherosclerosis

Year	Contributors	Contribution	Reference Publication
Late 17th century Early 18th century	Bellini Thebesius	First documented evidenceof coronary calcification	—
1761	Morgagni, John Baptist	Further studies of coronary artery calcification	1
1936	Leary and other pathologists	Established calcification as a hallmark of advanced atherosclerosis	3
1959	Blankenhorn et al	Detection of coronary calcification on fluoroscopy	4
1961	Lieber et al	Correlation of coronary calcification with clinical atherosclerotic disease	5
1965	Eggen et al	Correlation of coronary calcification on autopsy with increased CAD mortality	6
1988	Janowitz et al	Use of EBCT for detection of coronary calcium	9
1990	Agatston et al	Scoring system for quantifying coronary calcium	11
2002	Kopp et al	Use of MDCT for measuring coronary calcium	13

of bones.[17,18] The deposited mineral is calcium phosphate hydroxyapatite [$Ca_3PO_4 \cdot Ca(OH)_2$], similar to bone.[15,18] It is also proposed that in addition to dystrophic mineral deposition secondary to smooth muscle cell and macrophage death, vascular smooth muscle cells dedifferentiate and may express bone proteins and lay down mineralized matrix.[18,19] The evolutionary benefit of soft-tissue calcification hypothetically includes enwalling of areas of chronic inflammation,[19] and in the case of atherosclerotic calcification, it may add toward stabilization and biomechanical strength of a lipid-laden plaque.[20,21] On the other hand, the junction between calcified and noncalcified areas of a plaque is susceptible to increased stress due to differential stiffness. As such lesions with focal calcifications are more prone to dissection during balloon angioplasty,[15,22,23] and bulky plaques with spotty calcification are more prone to plaque rupture.[24] In theory, as a lesion becomes more uniformly calcified its vulnerability to rupture decreases.[15]

It may seem paradoxic that coronary calcium exerts a protective influence when numerous studies have shown worsened prognosis and an increased prevalence of cardiovascular disease with increasing coronary calcium. This contradiction may simply indicate that while the calcified plaque itself may not be the cause of an acute event, the extent of coronary arterial calcium is a marker of atherosclerosis and signifies higher burden of atherosclerosis in the coronary vasculature.

CORONARY ARTERY CALCIUM AND RELATION WITH AGE, GENDER, AND RACE

Pathologic studies alluding to a lower prevalence of coronary artery calcium have been described in African Americans,[6] even though the prevalence of most CAD risk factors and associated age-adjusted mortality is higher in African Americans.[25] Not only the prevalence but also the overall calcium burden, when present, is higher in Caucasians.[26] However, a handful of studies have refuted any significant difference in the prevalence of coronary artery calcium in Caucasians and African Americans.[27–29] The prevalence of coronary artery calcium in Asians and Hispanics, though not as well studied, also seems lower than in their Caucasian counterparts. Asian Indians, however, are an exception to this trend and show higher coronary artery calcium scores (CAC scores), closer to those of Caucasians.[30] **Table 2** shows some important studies in this field.

These interracial differences are more prominent in male gender and with increasing age.[26] There is some evidence that the rate of progression of CAC over time is slower in African Americans.[31] The prevalence of CAC in a study of unselected elderly aged 67 to 99 years showed that compared with African Americans, the Caucasian population was associated with an odds ratio of 2.131 ($P<.0001$) for having the highest quartile CAC score.[32] The reason for the ethnic differences in CAC is unclear, but could be related to differences in calcium and vitamin D metabolism and in bone mineralization.[33,34]

The MESA (Multi-Ethnic Study of Atherosclerosis) study, in a large multicenter population, correlated the prevalence and progression of subclinical cardiovascular disease in multiple ethnic groups, and offers important insights into racial differences of cardiovascular risk parameters. An interesting analysis of the MESA data revealed that acculturation and socioeconomic factors, such as being born in the United States, years of stay in the United States, and low education, were factors affecting CAC score.[35] The differences could not be explained by the presence of cardiovascular risk factors including smoking, diabetes, and hypertension.[35] The poor calcification of the atherosclerotic plaque in African Americans along with a higher incidence of CAD risk factors and possibly increased CAD mortality among African Americans is suggestive of a protective effect of plaque calcium burden.[25] The CAC in African Americans may thus seem to signify lower clinical correlation with CAD adverse events.[36]

On the other hand, a secondary analysis of the MESA cohort showed that despite the baseline differences in CAC score, a doubling of the CAC score in all 4 major racial groups was associated with a similar proportional increase in the incidence of coronary events.[37] It has been shown that for high CAC scores the relative prognosis is worse for African Americans followed by Hispanics and Asians in comparison with Caucasians, and that CAC was identified as the single greatest predictor of time to mortality regardless of ethnicity.[38] These studies reinforce the utility of measuring CAC score in all racial groups, noting that the predictive information provided by CAC was additive to the standard risk-factor stratification across all 4 groups. Therefore, after adjusting for a different baseline CAC score value, incremental coronary artery calcium burden is associated with a proportional increase in cardiovascular risk and mortality.

The prevalence of CAC has long been known to be higher in males and increases with advancing age.[11] The gender association of CAC often reflects the trends seen in atherosclerosis, and the prevalence of CAC in women starts

Table 2
Coronary artery calcium: relation with age, gender, and race

Authors	Study Population	Caucasians		AA		Hispanic		Asians	
		Male	Female	Male	Female	Male	Female	Male	Female
Bild et al[116] (MESA study)	Population based, excluded apparent CAD	70.4	44.6	52.1	36.5	56.5	34.9	59.2	41.9
Tang et al[117] using cine-fluoroscopy	Population based	60		36		—		60	
Budoff et al[118]	Referred symptomatic patients	84		62		71		73	
Lee et al[119] (PACC study)	Active army volunteers	19.2		10.3		—		—	
Jain et al[27] (Dallas Heart Study; CAC score >10)	Population based, included CAD	41		37		—		—	
Bild et al[28] (CARDIA study; CAC >2.05 mm³)	Population based, low-risk young volunteers	17.1	4.6	16.1	11.8	—		—	
Khurana et al[29] (CAC score >10)	Population based	—	32.33		31.25	—		—	
Doherty et al[43]	High-risk asymptomatic patients	59.9		35.5		—		—	
Hatwalkar et al[30]	Referred asymptomatic subjects	65		53		53		55 (for Asian Indians 62)	
Nasir et al[38]	High-risk asymptomatic patients	66		58		55		55	
Fair et al[120]	Presumed healthy 60–69-year-old subjects	78	39	62	44	75	38	68	58
Budoff et al[121]	Asymptomatic referred patients	78	44	69	36	72	34	69	42

Abbreviations: AA, African American; CAD, coronary artery disease; CARDIA, Coronary Artery Risk Development in Young Adults; EBCT, electron-beam computed tomography; MDCT, multirow detector computed tomography; MESA, Multi-Ethnic Study of Atherosclerosis; PACC, Prospective Army Coronary Calcium.

approaching that in men by age 60 years.[39] The MESA cohort also showed a lower CAC score for women across all age groups.[40] Despite the gender differences, the luminal narrowing predicted by the presence of coronary artery calcium seems to be similar for both men and women.[41] An interesting observation suggests a relation between high levels of bone loss from osteoporosis in women with increased CAC score. A substudy of the MESA showed that low volumetric bone mineral density at the lumbar spine was associated with presence and amounts of CAC and abdominal aortic calcium in women.[42]

The increase in CAC score with age is well established and is seen across both genders and all race groups.[40] In a study by Newman and colleagues,[32] 614 elderly subjects with a mean age of 80 years were evaluated and found to have increased CAC score with increasing age; it was also noted that patients older than 85 years had excessive CAC burden unusual for younger adults, but paradoxically without a significant history of CAD events. As such, a given level of calcium may have a different predictive value in the old than in the young; yet higher CAC is likely to have higher risk of discriminating ability over other risk factors.

DISTRIBUTION OF CORONARY ARTERY CALCIUM

The calcium deposition in coronary arteries is almost exclusively associated with atherosclerosis. However, the distribution does not completely parallel the distribution of atherosclerotic lesions, leading to speculation that atherosclerosis and calcification are related but distinct processes.[43] The distribution of CAC occurs closer to the origin of the coronary artery and can progress even as the atherosclerotic plaque itself regresses. Mautner and colleagues[44] showed that most calcific deposits were present within 5 cm of the aortic ostium of the right coronary artery (RCA) and within 3 cm of the left anterior descending artery (LAD) and left circumflex artery (LCxA) origins. The LAD (86%) was the most heavily calcified coronary artery, followed by RCA (62%) and LCxA (60%).[44] That calcification involves the proximal parts of coronaries has been shown earlier as well.[45] **Table 3** displays some important data reported by the investigators looking at this aspect of CAC.

Sangiorgi and colleagues[46] have showed an excellent correlation between calcium area and plaque area and also confirmed that calcification, along with atherosclerosis, involved LAD most extensively followed in decreasing order by RCA and LCxA. Rumberger and colleagues[47] reported a close correlation between CAC and increased plaque burden at whole heart, individual coronary artery, and segmental coronary artery levels. Analyzing the same autopsy specimens as Rumberger and colleagues, Simons and colleagues[48] observed a lower likelihood of obstructive disease in the absence of calcium. However, in contrast to the study by Sangiorgi and colleagues, they showed a correlation between CT-assessed coronary artery calcium burden and percent lumen stenosis although, as admitted by the investigators, the association was broad.[48] Simons and colleagues also noted a marginal correlation between plaque area and coronary artery calcium burden; LAD was noted to be the leading coronary artery in terms of having the highest calcium burden, atherosclerotic plaque area, and percent luminal stenosis, followed by the RCA and left coronary artery, respectively.

It has been reported that few large coronary calcium deposits and lesions in the left main coronary artery are associated with a particularly high mortality risk.[49]

RELATION OF CORONARY ARTERY CALCIUM WITH VALVULAR CALCIFICATION

Aortic valvular sclerosis has been demonstrated to share many of the risk factors and pathophysiologic features with atherosclerosis.[50,51] Takasu and colleagues[52] also showed a very close correlation between the presence of aortic valvular calcification (AVC) and coronary artery calcium. The amounts of elemental calcium, magnesium, and phosphorus as assessed by spectrometry on dissected specimens of the coronary artery, aortic valve, mitral valve, and ascending aorta were found to correlate in a of series of autopsies,[53] which further establishes some relationship between the calcification of the various cardiac structures.

Mitral annular calcification (MAC) is also thought to be closely related to the vascular atherosclerotic process.[54] Tenenbaum and colleagues[55] have shown a relation between advanced MAC as seen on 2-dimensional echocardiogram and severe coronary artery calcium as seen on spiral CT. The same investigators also discovered that although postmenopausal women had a higher prevalence of advanced MAC, the presence of advanced MAC was predictive of a high CAC score in both men and women.[56] Tenenbaum and colleagues subsequently concluded that MAC assessment has low sensitivity and specificity, and does not have any incremental diagnostic value over measuring CAC by CT.[57]

Table 3
Distribution of coronary artery calcium

Authors	Study Design	Methods	Results	Remarks
Mautner et al[44]	Evaluated 4298 paired 3-mm EBCT and histomorphometric segments	Amount of calcium on EBCT correlated highly with histomorphometric measures	Most calcium deposits noted close to origin of arteries, LAD noted to be most frequently calcified	Study gives more credibility to the use of CT for assessment of CAC
Sangiorgi et al[46]	Studied 13 consecutively obtained autopsied hearts	A total of 37 nondecalcified coronary arteries were processed, sectioned at 3-mm intervals (723 sections), and evaluated by computer planimetry and densitometry	CAC is correlated positively with coronary artery atherosclerotic plaque but not with lumen diameter. Most involved arteries were LAD followed by RCA and LCA	The noncorrelation with lumen diameter could be due to arterial remodeling after plaque formation
Rumberger at al[47]	Studied 13 autopsied hearts	Each artery was scanned and divided into corresponding 3-mm segments, with representative histologic sections quantified for atherosclerotic plaque area per segment	The CAC corresponded with hearts as a whole, for individual coronary arteries, and for individual coronary artery segments. Most involved arteries were LAD followed by RCA and LCA	The coronary plaque area was 5 times greater than calcium area; it seems the plaque area had to cross 5 mm^2 per segment for calcium area to achieve the detectable threshold of 1 mm^2
Simons et al[48]	Studied 13 consecutive autopsied (the same autopsy specimens as the Rumberger study)	The hearts were first scanned. Each artery dissected free, positioned longitudinally, and scanned free. 3-mm segments corresponding to CT scans were then histologically studied	The CAC burden correlated with total plaque area and also percent lumen stenosis. The correlation was linear but broad	In the absence of CAC on CT imaging, the atherosclerotic disease present was found to be nonobstructive

Abbreviations: CAC, coronary artery calcification; CT, computed tomography; LAD, left anterior descending artery; LCA, left coronary artery; RCA, right coronary artery.

Contrary to this evidence, Pohle and colleagues,[58] in a different study design looking at parameters influencing the progression of AVC and CAC, found a correlation between the progression of 2 but no correlation of baseline values. Yamamoto and colleagues,[59] while primarily looking at the relation of coronary and extracoronary calcification with obstructive CAD on angiography, also showed that CAC score correlates with MAC and AVC in a statistically significant fashion. **Table 4** displays the important studies under this subheading.

RELATION OF CORONARY ARTERY CALCIUM WITH AORTIC CALCIFICATION

As opposed to CAC, which is almost always atherosclerotic (intimal deposition), aortic calcification can be intimal, which is mostly atherosclerotic, or medial, which is nonatherosclerotic.[60] Aortic calcification is also independently related to risk of coronary heart disease (CHD).[61] Aortic calcification has been shown to be associated with increased severity of CAD.[59,62] The aortic calcification actually seen on EBCT scanning cannot be differentiated into intimal or medial.[63] However, there is also some evidence that even the medial vascular calcification is associated with increased risk of future cardiovascular events.[64] The prevalence of ascending aorta calcification is low, and was not even measured in the MESA cohort.[65] There is a correlation between coronary and thoracic aortic calcification; this association may be stronger for descending thoracic aortic calcification (TAC) compared with ascending TAC, for unclear reasons.[66] Wong and colleagues[67] also found a similar correlation between TAC, AVC, and CAC, and established the incremental value of measuring TAC and AVC over CAC in the estimation of 10-year risk of cardiovascular disease. Of interest, they also reported that whereas most cardiovascular risk factors like age, male gender, and low-density lipoprotein cholesterol were directly related to the likelihood of CAC, TAC, and AVC, the presence of high diastolic pressures correlated with high CAC, and low diastolic blood pressure correlated with increased TAC and AVC. This finding might just be reflective of the higher pulse pressures caused by increased aortic stiffness.[67] The association of higher TAC and AVC with increased cardiovascular risk and CAC may lie in its clinical utility as another measure of increased cardiovascular risk, which can be measured in the same scan as coronary artery calcium without additional expense. **Table 5** lists some significant studies showing the relationship between CAC and aortic calcification.

CORONARY ARTERY CALCIUM, CONVENTIONAL CARDIOVASCULAR RISK FACTORS, AND THE METABOLIC SYNDROME

CAC deposition is closely and almost exclusively related to atherosclerosis.[68] It thus might be expected that the risk factors associated with atherosclerosis would also be related to CAC. Several studies (see **Table 5**) have confirmed an association between conventional risk factors and CAC.

The majority of the studies demonstrate a correlation between increased CAC score with a higher number of traditional risk factors. The benefit of CAC score lies in its potential to add incremental information for the prediction of coronary events and mortality beyond traditional risk factors.[69–71] Some studies have argued for the use of CAC score in addition to the current Adult Treatment Panel III (ATP-III) defined risk strata to improve the use and administration of lipid-lowering therapy.[72] Hoffmann and colleagues[73] attempted to establish the distribution of CAC score across various age groups in healthy subjects of both sexes and derived normal CAC score values. These investigators also determined CAC distributions within Framingham Risk Score (FRS) categories and noted that the presence and quantity of CAC increased with higher FRS category for either gender. Application of the relative cutoff values derived from a healthy, risk-free population led to a 50% increase in identifying subjects with increased CAC, compared with if the standard cutoff were derived from the overall population. Also, the use of relative cutoff values instead of absolute cutoff values identified more subjects with increased CAC in women, younger persons, and intermediate FRS patients. However, it is unclear as to whether identifying subjects with low absolute CAC score, which are high for their age and sex, will help in prognostication of CAD.[74] In a recently published study, Polonsky and colleagues[75] followed for a median of 5.8 years a cohort of 5878 subjects drawn from the MESA. The study showed the incremental benefit of adding CAC score to conventional risk factors of age, sex, tobacco use, systolic blood pressure, antihypertensive medication use, total and high-density lipoprotein cholesterol, and race/ethnicity. Twenty-six percent of the subjects needed reclassification with the addition of CAC score to the prediction model. The inclusion of CAC score increased the area under the curve (AUC) for prediction of coronary events from 0.76 to 0.81. **Table 6** displays some the landmark trials establishing the relationship between CAC and conventional metabolic risk factors.

Table 4
Relation of coronary artery calcium to valvular calcification

Study	Methods	Results	Remarks
Takasu et al[52]	620 asymptomatic referred patients studied twice 12 months apart	Significant correlation between presence of AVC and CAC on initial studies and parallel increase in progression	Most participants with AVC and CC scores of 0 on initial scan did not have a significant calcium deposit on repeated scan
Adler et al[122]	376 patients with hypertension	Significant differences in the mean CAC, and number of vessels calcified between the groups with and without AVC	Strengthens the significant association between the presence of AVC and advanced CC on spiral CT
Tenenbaum et al[55]	522 patients with hypertension	Advanced MAC was correlated with very high CAC score and proven CAD	A role for echocardiogram in the indirect diagnosis of CAD is raised with this study
Cury et al[123]	420 subjects without known CAD underwent MDCT as part of another study	The presence of AVC and mitral valvular calcification (annular and on leaflets) and descending aortic calcification increased the likelihood of presence of CAC	Used a scoring system analogous to the Agatston scoring system due to poor applicability of latter to noncoronary calcium scoring
Pohle et al[58]	104 subjects with presence of AVC on EBCT done for CAC score. Performed 2 studies on a particular subject separated by a mean of 15.3 months	There was no significant correlation between the AVC and CAC on initial assessment	The temporal rate of progression of CAC and AVC had a significant correlation and rate of CAC progression predicted rate of AVC progression. High LDL levels predicted higher rates of progression of both CAC and AVC. treatment with statins decreased the progression of both
Walsh et al[124]	327 subjects drawn from the Framingham offspring study who had undergone EBCT between 1997 and 1999	Thoracic aortic calcification and CAC did not correlate with AVC with any statistical significance after adjustment for age and gender	Another aspect of the study revealed poor sensitivity of EBCT (with fair specificity) in detecting aortic valve degenerative disease

Abbreviations: AVC, aortic valvular calcification; CC, coronary calcium; MAC, mitral annular calcification; LDL, low-density lipoprotein.

Table 5
Relation of coronary artery calcium to aortic calcification

Authors	Methods	Results	Remarks
Adler et al[63]	405 patients with at least two risk factors for atherosclerosis were included, and underwent chest CT for CC and aortic calcification scoring	Demonstrated a strong association of CAC and calcification of the thoracic aorta on spiral CT	The study also sees the association between CAC and aortic calcification as a possible basis between CAD and cerebrovascular disease
Takasu et al[65]	Studied the MESA cohort of 6814 women and men ages 45–84 years old	Descending thoracic aortic calcification was found to be a strong predictor of CAC independent of cardiovascular risk factors	This is the largest such study, and studied the MESA cohort
Eisen et al[66]	361 stable angina pectoris patients	Significant correlation found between presence of aortic calcification with CAC	Study also noted significant correlation between aortic calcification and aortic valve calcification and mitral annular calcification
Wong et al[67]	2740 persons without known CHD aged 20–79 years	Significant correlation found among presence of aortic calcification, AVC, and CAC	Study found that TAC and AVC provide incremental value for predicting estimated 10-year risk of CHD over CAC
Raggi et al[125]	245 self-referred patients	Significant correlation between CAC and AVC	Out of all the conventional risk factors studied, only age, male gender, and Lp(a) were associated with CAC

Abbreviations: CHD, coronary heart disease; LP(a), lipoprotein(a); TAC, thoracic aortic calcification.

CORONARY ARTERY CALCIUM COMPARED WITH CONVENTIONAL ANGIOGRAPHY

The relation of coronary artery stenosis on angiography with coronary artery calcium as seen by fluoroscopy was demonstrated by Margolis and colleagues[8] as far back as 1980. This seemed intuitive, with the well-established link between CAC and coronary atherosclerosis on pathologic studies.[6] The relation of increased CAC with progression of obstructive CAD was described in 1991 by Janowitz and colleagues[76] in a pilot study of 25 patients, when ultrafast CT was used for the first time to follow the natural history of calcified plaque. Patients with obstructive CAD showed a significantly elevated baseline CAC score over asymptomatic patients, and also showed higher increases in CAC score when these patients were scanned again after a mean of about 406 days. **Table 7** enumerates the important studies looking at the relationship between CAC and conventional coronary angiography.

In a fairly big study of 1764 patients with suspected CAD who underwent both coronary angiography and EBCT for CAC scoring, Haberl and colleagues[77] showed a significantly positive correlation between increasing CAC scores and increased probability of finding angiographically significant stenosis. Budoff and colleagues,[78] in a study of 1861 patients, also reached a similar conclusion. These studies also showed the very low probability of coronary stenosis with undetectable coronary calcium, with negative predictive power approaching 99%, suggesting a role for CAC as a gatekeeper prior to coronary angiography. In a study of 100 patients, Breen and colleagues[79] showed that the absence of CAC had 100% negative predictive value for clinically significant CAD. On the other hand, in a study of exclusively Japanese patients who underwent EBCT for CAC scoring, Kajinami and colleagues[80] performed a site-by-site comparison of calcification as seen on EBCT with angiographic stenosis. The investigators analyzed a total of 2407 segments of coronary vasculature, and

Table 6
Relation of coronary artery calcium to conventional cardiovascular risk factors

Authors	Study Objective	Study Population	Results	Remarks
Karim et al[126]	To study subclinical atherosclerosis in the coronary arteries, aorta, and the common carotid artery, and its relation with the FRS	Total of 498 asymptomatic disease-free subjects chosen randomly underwent carotid artery ultrasound and coronary artery and aortic CT scans	With each percent increase in the 10-year FRS the risk of having CAC increased by 14%	CAC, aortic calcium, and CIMT were each independently related to the 10-year FRS
Wong et al[127]	To study the relationship of CAC with age and conventional risk factors	865 self referred subjects	A significant continuous graded relation between total CAC score with the number of risk factors noted	In men the parallel relation between risk factors and CAC was limited, with CAC prevalence approaching 80% regardless of risk factors
Mahoney et al[128]	To study FRS for predicting CAC	857 patients aged 29–43 years. Scores were compared in subjects with and without CAC and were also used to predict presence of CAC	Higher FRS corresponded with increased CAC	Relatively younger population studied. Adding BMI to the score improved its predictive value
Mahoney et al[129] (The Muscatine study)	To detect an association between childhood coronary risk factors and adult CAC score	384 patients had coronary risk factors measured in childhood (mean age 15 years) and twice during young adult life, and underwent an electron-beam computed tomographic study at their second young adult examination	Increased BMI, BP, and low HDL levels in childhood predict higher CAC in adulthood	First study linking childhood coronary risk factors to evidence of advanced atherosclerosis in asymptomatic adults
Goff et al[72]	To compare the ATP-III defined risk strata with CAC and prevalence and control of dyslipidemia	The MESA cohort of 6814 asymptomatic subjects	ATP-III defined risk categories broadly but imperfectly correlated with CAC. Suboptimal control of dyslipidemia seen in all ATP-III strata	CAC score assessment may additionally identify patients who currently do not qualify for hypolipidemic agents based on ATP-III risk factors

Study				
Sung et al[69]	Attempted to identify the factors that lead to a discordance between FRS and CAC	1653 asymptomatic Korean subjects	FRS corresponded with CAC score with a positive correlation with some discrepancy	Higher age associated with discrepancy between CAC and FRS. The investigators argue that CAC score can be used to improve the discriminatory ability of FRS in older adults
Kondos et al[70]	Role of CAC score over and above conventional risk factors	8855 asymptomatic individuals	Both the conventional risk factors and CAC are associated with cardiac events	CAC score provides incremental prognostic information above the conventional risk factors
Michos et al[130]	Cross-sectional study looking specifically at the question of whether multiple metabolic risk factors lead to high risk for CAC	6141 asymptomatic consecutive physician-referred patients without known CAD or DM	Increasing number of metabolic risk factors were associated with increased CAC	Family history of premature CAD was significantly associated with CAC, magnifying the effects of metabolic risk factors
Nasir et al[131]	Cross-sectional study looking at relation between family history of premature CAD with CAC	8549 asymptomatic individuals	Highly significant association between family history of premature CHD and the presence and extent of CAC	A sibling history was a more powerful predictor than parental history
Arad et al[132]	Study correlations of baseline CAC scores with CAD risk factors and insulin resistance parameters	5582 asymptomatic patients, without diagnosed CAD or insulin requiring DM excluded	CAC score was significantly correlated with most metabolic syndrome parameters	Establishes a direct relation between insulin resistance and CAC
Wong et al[133]	Compared the prevalence and extent of CAC in patients with metabolic syndrome	1823 persons who underwent screening for CAC, physician or self referred or part of another research study	A high prevalence of CAC in individuals with metabolic syndrome. The likelihood of CAC presence increased with increasing risk factors	A high prevalence of CAC noted in subjects with metabolic syndrome, calling for more aggressive intervention in this group

(continued on next page)

Table 6
(continued)

Authors	Study Objective	Study Population	Results	Remarks
Ho et al[71]	Study sought to explore the relation of CAC to MDCT-detected coronary stenosis and to detect any incremental benefit of measuring CAC over traditional risk factors	664 high-risk or symptomatic referred patients	CAC score significantly correlated with increased stenoses. The CAC score also positively correlated with traditional risk factors	Study showed an incremental value to CAC score in predicting stenotic lesions over traditional risk factor measurement
Hoffmann et al[73]	Study objective was to establish normal distributions of CAC for age and gender. It also provided CAC score distribution of overall cohort and that at intermediate FRS	3238 subjects from the offspring and third-generation cohorts of the community-based Framingham Heart Study, excluding those with apparent cardiovascular disease	The prevalence of CAC in the intermediate FRS risk population was 33.3% higher than in the healthy reference sample. The mean CAC score defining each percentile increased with age in both sexes	Applying the absolute cutoff underestimated the proportion of subjects with increased CAC, especially women, young persons, and those at intermediate CHD risk by FRS
Polonsky et al[75]	To determine whether adding CAC score to a prediction model based on traditional risk factors improves classification of risk	5878 subjects from the MESA cohort were followed for a median of 5.8 years	The inclusion of CAC score in prediction model led to an additional 8% subjects in the intermediate-risk group getting separated into high-risk and low-risk categories	There was significant improvement in the discriminatory ability of the prediction model when CAC score was added to the conventional risk factors

Abbreviations: ATP-III, Adult Treatment Panel III; BMI, body mass index; BP, blood pressure; CIMT, carotid intima-media thickness; DM, diabetes mellitus; FRS, Framingham Risk Score; HDL, high-density lipoprotein.

Table 7
Relation of coronary artery calcium to conventional angiography

Authors	Study Objective	Study Population	Results	Remarks
Haberl et al[77]	To correlate the CAC score with results of coronary angiography	1764 symptomatic patients with suspected CAD who underwent coronary angiography	Absence of CAC predicted a <1% chance of having angiographically significant stenosis	Higher CAC scores corresponded with decreased sensitivity and increased specificity of coronary stenosis
Budoff et al[102]	To evaluate the incorporation of CAC in a model for prediction of angiographic CAD	1851 patients with suspected CAD who underwent coronary angiography	Presence of CAC predicted angiographically significant CAD with a sensitivity of 95% and a specificity of 66%	Higher CAC scores improved the specificity of angiographically significant CAD and probability of finding multivessel disease
Breen et al[79]	To assess the relationship of coronary artery calcification to angiographically detectable disease	100 patients undergoing elective diagnostic angiography	Sensitivity of ultrafast CT in detecting angiographically detectable disease was 94% and the specificity was 72%	None of the patients without CAC had clinically significant angiographic disease
Gottlieb et al[82]	To evaluate the predictive value of absent CAC in ruling out obstructive CAD	Multicenter study of 291 patients undergoing conventional angiography were subjected to MDCT for CAC score	The positive predictive value of CAC = 0 in predicting the absence of obstructive CAD is 81%	The absence of CAC does not exclude obstructive CAD
Rubinshtein et al[83]	To compare CAC score with presence of obstructive CAD	668 consecutive patients with chest pain syndrome	7% of patients with CAC score = 0% and 17% of patients with low CAC score had obstructive CAD	The lesions missed by coronary calcium scoring were not insignificant and involved LAD in 66% of patients

found 666 (27%) segments with calcification. The positive predictive value of CAC for significant coronary stenosis was 0.36 and for any detectable atherosclerotic lesion was 0.80. Diffuse and wide lesions correlated strongly with the presence of atherosclerotic lesions. Kajinami and colleagues proposed using morphologic evaluation of CAC to improve the predictability of angiographically detectable coronary atherosclerosis. In another Japanese study by Yamamoto and colleagues,[59] 99 patients who underwent both conventional coronary angiography and EBCT were studied. Calcification of not only coronary arteries but also that of aortic valve, mitral annulus, and descending aorta was studied. The investigators noted a significant

correlation between CAC and increasing obstructive coronary disease. The addition of aortic calcification increased the specificity of CAC in detecting obstructive coronary disease. AVC and descending TAC was associated with the presence of advanced obstructive coronary disease; by contrast, MAC was not independently predictive of obstructive coronary disease in this study.

Thus although the absence of CAC in patients with obstructive CAD would be rare, it is possible and may have dire ramifications. In an interesting retrospective study by Marwan and colleagues,[81] 21 patients with symptomatic CAD with no detectable CAC but having obstructive CAD (on both CT angiography and invasive coronary angiography) were compared with 42 patients with CAC and obstructive CAD. The patients with stenosis but no calcification were younger and more frequently presented with unstable symptoms as compared with patients who had detectable CAC. This finding might be related to the fact that CAC is associated with mature plaques less likely to rupture and cause acute coronary syndrome (as discussed in the Pathophysiology section). Of note, this study was not designed to look at the value of CAC at predicting obstructive CAD.

Gottlieb and colleagues,[82] in a study that contradicts current understanding, showed that absence of CAC is poor at ruling out coronary artery stenosis of greater than 50% and does not obviate the use of coronary angiography. Rubinshtein and colleagues,[83] also had reached a similar conclusion in an earlier study, when they noted that in patients presenting with chest pain a CAC score of 0 does not completely exclude obstructive CAD as seen on conventional angiography. The reasons for the apparently contradictory findings of these studies could be the higher risk profiles of the patients in both studies, but they are not very clear and call for more caution when interpreting the finding of a negative CAC result.[84]

RELATION OF CORONARY ARTERY CALCIUM WITH OTHER TESTS FOR CORONARY ARTERY DISEASE

The purpose of CAC scoring, of course, is to improve our ability to diagnose and prognosticate CAD. It is thus important to determine its investigative role in relation to other currently available diagnostic tools. Shavelle and colleagues[85] published a study of 97 symptomatic patients who underwent both EBCT for CAC score and coronary angiography; 90% also underwent stress testing. This study showed that the sensitivity of coronary artery calcium in predicting obstructive CAD was 96%, with a positive predictive value of 80%. The specificity for predicting obstructive CAD was relatively low, at 46%, when compared with the specificity of exercise testing at 60%, and at 67% for radionuclide myocardial perfusion testing. The combined specificity of both EBCT and stress electrocardiogram (ECG) testing was higher at 83%. Lamont and colleagues[86] suggested that CAC measured by EBCT could identify patients with false-positive stress test results.

Schmermund and colleagues[87] proposed incremental values of CAC score over radionuclide perfusion imaging in predicting the extent of angiographic CAD. Most of the older studies compared the presence of obstructive CAD as predicted by CAC score by EBCT and stress testing. A few studies have also looked into CAC score for predicting myocardial ischemia on stress testing. In a study of asymptomatic patients, He and colleagues[88] showed that below a threshold CAC score of 10, no patient and below a threshold of 100, a very small proportion of patients have positive single-photon emission CT (SPECT) perfusion scans. Of interest, Ho and colleagues[89] showed in another study that patients with a low CAC score can still have CAD, albeit at a very low incidence, and in such cases AVC may identify patients with CAD.

Berman and colleagues[90] found a correlation between increasing CAC score and presence of ischemia on SPECT perfusion scans. Like He and colleagues, they too noted a threshold effect with almost no patients with a CAC score of less than 100 showing evidence of positive myocardial SPECT perfusion scan. Of note, 56% of subjects with a CAC score greater than 100 had a normal perfusion scan. Wong and colleagues[91] also showed that the presence of a metabolic abnormality (metabolic syndrome or diabetes) indicated a lower cut point for a CAC score of 100 compared with 400 without such an abnormality, above which the incidence of myocardial ischemia was increased.

It seems that results of CAC scores and inducible myocardial ischemia as seen on SPECT imaging parallel each other and are concordant. Discordant results of myocardial perfusion and calcium study in the same patient, such as when the stress test is positive in the presence of low CAC score, may pose a dilemma. It is unclear whether the prognosis of these patients is similar that of patients with negative stress test and low CAC score. In the opposite situation, where the stress test is negative but the CAC score is high, the magnitude of CAC exerted little influence on outcomes in a longitudinal study over a mean follow-up period of 32 months.[92] On this basis, Rozanski and colleagues proposed restraint from aggressive management of patients with high CAC scores in the presence of a normal myocardial perfusion scan.

In another similar study, Ramakrishna and colleagues[93] studied 835 asymptomatic patients who underwent both CAC score and myocardial perfusion imaging, and noted a correlation, albeit weak, between these two tests; both tests independently correlated with mortality. In a further study of the same cohort, Askew and colleagues[94] identified 69 asymptomatic patients with presence of coronary artery calcium who had undergone a baseline and a follow-up (up to 4 years) myocardial perfusion scan. The investigators reported that initially negative perfusion scan even in the presence of CAC portended a good prognosis, and even though repeat scans of 6% of the subjects turned positive, they were not associated with any adverse events.[94] **Table 8** lists the important trials on this topic.

PROGNOSIS OF CORONARY ARTERY CALCIUM SCORE: RELATION TO CARDIOVASCULAR EVENTS AND MORTALITY

The risk of cardiovascular risk increases almost linearly with increasing CAC score. This tenet has been established by many studies (**Table 9**). The main problem when comparing these studies is the lack of standardization in methodology of testing and assessment of results. The studies varied in how the EBCT scans were done with respect to thickness of slices, and how the CAC score data were categorized and cardiovascular events were measured. Nevertheless, there is generally a strong consistency between increased CAC score and risk of cardiovascular events.

The absence of CAC is associated with low annual event rates of between 0.06% and 0.11%.[95–97] It seems the mere presence of CAC does not provide much prognostic information, with relative risk of CAD noted to be as low 1.36 to as high as 10.75.[95,98] The relative risk in patients with high CAC burden seems to be significant, with relative risk up to 26 times in subjects with a CAC score of greater than 400 compared with subjects with no CAC.[96] For very high scores of 1000 or greater the risk of myocardial infarction of coronary death within 1 year was as high as 25%.[99]

This figure compares favorably with a relative risk varying between 1.5 and 3.4 conferred by traditional risk factors such as diabetes, smoking, hypertension, and extreme dyslipidemia.[100] Becker and colleagues[101] showed that the AUC was higher for CAC score than for ATP-III scores and PRO-CAM (Prospective Cardiovascular Münster Study) scores. The AUC was also significantly increased when the CAC score was added to traditional risk factors.[37] The CAC score provided incremental information over risk factors in most of the ethnic groups studied. Budoff and colleagues[102] reported a study incorporating the large sample size of 25,253 subjects and a long follow-up period of a mean of 6.8 years, and established a strong relationship between all-cause mortality and increasing CAC score.[102] These investigators also showed a worsening prognosis with increasing number of calcified vessels.

The prognostic value of CAC seems valid also for diabetics, as shown in a study by Raggi and colleagues,[98] where the effect of CAC on all-cause mortality was the same in diabetics and nondiabetics. In another study looking exclusively at asymptomatic diabetic subjects, Anand and colleagues[103] showed that the CAC score was superior to all conventional cardiovascular risk factors and had the best AUC even when compared with UKPDS (United Kingdom Prospective Diabetes Study Risk Score) and FRS. The CAC score also holds prognostic value for women; Raggi and colleagues[104] showed a higher all-cause mortality for women with increasing CAC score. Of interest, for a given stratum of calcification women had a greater probability of death compared with men in the same category. The prognostic implication of CAC in patients with renal disease, however, is unclear. Vascular calcification in these patients is not only related to the intimal calcification from atherosclerosis but also to the medial calcification related to ectopic calcium deposition seen in advanced renal failure, and may not always correlate with coronary arterial stenosis.[105] However, other studies do seem to show CAC to be related to coronary artery stenosis, as well as to myocardial infarction and angina.[106,107]

There exists a valid argument for the use of age-, sex-, and race/ethnicity-specific percentiles in CAC scoring, due to the significant variation in the presence of CAC among various age, race, and gender groups. In a recent analysis of the MESA cohort, however, Budoff and colleagues[108] showed that absolute CAC scores work better than the group-specific percentiles.

GUIDELINES AND RECOMMENDATIONS FOR CORONARY CALCIUM SCANNING

The United States Preventive Services Task Force, in its recommendations released in 2004, recommends against CAC scanning for detecting the "presence of severe coronary artery stenosis (CAS) or the prediction of CHD events in adults at low risk for CHD events."[109] From their perspective, the excessive costs and potential harm associated with additional testing exceeds putative advantages.

The potential benefits of coronary calcium scanning need to be weighed against the real costs of the procedure itself, and the further testing and therapy directed by the results of CAC scanning. The downstream financial costs such a scan would spark off can be substantial and prohibitive, especially in today's environment of cost consciousness in medicine. Shaw and colleagues[110] reported on a subset of the EISNER study population, which was specifically evaluated and followed up for cardiovascular resource

Table 8
Relation of coronary artery calcium to cardiac stress testing

Authors	Study Objective	Study Population	Results	Remarks
Shavelle et al[85]	Comparison of CAC score and cardiac stress testing with coronary angiography	97 symptomatic patients. All patients underwent coronary angiography within 3 months of EBCT. 90% underwent stress testing	The relative risk of obstructive CAD as seen on angiography was higher (4.53) for patients who had CAC on EBCT, compared with an RR of 1.72–1.96 for stress test + patients	The investigators conclude superior diagnostic ability of CAC score over stress testing in detecting CAD. However, the specificity of CAC score is lower than stress testing
Kajinami et al[134]	Comparison of CAC score with ECG and Thallium stress test	251 consecutive patients with suspected CAD. All patients underwent EBCT, stress test, and angiography	A cutoff calcification score for prediction of significant stenosis, determined by receiver operating characteristic curve analysis, showed high sensitivity and specificity for presence of obstructive CAD	In this study the sensitivity and specificity of the EBCT was higher than both ECG stress testing and Thallium stress testing
Spadaro et al[135]	Comparison of EBCT and Thallium stress test with coronary angiography	150 patients who underwent thallium stress tests, EBCT, and coronary angiography	RR for obstructive CAD was 14.9 for patients with CAC compared with 3.5 for patients with positive thallium stress	EBCT when combined with thallium stress testing yielded an odds ratio of 15.8 and was superior to either test alone
Lamont et al[86]	Assessing the additive value of CAC score over treadmill stress testing	153 symptomatic patients with positive stress test. All underwent CAC scoring and angiography	The false-positive rate of the treadmill stress test compared with angiography was 27%. The sensitivity of a nonzero coronary calcium score for obstructive CAD was 98%	EBCT can potentially be used to identify patients with false-positive stress test results and decrease the number of invasive catheterization procedures
Schmermund et al[87]	Assessing the value of CAC score in predicting the angiographic extent of CAD	308 patients with suspected CAD underwent angiography. EBCT and NCEP risk-factor assessment was done in most of these patients. SPECT scans were performed in about half of the patients	CAC score was better at predicting the extent of CAD compared with either risk factor scores or SPECT derived radionuclide perfusion score	EBCT-derived CAC score is the best noninvasive tool to quantify plaque burden

Study	Purpose	Methods	Results	Conclusion
He et al[88]	Assessing the value of CAC score in detecting silent ischemia	3895 asymptomatic subjects had EBCT. 411 underwent SPECT perfusion scans	CAC poorly predicted positive stress tests, with only 22% patients with CAC having positive stress test results. The negative predictive value of CAC score was very high, with no subjects with a score <10 having a positive stress test	CAC score may be used to determine which patients are subjected to stress test
Berman et al[90]	Assessing the relation between SPECT perfusion scan and CAC	1195 patients without known CAD underwent SPECT perfusion scans and CAC tomography	The frequency of detected ischemia on SPECT perfusion scan increased progressively with increasing CAC score	Almost no subject with a CAC score <100 had ischemia. Of note, 56% subjects with CAC >100 had normal perfusion scan
Alan et al[92]	Assessing the prognosis in patients undergoing both CAC scanning and exercise MPS	1153 patients undergoing both CAC scanning and MPS. Patients followed for a mean period of 32 months	High CAC score correlated with ischemia on perfusion scanning. Negative perfusion scans predicted low mortality across all CAC score subgroups	Among patients with nonischemic MPS studies, high CAC scores do not confer an increased risk for cardiac events
Ramakrishna et al[93]	Assessing the relation and prognostic value between CAC score and perfusion imaging	835 patients underwent both EBCT and stress SPECT within a 3-month period, and were followed for an average of 4.8 years	There was a weak but statistically significant correlation between CAC score and SSS	Both CAC score and high SSS independently predicted mortality and nonfatal cardiovascular events. Only CAC score predicted mortality in asymptomatic subjects

Abbreviations: ECG, electrocardiogram; MPS, myocardial perfusion scintigraphy; NCEP, National Cholesterol Education Program; RR, relative risk; SPECT, single-photon emission computed tomography; SSS, summated stress score; TMST, treadmill stress test.

Table 9
Relation of coronary artery calcium to cardiovascular prognosis

Authors	Measured End Point	Number of Patients Studied	Follow-Up Period	CAC score	Relative Risk (95% CI)	Comments
Arad et al[136]	Coronary deaths, nonfatal MI, and revascularization	1172 asymptomatic persons	3.6 years (mean)	≥80 ≥160 ≥600	Odds ratio 22.3 (5.1–97.4) 22.2 (6.4–77.4) 20.3 (7.8–53.1)	The positive predictive value, negative predictive value, and specificity were progressively higher with increasing CAC score category even though the odds ratios were maximized by CAC score of 80–160
Wong et al[137]	Cardiovascular events including MI, stroke, revascularization	926 asymptomatic subjects	3.3 years (mean)	1–15 16–80 81–270 >271	0.72 3.29 4.5 8.8	The CAC score was divided by quartiles. There was a graded relation between the CAC score and future cardiovascular events
Pletcher et al[138]	MI + CHD death	3970 patients	32–43 months (mean)	0 1–100 101–400 >400	1 2.1 (1.6–2.9) 5.4 (2.2–13) 10 (3.1–34)	Standardized results of 4 studies (including the above 2 studies). Adjustment for established CHD risk factors done
Greenland et al[139]	MI + CHD death	1029 asymptomatic patients	84 months (median)	0 1–100 101–300 >300	1 1.5 (0.7–2.9) 2.1 (1.0–4.3) 3.9 (2.1–7.3)	Confirms the prognostic value of high CAC score
Taylor et al[95]	Unstable angina, MI, CHD death	1607 asymptomatic young men (40–50 years, mean 42.9 years)	36 months (12–72 months)	No CAC CAC present	1 10.75 (2.23–51.84)	Both groups controlled for FRS and family history of CAD

Study	Endpoint	Population	Follow-up	CAC category	HR (95% CI)	Comments
Kondos et al[70]	MI + CHD death	4151 asymptomatic men (30–76 years, mean 50 years) 1484 asymptomatic women (30–76 years, mean 54 years)	37 ± 12 months 37 ± 12 months	No CAC CAC present No CAC CAC present	1 3.86 (1.17–12.70) 1 1.53 (0.23–10.09)	Cox proportional hazards regression models included age, smoking history, diabetes, hypercholesterolemia, and hypertension
Shaw et al[140]	All-cause mortality	10,377 asymptomatic individuals	5 years (mean)	11–100 101–400 401–1000 >1000	1.64 (1.12–2.41) 1.74 (1.16–2.61) 2.54 (1.62, 3.99) 4.03 (2.52, 6.40)	On the Cox proportional hazards analysis, age and CAC score were the strongest predictors of mortality. The CAC score when applied to the Framingham risk scores further stratified individuals for increased mortality with increasing CAC score at the same Framingham category
Vliegenthart et al[141]	MI + CHD death	1795 asymptomatic elderly subjects (71.1 years, 62–85 years)	3.3 years	0–100 101–400 401–1000 >1000	1 2.7 (1.0–7.7) 4.1 (1.4–11.6) 8.1 (2.9–22.3)	Adjusted for body mass index, hypertension, total cholesterol, HDL cholesterol, smoking, diabetes mellitus, and family history of myocardial infarction
Arad et al[96]	MI + CHD death + revascularization	4613 asymptomatic subjects (59 ± 6 years)	4.3 years	0 1–99 100–399 ≥400	1 1.9 (0.8–4.2) 10.2 (4.8–21.6) 26.2 (12.6–53.7)	Confirms the prognostic value of high CAC score
Folsom et al[142]	MI, angina, stroke, and fatal CVD	6698 asymptomatic (45–84 years)	5.3 years	0 1–88 88–6315	1 2.6 (1.6–4.0) 6.0 (3.9–71)	Age-, race-, and sex-adjusted HR

(continued on next page)

Table 9
(continued)

Authors	Measured End Point	Number of Patients Studied	Follow-Up Period	CAC score	Relative Risk (95% CI)	Comments
Lakoski et al[143]	MI + CHD death + revascularization + angina	3601 asymptomatic women (60 ± 9 years, 45–84 years)	3.75 years	0 1–99 100–299 ≥300	1 2.4 (0.8–7.3) 1.5 (0.3–8.3) 8.3 (2.3–30.0)	Adjusted for age, ethnicity, body mass index, LDL cholesterol, hypertension, smoking, family history, estrogen use, and statin
Budoff et al[102]	All-cause mortality	25,253 asymptomatic individuals	6.8 years (mean)	1–10 11–100 101–399 400–699 700–999 ≥1000	1.31 (1.23–1.39) 1.48 (0.71–3.07) 3.84 (2.20–6.68) 5.78 (3.00–11.16) 6.47 (3.37–12.43) 9.36 (5.36–16.33)	Constitutes the largest and longest follow-up after CAC scanning. The prognostic value was incremental to Framingham risk model
Raggi et al[98]	All-cause mortality	9474 asymptomatic nondiabetic subjects (53 ± 10 years) 903 diabetic subjects (57 ± 10 years)	5 ± 3.5 years 5 ± 3.5 years	No CAC CAC present No CAC CAC present	1 1.44 (1.16–1.80) 1 1.36 (1.21–1.54)	Diabetic and nondiabetic with no CAC showed similar survival. Those without calcium had a low short-term risk of death even in presence of diabetes

Study	Endpoint	Population	Follow-up	CAC score	M	F	Comments
Becker et al[101]	MI + CHD death	1726 asymptomatic adults	40.3 ± 7.3 months	0–10	1	1	CAC was more sensitive than traditional risk factors in predicting events, especially discriminatory in individuals with intermediate risk
				11–100	1.7	1.9	
				101–400	4.1	4.5	
				>400	6.8	7.9	
Detrano et al[37] MESA study	MI + CHD death	6722 subjects with no known cardiac disease	3.9 years (median)	0	1		The study had a higher representation of nonwhite subjects and demonstrated equivalent prognostic value of CAC score in all major racial groups
				1–100	3.89		
				101–300	7.08		
				>300	6.84		

Abbreviations: CVD, cardiovascular disease; HR, heart rate; MI, myocardial infarction.

consumption, procedural costs, and clinical outcomes after CAC scanning. The investigators followed 1361 patients for a total of 4 years after CAC scanning, and reported increasing use of further noninvasive and invasive testing with increasing CAC scores.[110] The majority of the patients (78%) had a CAC score of 100 or less and had annual cardiovascular disease costs between $25 and $35. Fewer than 1% of subjects with a CAC score of 1000 or less had invasive coronary angiograms and only 19.4% of those with a CAC score greater than 1000 had the angiogram. Another study reported a drop of 15.4% in the number of invasive coronary angiograms performed with the application of CT scanning for cardiovascular disease.[111] Shaw and colleagues also note that the differential in costs among high-risk and low-risk subjects undergoing CAC scans would be much wider than those stratified by FRS or unconventional methods such as high-sensitivity C-reactive protein.

The American Heart Association (AHA) statement from 2006 authored by Budoff and colleagues[112] acknowledges MDCT for CAC scanning as a promising tool most relevant for the testing of asymptomatic individuals at risk for CAD, who may be led to effective lifestyle-based and pharmacotherapeutic interventions to reduce their risk of developing manifest CAD. The AHA did not recommend serial measurement of CAC score for the purposes of evaluating therapies. The 2007 American College of Cardiology/AHA statement taking into account complicated cost-benefit analysis did not recommend for or against the CAC scoring of patients for cardiovascular prognostication. It discouraged the measurement of CAC score in low-risk persons (eg, <10% 10-year risk of CHD) or "population screening."[113] It does, however, advise its judicious use in patients with intermediate risk, noting the following:

> The Committee judged that it may be reasonable to consider use of CAC measurement in such patients based on available evidence that demonstrates incremental risk prediction information in this selected (intermediate risk) patient group. This conclusion is based on the possibility that such patients might be reclassified to a higher risk status based on high CAC score, and subsequent patient management may be modified.

The investigators went on to note that screening may also be appropriate for special purposes such as determining the cause of cardiomyopathy (ischemic vs nonischemic) and in the setting of equivocal exercise testing results.

HYPOTHETICAL COST MODELS OF CORONARY ARTERY CALCIUM SCORING: THE EMERGENCY ROOM AND OUTPATIENT SETTING

In pursuit of analyzing the economic impact of CAC scanning, the authors have devised two simple decision models (**Table 10**). The first model evaluates the role of CAC scanning in the acute evaluation of chest pain. The base case scenario included a 50-year-old patient presenting to the Emergency Department with acute onset of chest pain. Initial enzymes and presenting electrocardiogram were negative/inconclusive for acute myocardial infarction. This patient subset includes patients with 30% prevalence of CAC scores of 100 or greater. The cost model evaluated the cost to identify significant obstructive CAD as compared with the usual care approach that included coronary computed tomographic angiography (CCTA). The total cost of CAC was set at $150 and the cost of a CCTA was set at $290. The end point of this analysis included: (1) obstructive CAD defined as 50% or greater coronary stenosis and (2) an acute coronary syndrome (ACS). The prevalence of CAD was set at 10% and the prevalence of ACS at 3%, based on the analysis by Goldstein and colleagues[114] and the ROMICAT study.[115]

The results of this model revealed that the use of CAC was more costly because downstream testing was more often recommended because of a higher prevalence of significant CAC of 100 or greater, in comparison with the lower prevalence of obstructive CAD by CCTA. The result is a total higher cost and a delta cost of $5200 to identify one more patient with obstructive CAD using CAC as compared with CCTA. Applying the same costs to the second model, the total cost to identify one more patient with ACS was $13,000 for CAC compared with CCTA.

For the patient presenting in the outpatient setting, a decision model was devised to examine detection of high-risk asymptomatic patients when comparing CAC with carotid intima-media thickness (CIMT). Based on the results of the MESA registry and related data analysis, CAC resulted in an improved risk classification within the range of 5% to 10%. Procedural costs were assigned to CAC at $150 and to CIMT at $100. Defining a simple cost model to identify one additional correctly classified patient at risk for major adverse cardiovascular events, the results revealed a cost of $1000 to identify one additional patient with CAC in comparison with CIMT.

The presence of coronary artery calcium is closely associated with the presence of

Table 10
Hypothetical cost model of CAC score

A. Use of CAC vs CCTA in the ED Evaluation of Acute Onset Chest Pain

Population: 10 million acute pain patients in the ED

		Cost (US$)	No. with CAD	Incremental Cost-Effectiveness Ratio (US$)
		6,900,000,000.00	1,000,000	
#1	CAD Model			5200.00
	(Prevalence = 10%)	5,600,000,000.00	750,000	
			No. with ACS	
Cost to Identify Significant CAD Using CAC vs Usual Care =				
		6,900,000,000.00	400,000	
#2	ACS Model			13,000.00
	(Prevalence = 3%–5%)	5,600,000,000.00	300,000	

B. Use of CAC vs CIMT in the Detection of High-Risk Asymptomatics

			No. with Correctly Identified Cardiovascular Event	
Population: 40 million patients with an intermediate Framingham risk score				
#3	Risk Classification	6,000,000,000.00	12,000,000	
	(Delta Improvement with CAC 5%–10%)			1000.00
		4,000,000,000.00	9,000,000	

Abbreviations: ACS, acute coronary syndrome; CCTA, coronary computed tomographic angiography; ED, Emergency Department.

atherosclerotic lesions in the coronary vasculature. Detection of coronary calcium by imaging techniques has evolved over the last few decades and has become especially more sophisticated with advanced imaging technology. Whereas the status of coronary artery calcium as a marker of increased cardiovascular risk is well established, the indication for testing continues to be a topic of debate.

REFERENCES

1. Morgagni GB. De Sedibus et Causis Morborum per Anatomen Indagatis. 1769.
2. Blankenhorn DH. Coronary arterial calcification a review. Am J Med Sci 1961;242(2):1–10.
3. Leary T. Atherosclerosis: special consideration of aortic lesions. Arch Pathol 1936;21:419–58.
4. Blankenhorn DH, Stern D. Calcification of the coronary arteries. Am J Roentgenol Radium Ther Nucl Med 1959;81(5):772–7.
5. Lieber A, Jorgens J. Cinefluorography of coronary artery calcification. Correlation with clinical arteriosclerotic heart disease and autopsy findings. Am J Roentgenol Radium Ther Nucl Med 1961;86:1063–72.
6. Eggen DA, Strong JP, McGill HC Jr. Coronary calcification. Relationship to clinically significant coronary lesions and race, sex, and topographic distribution. Circulation 1965;32(6):948–55.
7. Bartel AG, Chen JT, Peter RH, et al. The significance of coronary calcification detected by fluoroscopy. A report of 360 patients. Circulation 1974;49(6):1247–53.
8. Margolis JR, Chen JT, Kong Y, et al. The diagnostic and prognostic significance of coronary artery calcification. A report of 800 cases. Radiology 1980;137(3):609–16.
9. Janowitz WR, Agatston AS, King D, et al. High-resolution ultrafast CT of the coronary arteries: new technique for visualizing coronary artery anatomy. Radiology 1988;169:345.
10. Tanenbaum SR, Kondos GT, Veselik KE, et al. Detection of calcific deposits in coronary arteries by ultrafast computed tomography and correlation with angiography. Am J Cardiol 1989;63(12):870–2.
11. Agatston A, Janowitz W, Hildner F, et al. Quantification of coronary artery calcium using ultrafast computed tomography. J Am Coll Cardiol 1990;15(4):827–32.
12. Callister TQ, Cooil B, Raya SP, et al. Coronary artery disease: improved reproducibility of calcium scoring with an electron-beam CT volumetric method. Radiology 1998;208(3):807–14.
13. Kopp AF, Ohnesorge B, Becker C, et al. Reproducibility and accuracy of coronary calcium

measurements with multi-detector row versus electron-beam CT. Radiology 2002;225(1):113–9.

14. Stary HC. The sequence of cell and matrix changes in atherosclerotic lesions of coronary arteries in the first forty years of life. Eur Heart J 1990;11(Suppl E):3–19.

15. Wexler L, Brundage B, Crouse J, et al. Coronary artery calcification: pathophysiology, epidemiology, imaging methods, and clinical implications. A statement for health professionals from the American Heart Association. Writing Group. Circulation 1996;94(5):1175–92.

16. Bolick LE, Blankenhorn DH. A quantitative study of coronary arterial calcification. Am J Pathol 1961;39: 511–9.

17. Shao JS, Cai J, Towler DA. Molecular mechanisms of vascular calcification: lessons learned from the aorta. Arterioscler Thromb Vasc Biol 2006;26(7): 1423–30.

18. Bostrom K, Watson KE, Horn S, et al. Bone morphogenetic protein expression in human atherosclerotic lesions. J Clin Invest 1993;91(4):1800–9.

19. Abedin M, Tintut Y, Demer LL. Vascular calcification: mechanisms and clinical ramifications. Arterioscler Thromb Vasc Biol 2004;24(7):1161–70.

20. Lee RT, Grodzinsky AJ, Frank EH, et al. Structure-dependent dynamic mechanical behavior of fibrous caps from human atherosclerotic plaques. Circulation 1991;83(5):1764–70.

21. Cheng GC, Loree HM, Kamm RD, et al. Distribution of circumferential stress in ruptured and stable atherosclerotic lesions. A structural analysis with histopathological correlation. Circulation 1993; 87(4):1179–87.

22. Hodgson JM, Reddy KG, Suneja R, et al. Intracoronary ultrasound imaging: correlation of plaque morphology with angiography, clinical syndrome and procedural results in patients undergoing coronary angioplasty. J Am Coll Cardiol 1993; 21(1):35–44.

23. Fitzgerald PJ, Ports TA, Yock PG. Contribution of localized calcium deposits to dissection after angioplasty. An observational study using intravascular ultrasound. Circulation 1992;86(1):64–70.

24. Motoyama S, Kondo T, Sarai M, et al. Multislice computed tomographic characteristics of coronary lesions in acute coronary syndromes. J Am Coll Cardiol 2007;50(4):319–26.

25. Health NIo, editor. 2004 NHLBI morbidity and mortality chart book. National Heart, Lung, and Blood Institute; 2004.

26. Newman AB, Naydeck BL, Whittle J, et al. Racial differences in coronary artery calcification in older adults. Arterioscler Thromb Vasc Biol 2002;22(3): 424–30.

27. Jain T, Peshock R, McGuire DK, et al. African Americans and Caucasians have a similar prevalence of

coronary calcium in the Dallas Heart Study. J Am Coll Cardiol 2004;44(5):1011–7.

28. Bild DE, Folsom AR, Lowe LP, et al. Prevalence and correlates of coronary calcification in black and white young adults: the Coronary Artery Risk Development in Young Adults (CARDIA) Study. Arterioscler Thromb Vasc Biol 2001;21(5):852–7.

29. Khurana C, Rosenbaum CG, Howard BV, et al. Coronary artery calcification in black women and white women. Am Heart J 2003;145(4):724–9.

30. Hatwalkar A, Agrawal N, Reiss DS, et al. Comparison of prevalence and severity of coronary calcium determined by electron beam tomography among various ethnic groups. Am J Cardiol 2003; 91(10):1225–7.

31. Kawakubo M, LaBree L, Xiang M, et al. Race-ethnic differences in the extent, prevalence, and progression of coronary calcium. Ethn Dis 2005; 15(2):198–204.

32. Newman AB, Naydeck BL, Sutton-Tyrrell K, et al. Coronary artery calcification in older adults to age 99: prevalence and risk factors. Circulation 2001; 104(22):2679–84.

33. Tejada C, Strong JP, Montenegro MR, et al. Distribution of coronary and aortic atherosclerosis by geographic location, race, and sex. Lab Invest 1968;18(5):509–26.

34. Orakzai SH, Orakzai RH, Nasir K, et al. Subclinical coronary atherosclerosis: racial profiling is necessary! Am Heart J 2006;152(5):819–27.

35. Diez Roux AV, Detrano R, Jackson S, et al. Acculturation and socioeconomic position as predictors of coronary calcification in a multiethnic sample. Circulation 2005;112(11):1557–65.

36. Doherty TM, Tang W, Detrano RC. Racial differences in the significance of coronary calcium in asymptomatic black and white subjects with coronary risk factors. J Am Coll Cardiol 1999;34(3):787–94.

37. Detrano R, Guerci AD, Carr JJ, et al. Coronary calcium as a predictor of coronary events in four racial or ethnic groups. N Engl J Med 2008; 358(13):1336–45.

38. Nasir K, Shaw LJ, Liu ST, et al. Ethnic differences in the prognostic value of coronary artery calcification for all-cause mortality. J Am Coll Cardiol 2007; 50(10):953–60.

39. Janowitz WR, Agatston AS, Kaplan G, et al. Differences in prevalence and extent of coronary artery calcium detected by ultrafast computed tomography in asymptomatic men and women. Am J Cardiol 1993;72(3):247–54.

40. McClelland RL, Chung H, Detrano R, et al. Distribution of coronary artery calcium by race, gender, and age: results from the Multi-Ethnic Study of Atherosclerosis (MESA). Circulation 2006;113(1):30–7.

41. Rumberger JA, Schwartz RS, Simons DB, et al. Relation of coronary calcium determined by

electron beam computed tomography and lumen narrowing determined by autopsy. Am J Cardiol 1994;73(16):1169–73.

42. Hyder JA, Allison MA, Wong N, et al. Association of coronary artery and aortic calcium with lumbar bone density: the MESA Abdominal Aortic Calcium Study. Am J Epidemiol 2009;169(2):186–94.

43. Doherty TM, Detrano RC, Mautner SL, et al. Coronary calcium: the good, the bad, and the uncertain. Am Heart J 1999;137(5):806–14.

44. Mautner GC, Mautner SL, Froehlich J, et al. Coronary artery calcification: assessment with electron beam CT and histomorphometric correlation. Radiology 1994;192(3):619–23.

45. Young W, Gofman JW, Tandy R, et al. The quantitation of atherosclerosis. II. Quantitative aspects of the relationship of blood pressure and atherosclerosis. Am J Cardiol 1960;6:294–9.

46. Sangiorgi G, Rumberger JA, Severson A, et al. Arterial calcification and not lumen stenosis is highly correlated with atherosclerotic plaque burden in humans: a histologic study of 723 coronary artery segments using nondecalcifying methodology. J Am Coll Cardiol 1998;31(1):126–33.

47. Rumberger JA, Simons DB, Fitzpatrick LA, et al. Coronary artery calcium area by electron-beam computed tomography and coronary atherosclerotic plaque area. A histopathologic correlative study. Circulation 1995;92(8):2157–62.

48. Simons DB, Schwartz RS, Edwards WD, et al. Noninvasive definition of anatomic coronary artery disease by ultrafast computed tomographic scanning: a quantitative pathologic comparison study. J Am Coll Cardiol 1992;20(5):1118–26.

49. Williams M, Shaw LJ, Raggi P, et al. Prognostic value of number and site of calcified coronary lesions compared with the total score. JACC Cardiovasc Imaging 2008;1(1):61–9.

50. Stewart BF, Siscovick D, Lind BK, et al. Clinical factors associated with calcific aortic valve disease. Cardiovascular Health Study. J Am Coll Cardiol 1997;29(3):630–4.

51. O'Brien KD, Reichenbach DD, Marcovina SM, et al. Apolipoproteins B, (a), and E accumulate in the morphologically early lesion of 'degenerative' valvular aortic stenosis. Arterioscler Thromb Vasc Biol 1996;16(4):523–32.

52. Takasu J, Shavelle DM, O'Brien KD, et al. Association between progression of aortic valve calcification and coronary calcification: assessment by electron beam tomography1. Acad Radiol 2005; 12(3):298–304.

53. Tohno Y, Tohno S, Mahakkanukrauh P, et al. Earlier accumulation of calcium, phosphorus, and magnesium in the coronary artery in comparison with the ascending aorta, aortic valve, and mitral valve. Biol Trace Elem Res 2006;112(1):31–42.

54. Adler Y, Fink N, Spector D, et al. Mitral annulus calcification—a window to diffuse atherosclerosis of the vascular system. Atherosclerosis 2001;155(1):1–8.

55. Tenenbaum A, Shemesh J, Fisman EZ, et al. Advanced mitral annular calcification is associated with severe coronary calcification on fast dual spiral computed tomography. Invest Radiol 2000; 35(3):193–8.

56. Tenenbaum A, Fisman EZ, Pines A, et al. Gender paradox in cardiac calcium deposits in middle-aged and elderly patients: mitral annular and coronary calcifications interrelationship. Maturitas 2000; 36(1):35–42.

57. Tenenbaum A, Fisman EZ, Shemesh J, et al. Combined coronary and mitral annulus calcium detection in the non-invasive diagnosis of coronary artery disease in patients with systemic hypertension. Coron Artery Dis 2002;13(2):113–7.

58. Pohle K, Maffert R, Ropers D, et al. Progression of aortic valve calcification: association with coronary atherosclerosis and cardiovascular risk factors. Circulation 2001;104(16):1927–32.

59. Yamamoto H, Shavelle D, Takasu J, et al. Valvular and thoracic aortic calcium as a marker of the extent and severity of angiographic coronary artery disease. Am Heart J 2003;146(1):153–9.

60. Shanahan CM, Proudfoot D, Farzaneh-Far A, et al. The role of Gla proteins in vascular calcification. Crit Rev Eukaryot Gene Expr 1998;8(3–4):357–75.

61. Iribarren C, Sidney S, Sternfeld B, et al. Calcification of the aortic arch: risk factors and association with coronary heart disease, stroke, and peripheral vascular disease. JAMA 2000;283(21):2810–5.

62. Watanabe K, Hiroki T, Koga N. Relation of thoracic aorta calcification on computed tomography and coronary risk factors to obstructive coronary artery disease on angiography. Angiology 2003;54(4): 433–41.

63. Adler Y, Fisman EZ, Shemesh J, et al. Spiral computed tomography evidence of close correlation between coronary and thoracic aorta calcifications. Atherosclerosis 2004;176(1):133–8.

64. Lehto S, Niskanen L, Suhonen M, et al. Medial artery calcification. A neglected harbinger of cardiovascular complications in non-insulin-dependent diabetes mellitus. Arterioscler Thromb Vasc Biol 1996;16(8):978–83.

65. Takasu J, Budoff MJ, O'Brien KD, et al. Relationship between coronary artery and descending thoracic aortic calcification as detected by computed tomography: the Multi-Ethnic Study of Atherosclerosis. Atherosclerosis 2009;204(2):440–6.

66. Eisen A, Tenenbaum A, Koren-Morag N, et al. Calcification of the thoracic aorta as detected by spiral computed tomography among stable angina pectoris patients: association with cardiovascular events and death. Circulation 2008;118(13):1328–34.

67. Wong ND, Sciammarella M, Arad Y, et al. Relation of thoracic aortic and aortic valve calcium to coronary artery calcium and risk assessment. Am J Cardiol 2003;92(8):951–5.

68. Ross R. The pathogenesis of atherosclerosis: a perspective for the 1990s. Nature 1993;362(6423): 801–9.

69. Sung J, Lim SJ, Choe Y, et al. Comparison of the coronary calcium score with the estimated coronary risk. Coron Artery Dis 2008;19(7):475–9.

70. Kondos GT, Hoff JA, Sevrukov A, et al. Electron-beam tomography coronary artery calcium and cardiac events: a 37-month follow-up of 5635 initially asymptomatic low- to intermediate-risk adults. Circulation 2003;107(20):2571–6.

71. Ho JS, FitzGerald SJ, Stolfus LL, et al. Relation of a coronary artery calcium score higher than 400 to coronary stenoses detected using multidetector computed tomography and to traditional cardiovascular risk factors. Am J Cardiol 2008;101(10): 1444–7.

72. Goff DC Jr, Bertoni AG, Kramer H, et al. Dyslipidemia prevalence, treatment, and control in the Multi-Ethnic Study of Atherosclerosis (MESA): gender, ethnicity, and coronary artery calcium. Circulation 2006;113(5):647–56.

73. Hoffmann U, Massaro JM, Fox CS, et al. Defining normal distributions of coronary artery calcium in women and men (from the Framingham Heart Study). Am J Cardiol 2008;102(9):1136–41, 1141.e1131.

74. Akram K, Voros S. Absolute coronary artery calcium scores are superior to MESA percentile rank in predicting obstructive coronary artery disease. Int J Cardiovasc Imaging 2008;24(7):743–9.

75. Polonsky TS, McClelland RL, Jorgensen NW, et al. Coronary artery calcium score and risk classification for coronary heart disease prediction. JAMA 2010;303(16):1610–6.

76. Janowitz WR, Agatston AS, Viamonte M Jr. Comparison of serial quantitative evaluation of calcified coronary artery plaque by ultrafast computed tomography in persons with and without obstructive coronary artery disease. Am J Cardiol 1991;68(1):1–6.

77. Haberl R, Becker A, Leber A, et al. Correlation of coronary calcification and angiographically documented stenoses in patients with suspected coronary artery disease: results of 1,764 patients. J Am Coll Cardiol 2001;37(2):451–7.

78. Budoff MJ, Diamond GA, Raggi P, et al. Continuous probabilistic prediction of angiographically significant coronary artery disease using electron beam tomography. Circulation 2002;105(15):1791–6.

79. Breen JF, Sheedy PF 2nd, Schwartz RS, et al. Coronary artery calcification detected with ultrafast CT as an indication of coronary artery disease. Radiology 1992;185(2):435–9.

80. Kajinami K, Seki H, Takekoshi N, et al. Coronary calcification and coronary atherosclerosis: site by site comparative morphologic study of electron beam computed tomography and coronary angiography. J Am Coll Cardiol 1997;29(7):1549–56.

81. Marwan M, Ropers D, Pflederer T, et al. Clinical characteristics of patients with obstructive coronary lesions in the absence of coronary calcification: an evaluation by coronary CT angiography. Heart 2009;95(13):1056–60.

82. Gottlieb I, Miller JM, Arbab-Zadeh A, et al. The absence of coronary calcification does not exclude obstructive coronary artery disease or the need for revascularization in patients referred for conventional coronary angiography. J Am Coll Cardiol 2010;55(7):627–34.

83. Rubinshtein R, Gaspar T, Halon DA, et al. Prevalence and extent of obstructive coronary artery disease in patients with zero or low calcium score undergoing 64-slice cardiac multidetector computed tomography for evaluation of a chest pain syndrome. Am J Cardiol 2007;99(4):472–5.

84. Redberg RF. What is the prognostic value of a zero calcium score? J Am Coll Cardiol 2010;55(7): 635–6.

85. Shavelle DM, Budoff MJ, LaMont DH, et al. Exercise testing and electron beam computed tomography in the evaluation of coronary artery disease. J Am Coll Cardiol 2000;36(1):32–8.

86. Lamont DH, Budoff MJ, Shavelle DM, et al. Coronary calcium scanning adds incremental value to patients with positive stress tests. Am Heart J 2002;143(5):861–7.

87. Schmermund A, Denktas AE, Rumberger JA, et al. Independent and incremental value of coronary artery calcium for predicting the extent of angiographic coronary artery disease: comparison with cardiac risk factors and radionuclide perfusion imaging. J Am Coll Cardiol 1999;34(3): 777–86.

88. He ZX, Hedrick TD, Pratt CM, et al. Severity of coronary artery calcification by electron beam computed tomography predicts silent myocardial ischemia. Circulation 2000;101(3):244–51.

89. Ho J, FitzGerald S, Cannaday J, et al. Relation of aortic valve calcium to myocardial ischemic perfusion in individuals with a low coronary artery calcium score. Am J Cardiol 2007;99(11):1535–7.

90. Berman DS, Wong ND, Gransar H, et al. Relationship between stress-induced myocardial ischemia and atherosclerosis measured by coronary calcium tomography. J Am Coll Cardiol 2004;44(4):923–30.

91. Wong ND, Rozanski A, Gransar H, et al. Metabolic syndrome and diabetes are associated with an increased likelihood of inducible myocardial ischemia among patients with subclinical atherosclerosis. Diabetes Care 2005;28(6):1445–50.

92. Rozanski A, Gransar H, Wong ND, et al. Clinical outcomes after both coronary calcium scanning and exercise myocardial perfusion scintigraphy. J Am Coll Cardiol 2007;49(12):1352–61.

93. Ramakrishna G, Miller TD, Breen JF, et al. Relationship and prognostic value of coronary artery calcification by electron beam computed tomography to stress-induced ischemia by single photon emission computed tomography. Am Heart J 2007;153(5): 807–14.

94. Askew JW, Miller TD, Araoz PA, et al. Abnormal electron beam computed tomography results: the value of repeating myocardial perfusion single-photon emission computed tomography in the ongoing assessment of coronary artery disease. Mayo Clin Proc 2008;83(1):17–22.

95. Taylor AJ, Bindeman J, Feuerstein I, et al. Coronary calcium independently predicts incident premature coronary heart disease over measured cardiovascular risk factors: mean three-year outcomes in the Prospective Army Coronary Calcium (PACC) project. J Am Coll Cardiol 2005;46(5):807–14.

96. Arad Y, Goodman KJ, Roth M, et al. Coronary calcification, coronary disease risk factors, C-reactive protein, and atherosclerotic cardiovascular disease events: the St. Francis Heart Study. J Am Coll Cardiol 2005;46(1):158–65.

97. Raggi P, Cooil B, Callister TQ. Use of electron beam tomography data to develop models for prediction of hard coronary events. Am Heart J 2001;141(3):375–82.

98. Raggi P, Shaw LJ, Berman DS, et al. Prognostic value of coronary artery calcium screening in subjects with and without diabetes. J Am Coll Cardiol 2004;43(9):1663–9.

99. Wayhs R, Zelinger A, Raggi P. High coronary artery calcium scores pose an extremely elevated risk for hard events. J Am Coll Cardiol 2002;39(2): 225–30.

100. Wilson PW, D'Agostino RB, Levy D, et al. Prediction of coronary heart disease using risk factor categories. Circulation 1998;97(18):1837–47.

101. Becker A, Leber A, Becker C, et al. Predictive value of coronary calcifications for future cardiac events in asymptomatic individuals. Am Heart J 2008; 155(1):154–60.

102. Budoff MJ, Shaw LJ, Liu ST, et al. Long-term prognosis associated with coronary calcification: observations from a registry of 25,253 patients. J Am Coll Cardiol 2007;49(18):1860–70.

103. Anand DV, Lim E, Hopkins D, et al. Risk stratification in uncomplicated type 2 diabetes: prospective evaluation of the combined use of coronary artery calcium imaging and selective myocardial perfusion scintigraphy. Eur Heart J 2006;27(6):713–21.

104. Raggi P, Shaw LJ, Berman DS, et al. Gender-based differences in the prognostic value of coronary calcification. J Womens Health (Larchmt) 2004; 13(3):273–83.

105. Sharples EJ, Pereira D, Summers S, et al. Coronary artery calcification measured with electron-beam computerized tomography correlates poorly with coronary artery angiography in dialysis patients. Am J Kidney Dis 2004;43(2):313–9.

106. Haydar AA, Hujairi NM, Covic AA, et al. Coronary artery calcification is related to coronary atherosclerosis in chronic renal disease patients: a study comparing EBCT-generated coronary artery calcium scores and coronary angiography. Nephrol Dial Transplant 2004;19(9):2307–12.

107. Raggi P, Boulay A, Chasan-Taber S, et al. Cardiac calcification in adult hemodialysis patients. A link between end-stage renal disease and cardiovascular disease? J Am Coll Cardiol 2002;39(4): 695–701.

108. Budoff MJ, Nasir K, McClelland RL, et al. Coronary calcium predicts events better with absolute calcium scores than age-sex-race/ethnicity percentiles: MESA (Multi-Ethnic Study of Atherosclerosis). J Am Coll Cardiol 2009;53(4):345–52.

109. Force UPST. Screening for coronary heart disease. US Department of Health & Human Services; 2004.

110. Shaw LJ, Min JK, Budoff M, et al. Induced cardiovascular procedural costs and resource consumption patterns after coronary artery calcium screening: results from the EISNER (Early Identification of Subclinical Atherosclerosis by Noninvasive Imaging Research) study. J Am Coll Cardiol 2009;54(14):1258–67.

111. Baker LC, Atlas SW, Afendulis CC. Expanded use of imaging technology and the challenge of measuring value. Health Aff 2008;27(6):1467–78.

112. Budoff MJ, Achenbach S, Blumenthal RS, et al. Assessment of coronary artery disease by cardiac computed tomography: a scientific statement from the American Heart Association Committee on Cardiovascular Imaging and Intervention, Council on Cardiovascular Radiology and Intervention, and Committee on Cardiac Imaging, Council on Clinical Cardiology. Circulation 2006;114(16): 1761–91.

113. Greenland P, Bonow RO, Brundage BH, et al. ACCF/AHA 2007 clinical expert consensus document on coronary artery calcium scoring by computed tomography in global cardiovascular risk assessment and in evaluation of patients with chest pain: a report of the American College of Cardiology Foundation Clinical Expert Consensus Task Force (ACCF/AHA Writing Committee to Update the 2000 Expert Consensus Document on Electron Beam Computed Tomography). Circulation 2007;115(3):402–26.

114. Goldstein JA, Gallagher MJ, O'Neill WW, et al. A randomized controlled trial of multi-slice

coronary computed tomography for evaluation of acute chest pain. J Am Coll Cardiol 2007;49(8): 863–71.

115. Hoffmann U, Bamberg F, Chae CU, et al. Coronary computed tomography angiography for early triage of patients with acute chest pain: the ROMICAT (Rule Out Myocardial Infarction using Computer Assisted Tomography) trial. J Am Coll Cardiol 2009;53(18):1642–50.

116. Bild DE, Detrano R, Peterson D, et al. Ethnic differences in coronary calcification: the Multi-Ethnic Study of Atherosclerosis (MESA). Circulation 2005;111(10):1313–20.

117. Tang W, Detrano RC, Brezden OS, et al. Racial differences in coronary calcium prevalence among high-risk adults. Am J Cardiol 1995;75(16):1088–91.

118. Budoff MJ, Yang TP, Shavelle RM, et al. Ethnic differences in coronary atherosclerosis. J Am Coll Cardiol 2002;39(3):408–12.

119. Lee TC, O'Malley PG, Feuerstein I, et al. The prevalence and severity of coronary artery calcification on coronary artery computed tomography in black and white subjects. J Am Coll Cardiol 2003;41(1): 39–44.

120. Fair JM, Kiazand A, Varady A, et al. Ethnic differences in coronary artery calcium in a healthy cohort aged 60 to 69 years. Am J Cardiol 2007; 100(6):981–5.

121. Budoff MJ, Nasir K, Mao S, et al. Ethnic differences of the presence and severity of coronary atherosclerosis. Atherosclerosis 2006;187(2):343–50.

122. Adler Y, Shemesh J, Tenenbaum A, et al. Aortic valve calcium on spiral computed tomography (dual slice mode) is associated with advanced coronary calcium in hypertensive patients. Coron Artery Dis 2002;13(4):209–13.

123. Cury RC, Ferencik M, Hoffmann U, et al. Epidemiology and association of vascular and valvular calcium quantified by multidetector computed tomography in elderly asymptomatic subjects. Am J Cardiol 2004;94(3):348–51.

124. Walsh CR, Larson MG, Kupka MJ, et al. Association of aortic valve calcium detected by electron beam computed tomography with echocardiographic aortic valve disease and with calcium deposits in the coronary arteries and thoracic aorta. Am J Cardiol 2004;93(4):421–5.

125. Raggi P, Cooil B, Hadi A, et al. Predictors of aortic and coronary artery calcium on a screening electron beam tomographic scan. Am J Cardiol 2003; 91(6):744–6.

126. Karim R, Hodis HN, Detrano R, et al. Relation of Framingham risk score to subclinical atherosclerosis evaluated across three arterial sites. Am J Cardiol 2008;102(7):825–30.

127. Wong ND, Kouwabunpat D, Vo AN, et al. Coronary calcium and atherosclerosis by ultrafast computed tomography in asymptomatic men and women: relation to age and risk factors. Am Heart J 1994; 127(2):422–30.

128. Mahoney LT, Burns TL, Stanford W, et al. Usefulness of the Framingham risk score and body mass index to predict early coronary artery calcium in young adults (Muscatine Study). Am J Cardiol 2001;88(5):509–15.

129. Mahoney LT, Burns TL, Stanford W, et al. Coronary risk factors measured in childhood and young adult life are associated with coronary artery calcification in young adults: the Muscatine Study. J Am Coll Cardiol 1996;27(2):277–84.

130. Michos ED, Nasir K, Rumberger JA, et al. Relation of family history of premature coronary heart disease and metabolic risk factors to risk of coronary arterial calcium in asymptomatic subjects. Am J Cardiol 2005;95(5):655–7.

131. Nasir K, Michos ED, Rumberger JA, et al. Coronary artery calcification and family history of premature coronary heart disease: sibling history is more strongly associated than parental history. Circulation 2004;110(15):2150–6.

132. Arad Y, Newstein D, Cadet F, et al. Association of multiple risk factors and insulin resistance with increased prevalence of asymptomatic coronary artery disease by an electron-beam computed tomographic study. Arterioscler Thromb Vasc Biol 2001;21(12):2051–8.

133. Wong ND, Sciammarella MG, Polk D, et al. The metabolic syndrome, diabetes, and subclinical atherosclerosis assessed by coronary calcium. J Am Coll Cardiol 2003;41(9):1547–53.

134. Kajinami K, Seki H, Takekoshi N, et al. Noninvasive prediction of coronary atherosclerosis by quantification of coronary artery calcification using electron beam computed tomography: comparison with electrocardiographic and thallium exercise stress test results. J Am Coll Cardiol 1995;26(5): 1209–21.

135. Spadaro LA, Sherman S, Roth M, et al. Comparison of thallium stress testing and electron beam computed tomography in the prediction of coronary artery disease. J Am Coll Cardiol 1996; 27(Suppl):175A.

136. Arad Y, Spadaro LA, Goodman K, et al. Prediction of coronary events with electron beam computed tomography. J Am Coll Cardiol 2000;36(4):1253–60.

137. Wong ND, Hsu JC, Detrano RC, et al. Coronary artery calcium evaluation by electron beam computed tomography and its relation to new cardiovascular events. Am J Cardiol 2000;86(5):495–8.

138. Pletcher MJ, Tice JA, Pignone M, et al. Using the coronary artery calcium score to predict coronary heart disease events: a systematic review and meta-analysis. Arch Intern Med 2004;164(12): 1285–92.

139. Greenland P, LaBree L, Azen SP, et al. Coronary artery calcium score combined with Framingham score for risk prediction in asymptomatic individuals. JAMA 2004;291(2):210–5.

140. Shaw LJ, Raggi P, Schisterman E, et al. Prognostic value of cardiac risk factors and coronary artery calcium screening for all-cause mortality. Radiology 2003;228(3):826–33.

141. Vliegenthart R, Oudkerk M, Hofman A, et al. Coronary calcification improves cardiovascular risk prediction in the elderly. Circulation 2005;112(4):572–7.

142. Folsom AR, Kronmal RA, Detrano RC, et al. Coronary artery calcification compared with carotid intima-media thickness in the prediction of cardiovascular disease incidence: the Multi-Ethnic Study of Atherosclerosis (MESA). Arch Intern Med 2008;168(12):1333–9.

143. Lakoski SG, Greenland P, Wong ND, et al. Coronary artery calcium scores and risk for cardiovascular events in women classified as "low risk" based on Framingham risk score: the multi-ethnic study of atherosclerosis (MESA). Arch Intern Med 2007;167(22):2437–42.

Coronary Artery Calcium Testing: Dos and Don'ts

Tamar S. Polonsky, MD, MSCI[a],*,
Donald M. Lloyd-Jones, MD, ScM[b]

KEYWORDS

- Coronary artery calcium • Risk prediction • Atherosclerosis
- Epidemiology

Measurement of traditional risk factors remains the foundation of current clinical practice guidelines when screening for coronary heart disease (CHD) risk.[1,2] Observational studies including thousands of individuals have shown that more than 90% of patients presenting with their first CHD event have antecedent elevation of at least 1 traditional risk factor.[3,4] However, individual risk factors by themselves do not function well as screening tools because of substantial overlap between the levels of risk factors among people who do and do not experience events.[5,6] Combining multiple risk factors into algorithms that provide a more comprehensive estimate of risk, such as the Framingham risk score (FRS), substantially improves the ability to recognize individuals who are at higher risk of an event.[7] However, once clinical treatment thresholds are applied to these risk estimates, many adults who experience events are not classified as high risk. A substantial body of literature has therefore been devoted to finding novel markers that will enhance risk prediction.

A special panel from the American College of Cardiology Foundation/American Heart Association (ACCF/AHA) recently outlined the phases of evaluation that should occur when trying to determine the clinical utility of a novel risk marker.[8] There should be a statistical association between the risk marker and the outcome of interest. The marker should add incremental information beyond traditional risk factors and should change predicted risk sufficiently to alter therapeutic decisions. Also, use of a novel marker should change outcomes when tested in a randomized clinical trial and should be shown to be cost effective.

The coronary artery calcium (CAC) score has emerged as a powerful adjunct to risk assessment and has satisfied several of the criteria described earlier. Numerous studies have shown convincingly that the CAC score is predictive of future coronary events over and above traditional risk factors.[9–11] Results have been confirmed both in men and women in several different study populations, including the Multi-Ethnic Study of Atherosclerosis (MESA; white, black, Hispanic, and Chinese Americans), the Heinz-Nixdorf Recall Study (from Germany), and the Rotterdam Study (from the Netherlands).[12–14] CAC has also been shown to be predictive of all-cause mortality.[15,16] Further, when CAC is included in a prediction model based on traditional risk factors, risk classification is improved; a greater number of individuals who experience events are classified as high risk and more individuals who do not experience events are classified as low risk.[12–14]

There are many aspects of CAC testing that make it a potentially attractive test for CHD screening. Because calcification in the coronary arteries is pathognomonic for atherosclerosis, CAC testing is a direct measure of subclinical

Disclosures: The authors have nothing to disclose.
[a] Section of Cardiology, Department of Medicine, University of Chicago Medical Center, 5841 South Maryland Avenue, MC 6080, Chicago, IL 60637, USA
[b] Department of Preventive Medicine, Northwestern University Feinberg School of Medicine, 680 North Lakeshore Drive, Suite 1400, Chicago, IL 60611, USA
* Corresponding author.
E-mail address: tpolonsky@medicine.bsd.uchicago.edu

Cardiol Clin 30 (2012) 49–55
doi:10.1016/j.ccl.2011.11.004
0733-8651/12/$ – see front matter © 2012 Elsevier Inc. All rights reserved

CHD, whereas risk factors and biomarkers reflect more nonspecific predisposition to disease. The test can be performed using standard computed tomography (CT) scanners that are widely available; it does not require a technician with advanced training and is highly reproducible.[17]

However, there are several potential harms associated with widespread use of CAC testing. There may be substantial downstream testing (much of which may not be indicated), both for evaluation of high CAC scores and incidental findings. Additional testing adds both to the cost and radiation exposure that patients might experience. CAC testing can typically be performed with low levels of radiation exposure in experienced centers that use prospective triggering[18]; however, this may be more difficult to regulate with broader use.

It is also important to consider that CAC testing as a screening strategy per se has not been evaluated in a randomized clinical trial, and so it is not clear how the potential benefits of early detection of subclinical CHD measure directly against the potential harms. Because of the lack of trial data, groups such as the United States Preventive Services Task Force have argued against routine use of CAC testing as well as several other novel risk markers (carotid intima-media thickness, ankle-brachial index, and high-sensitivity C-reactive protein level).[19] Others have argued against waiting for clinical trial evidence, given the urgent need for more effective strategies to identify individuals at higher risk of CHD.[20] A trial of CAC testing would require a very large sample size and multiple years of follow-up, so data would not be available for many years.

In the following sections, the authors have outlined several principles of CAC testing into a list of dos and don'ts to help guide its clinical use based on available evidence.

DOs

Box 1 provides a summary of dos.

Do Reserve CAC Testing for Patients in Whom the Results are Most Likely to Alter Clinical Management

Patient selection is one of the most important considerations when considering CAC testing. In the 2010 Guideline for Risk Assessment in Asymptomatic Adults, the ACCF/AHA gave CAC testing a class IIa recommendation for patients who are at intermediate Framingham risk (estimated 10-year CHD risk of 10%–20%), meaning that use of CAC testing in this group is reasonable and that the benefits likely outweigh the risks.[2]

Box 1
Dos

1. Do reserve CAC testing for patients in whom the results are most likely to alter clinical management.
2. Do discuss the CAC score in a way that is meaningful for patients.
3. Do encourage patients to continue lifestyle modification, even if their CAC equals 0.
4. Do discuss the small risk of radiation.
5. Do warn patients that they will likely have to pay for CAC testing out-of-pocket.

The recommendation was rated as IIb for patients with an estimated 10-year risk of 6% to less than 10%, meaning that the test may be considered but the benefit is less well established. In contrast, a class III recommendation was given (not recommended) to patients whose 10-year estimated risk is less than 6%.

Data from large cohort studies clarify why CAC testing is less helpful in low- and high-risk individuals. In the South Bay Heart Watch Study, low-risk individuals (FRS, 0%–9%) with a high CAC score (ie, >300) experienced an event rate that was higher than low-risk individuals with a CAC score of 0, but the absolute event rate was still low.[10] Likewise, a low CAC score among high-risk adults did not eliminate their risk of a coronary event. In MESA, when the CAC score was added to a prediction model based on traditional risk factors, only 6 of 3746 low-risk participants were subsequently reclassified to high predicted risk.[12] Of 285 participants who were classified as high risk based on traditional risk factors, only 32 were reclassified as low risk based on their CAC scores. For most low- and high-risk individuals, CAC testing is unlikely to provide information that would substantially alter their treatment goals.

In contrast, the potential utility of CAC is quite different among intermediate-risk individuals. In MESA, 115 of 1847 intermediate-risk participants experienced events. More than 40% (48/115) occurred among individuals who were reclassified to high risk based on their CAC scores. Among the 712 individuals reclassified to low risk (based on a CAC score = 0 or very low scores), 15 experienced events (2.1%), suggesting that a low CAC score is predictive of a lower risk of events. Put another way, CAC testing needed to be performed on 4 to 6 intermediate-risk individuals to identify 1 person with a CAC score greater than 100, compared with almost 60 individuals in the lowest risk group (10-year risk of 0.0%–2.5%).[21]

Women represent another subgroup that might benefit from CAC testing when targeted carefully.[22] Because age and sex are the most dominant risk factors in the FRS, most women younger than 70 years have an estimated 10-year CHD risk of less than 10%.[23] Yet CVD is one of the leading causes of death for women in this age group.[24] In a study of 2447 asymptomatic women, 20% had CAC scores above the 75th percentile for their age and sex.[25] However, 84% were classified as low Framingham risk. The prevalence of CAC was particularly high (48%) among women with 2 or more risk factors and a family history of premature CHD (defined as having an immediate family member with a myocardial infarction or revascularization before age 55 years). This subgroup of women may warrant special consideration regarding the use of CAC testing.

Men and women with a family history of premature CHD often pose a management dilemma. They may not qualify for medical therapy based on their traditional risk factors according to guidelines, and yet they are at increased risk for future events. Several observational studies have shown that a family history is associated with a higher burden of subclinical CHD. Specific aspects of the family history may help identify those who would benefit from CAC testing. For example, in a study of 8549 individuals referred for CAC testing, the odds ratio for a CAC score greater than 0 was 1.3 among people with a parental history of CHD but 2.3 for individuals who had a sibling with CHD.[26] One potential explanation is that siblings are more likely to share a common environment (in addition to 50% of their genome) that fosters the development of CHD risk factors. In addition, events experienced by siblings may be less subject to recall bias than events in a parent occurring years prior.

The association of family history with CAC score may also be dependent on an individual's age.[27] In the Framingham Heart Study, the association of family history with CAC score was nonsignificant among the Offspring cohort (mean age, 63 years), but the odds ratio for CAC score greater than 0 was 2.17 among the Third Generation cohort (mean age, 47 years).[28]

Do Discuss the CAC Score in a Way that is Meaningful for Patients

Motivating patients to adopt lifestyle changes and to adhere to medications can be a major clinical challenge. To date, providing patients with information about their global CHD risk estimate has not been associated with long-lasting behavior changes, particularly if the information is only provided once.[29] CAC testing could serve as a powerful source of motivation because it provides objective evidence of atherosclerosis. Kalia and colleagues[30] studied 505 individuals treated with statins. Study investigators showed each participant sample images from their CT and described the degree of atherosclerosis as none, mild, moderate, or severe. After 3 years of follow-up, 44% of individuals with a CAC score of 0 reported taking a statin, compared with 75% with a CAC score of 100 to 399 and 90% with a CAC score of 400 or more. In the Early Identification of Subclinical Atherosclerosis by Noninvasive Imaging Research (EISNER) study, adults who underwent CAC testing met individually with a nurse to see sample images and receive counseling on risk factor modification.[31] After 4 years of follow-up, adults with any CAC score achieved significantly greater reductions in systolic blood pressure (SBP) and low-density lipoprotein (LDL) cholesterol than adults with a CAC score of 0. In a third study, Schwartz and colleagues[32] evaluated the association of CAC testing with health behavior modification. After a mean of 6 years, those with a CAC score greater than 0 were more likely to increase their exercise (19% vs 12%, P<.01) and change their diet (33% vs 21%, P<.01).

Although the association of CAC with medication adherence and behavior change is significant, many of the changes discussed earlier were modest. How CAC results are conveyed is likely an important factor in whether individuals are motivated to adopt aggressive preventive strategies. Another potentially useful tool is the arterial age calculator, found on the MESA Web site http://www.mesa-nhlbi.org/Calcium/ArterialAge.aspx. Patients or providers can enter the CAC score to calculate an arterial age, which is the age at which the estimated CHD risk is the same as that for the observed CAC score. Arterial age can then be used to revise the estimated 10-year CHD risk.

Take, for example, a 60-year-old woman with a total cholesterol level of 220 mg/dL, with a high-density lipoprotein (HDL) cholesterol level of 40 mg/dL, who is a nonsmoker, whose SBP is 140 mm Hg, and who is currently taking antihypertensive medication. Her 10-year estimated risk of CHD by FRS is 6%. With a CAC score of 50, her arterial age is 68 years (she is 60 years old, but her arteries resemble those of a 68-year-old person). Replacing age 60 years with age 68 years almost doubles her 10-year risk to 11%. With a CAC score of 75, her arterial age is 70 years and her estimated risk almost triples to 17%.

Alternatively, consider a 55-year-old man whose total cholesterol level is 210 mg/dL, HDL level is 35 mg/dL, and SBP is 140 mm Hg and who is on antihypertensive medication, is a current smoker, and has a CAC score of 10. His estimated CHD risk based on risk factors alone is 30%, which does not change after CAC testing, even though his score is low. If his CAC score was 0, his revised 10-year risk would decrease to 12%. However, the man would still qualify for lipid-lowering therapy, given that he has 2 risk factors and an FRS of 10% to 20%. In this situation, the CAC score would not provide useful information to guide management, and so testing would not be recommended.

Do Encourage Patients to Continue Lifestyle Modification, Even if Their CAC Score = 0

There is a theoretical concern that patients whose CAC score is 0 may use that to justify an unhealthy lifestyle. Observational studies have not supported that notion. For example, participants in the EISNER study with a CAC score of 0 did not experience an increase in their mean FRS, waist circumference, or weight over 4 years of follow-up.[31]

There are 2 important messages that health care providers can give patients with a CAC score of 0. First, the result is reassuring that an individual's risk of a CHD event over the next 10 years is very low, about 1%.[15] Second, however, patients should also understand that the absence of CAC does not guarantee the absence of atherosclerosis because they may have exclusively noncalcified plaque that is not identified by CAC testing. As a result, patients should still be encouraged to make appropriate therapeutic lifestyle changes to decrease their longer-term risk.

Do Discuss the Small Risk of Radiation

Ionizing radiation can be found throughout the environment. The average background exposure in the United States is approximately 3 mSv/y, with a range of 1 to 10 mSv.[33] When the CT is performed using prospective triggering, the radiation exposure is typically 0.9 to 1.1 mSv, compared with 165-mSv cumulative average background exposure for a 55-year-old adult.[34] All current recommendations suggest prospective triggering.[18] The exposure from one CAC test is about the same amount of radiation as 1 to 2 mammograms performed on each breast.

Using statistical modeling, Kim and colleagues[35] estimated the radiation-induced cancer incidence attributed to CAC testing. The investigators assumed a radiation dosage of 2.3 mSv per scan. Cancer incidence rates were 8 and 20 per 100,000 scans for men and women, respectively. Incidence rates were lower for protocols that

achieved a radiation dose closer to 1 mSv but were higher if CAC testing was performed in younger patients, because they are more sensitive to radiation. If screening was performed every 5 years in men from ages 45 to 75 years and in women from ages 55 to 75 years, the estimated risk increased to 42 and 62 per 100,000 in men and women, respectively. It is important to consider that these risks are averaged over a person's lifetime and are much smaller than the 10-year risk of a CHD event for many patients. However, given the radiation exposure and low prevalence of CAC, the ACCF/AHA recommend that CAC testing should generally not be done in younger patients.[2]

Do Warn Patients that they will Likely have to Pay for CAC Testing Out-of-Pocket

Most insurance plans do not cover CAC testing. The cost varies based on practice setting and geography, and so patients should be advised to confirm the cost beforehand. Most CAC tests cost between $100 and $400.

DON'Ts

A summary of the don'ts is shown in **Box 2**.

Don't Use CAC Testing to Evaluate Outpatients with Symptoms Suggestive of CHD

The CAC score is a reliable correlate of the overall atherosclerotic burden. However, sites of calcification on CT do not correlate well with regions of stenosis.[36,37] Further, among patients with a high clinical suspicion of CHD, a CAC score of 0 only has a negative predictive value of 68% for the absence of 1 or more stenoses greater than 50%.[37]

Box 2
Don'ts

1. Don't use CAC testing to evaluate outpatients with symptoms suggestive of CHD.
2. Don't screen frequently for development or progression of CAC.
3. Don't use CAC testing to monitor response to therapy.
4. Don't forget to warn patients about the potential for incidental findings.
5. Don't use the CAC score as an indication for an angiogram.

Don't Screen Frequently for Development or Progression of CAC

Several observational studies have shown that the development of new CAC is a relatively slow process. In a study of 422 individuals referred for CAC testing, the rate of conversion from a CAC score of 0 to a CAC score greater than 0 was nonlinear, occurring in 2 (0.5%), 5 (1.2%), 24 (5.7%), 26 (6.2%), and 49 (11.6%) individuals at follow-up years 1, 2, 3, 4, and 5, respectively.[38] The average CAC score at the time of conversion was 19 ± 19. In a multivariable analysis, only age greater than 40 years, diabetes, and smoking were predictive of newly incident CAC. By far, one of the strongest predictors is the baseline CAC score. Among individuals with a CAC score greater than 0 at baseline, annual changes are usually modest. In MESA, the annualized increase in CAC score was 0 to 99 units among 75% of participants.[39]

There is currently no established threshold that signifies a clinically meaningful progression. In a study of 495 asymptomatic individuals with annual imaging, those who suffered a myocardial infarction over 3 years of follow-up had had significantly greater percentage increases in CAC scores than those who remained event free (42% ± 23% vs 17% ± 25%, P<.001).[40] However, there was substantial overlap between the amounts of progression between the 2 groups. Progression of CAC likely represents, in part, calcification of existing noncalcified plaque. CAC progression could also represent accumulation of additional plaque, healing of small areas of plaque rupture, and worsening of atherosclerosis. It is impossible to distinguish between the different processes with CAC testing, making it difficult to know how to interpret the results. Given the associated radiation exposure, cost, and potential for incidental findings (see later), CAC testing should only be repeated if there are clear indications that the results would change dramatically from the prior examination.

Don't Use CAC Testing to Monitor Response to Therapy

Clinical trial data suggest that the CAC score is relatively insensitive to lipid-lowering therapy. In a study by Arad and colleagues,[41] 1005 asymptomatic adults with CAC scores above the 80th percentile for age and sex were randomized to atorvastatin, 20 mg, versus placebo. After 4 years, there was no difference in CAC scores between the 2 arms, despite a 43% reduction in LDL among those taking atorvastatin. In a subsequent study, 615 postmenopausal women with hyperlipidemia were randomized to atorvastatin, 80 mg, or pravastatin, 40 mg.[42] Women in both arms experienced an approximately 20% increase in CAC after 1 year, despite a 47% reduction in mean LDL with atorvastatin and a 25% reduction with pravastatin. Therefore, it seems most appropriate to follow patients' clinical response to therapy rather than repeat the CT scan.

Don't Forget to Warn Patients about the Potential for Incidental Findings

Noncardiac incidental findings are extremely common. Few are clinically significant, and yet they often lead to additional testing and procedures. In one study of 966 patients, 41.5% were found to have an incidental finding, 1.2% were deemed clinically significant, and 7% were indeterminate, requiring clinical or radiologic follow-up.[43] During follow-up, none of the indeterminate findings became clinically significant. However, 76 CT scans (71 thorax, 4 abdomen/pelvis, and 1 head) were performed for surveillance of the findings.

Pulmonary abnormalities are the most common source of incidental findings. In a study of 459 individuals, 81 (18%) were found to have pulmonary nodules and 63 had subsequent surveillance with at least 1 chest CT.[44] The original lesion was not identified in 22 participants (35%), the lesion had decreased or remained stable in 39 participants (62%), and there was interval growth in 2 participants (3%).

Don't Use the CAC Score as an Indication for an Angiogram

There is currently no evidence to support proceeding straight to invasive (or even noninvasive) coronary angiography based on a high CAC score, even if it is greater than 1000. Decisions about cardiac testing and procedures should be based overwhelmingly on the whole clinical picture, particularly symptoms and traditional risk factors. It may be reasonable to consider stress testing for a patient with a CAC greater than 400 and poor exercise tolerance because in these patients it is difficult to assess whether they are truly asymptomatic. However, there are no prospective data to show that this improves outcomes.

REFERENCES

1. Expert Panel on Detection, Evaluation, and Treatment of High Blood Cholesterol in Adults. Executive summary of the Third Report of the National Cholesterol Education Program (NCEP) Expert Panel on

Detection, Evaluation, and Treatment of High Blood Cholesterol in Adults (Adult Treatment Panel III). JAMA 2001;285:2486–97.

2. Greenland P, Alpert JS, Beller GA, et al. 2010 ACCF/AHA guideline for assessment of cardiovascular risk in asymptomatic adults: a report of the American College of Cardiology Foundation/American Heart Association Task Force on Practice Guidelines. Circulation 2010;122:e584–636.

3. Khot UN, Khot MB, Bajzer CT, et al. Prevalence of conventional risk factors in patients with coronary heart disease. JAMA 2003;290:898–904.

4. Greenland P, Knoll MD, Stamler J, et al. Major risk factors as antecedents of fatal and nonfatal coronary heart disease events. JAMA 2003;290:891–7.

5. Law MR, Wald NJ. Risk factor thresholds: their existence under scrutiny. BMJ 2002;324:1570–6.

6. Wald NJ, Hackshaw AK, Frost CD. When can a risk factor be used as a worthwhile screening test? BMJ 1999;319:1562–5.

7. Wilson PW, D'Agostino RB, Levy D, et al. Prediction of coronary heart disease using risk factor categories. Circulation 1998;97:1837–47.

8. Hlatky MA, Greenland P, Arnett DK, et al. Criteria for evaluation of novel markers of cardiovascular risk: a scientific statement from the American Heart Association. Circulation 2009;119:2408–16.

9. Detrano R, Guerci AD, Carr JJ, et al. Coronary calcium as a predictor of coronary events in four racial or ethnic groups. N Engl J Med 2008;358:1336–45.

10. Greenland P, LaBree L, Azen SP, et al. Coronary artery calcium score combined with Framingham score for risk prediction in asymptomatic individuals. JAMA 2004;291:210–5.

11. Raggi P, Callister TQ, Cooil B, et al. Identification of patients at increased risk of first unheralded acute myocardial infarction by electron-beam computed tomography. Circulation 2000;101:850–5.

12. Polonsky TS, McClelland RL, Jorgensen NW, et al. Coronary artery calcium score and risk classification for coronary heart disease prediction. JAMA 2010;303:1610–6.

13. Erbel R, Mohlenkamp S, Moebus S, et al. Coronary risk stratification, discrimination, and reclassification improvement based on quantification of subclinical coronary atherosclerosis: the Heinz Nixdorf Recall study. J Am Coll Cardiol 2010;56:1397–406.

14. Elias-Smale SE, Proenca RV, Koller MT, et al. Coronary calcium score improves classification of coronary heart disease risk in the elderly: the Rotterdam study. J Am Coll Cardiol 2010;56:1407–14.

15. Budoff MJ, Shaw LJ, Liu ST, et al. Long-term prognosis associated with coronary calcification: observations from a registry of 25,253 patients. J Am Coll Cardiol 2007;49:1860–70.

16. Raggi P, Gongora MC, Gopal A, et al. Coronary artery calcium to predict all-cause mortality in elderly men and women. J Am Coll Cardiol 2008;52:17–23.

17. Detrano RC, Anderson M, Nelson J, et al. Coronary calcium measurements: effect of CT scanner type and calcium measure on rescan reproducibility—MESA study. Radiology 2005;236:477–84.

18. Voros S, Rivera JJ, Berman DS, et al. Guideline for minimizing radiation exposure during acquisition of coronary artery calcium scans with the use of multidetector computed tomography: a report by the Society for Atherosclerosis Imaging and Prevention Tomographic Imaging and Prevention Councils in collaboration with the Society of Cardiovascular Computed Tomography. J Cardiovasc Comput Tomogr 2011;5:75–83.

19. U.S. Preventive Services Task Force. Using nontraditional risk factors in coronary heart disease risk assessment: U.S. Preventive Services Task Force recommendation statement. Ann Intern Med 2009;151:474–82.

20. Naghavi M, Falk E, Hecht HS, et al. From vulnerable plaque to vulnerable patient—part III: executive summary of the Screening for Heart Attack Prevention and Education (SHAPE) Task Force report. Am J Cardiol 2006;98:2H–15H.

21. Okwuosa TM, Greenland P, Ning H, et al. Distribution of coronary artery calcium scores by Framingham 10-year risk strata in the MESA (Multi-Ethnic Study of Atherosclerosis) potential implications for coronary risk assessment. J Am Coll Cardiol 2011;57:1838–45.

22. Lakoski SG, Greenland P, Wong ND, et al. Coronary artery calcium scores and risk for cardiovascular events in women classified as "low risk" based on Framingham risk score: the Multi-Ethnic Study of Atherosclerosis (MESA). Arch Intern Med 2007;167:2437–42.

23. Ford ES, Giles WH, Mokdad AH. The distribution of 10-year risk for coronary heart disease among US adults: findings from the National Health and Nutrition Examination Survey III. J Am Coll Cardiol 2004;43:1791–6.

24. Roger VL, Go AS, Lloyd-Jones DM, et al. Heart disease and stroke statistics-2011 update. Circulation 2011;123:e18–e209.

25. Michos ED, Nasir K, Braunstein JB, et al. Framingham risk equation underestimates subclinical atherosclerosis risk in asymptomatic women. Atherosclerosis 2006;184:201–6.

26. Nasir K, Michos ED, Rumberger JA, et al. Coronary artery calcification and family history of premature coronary heart disease: sibling history is more strongly associated than parental history. Circulation 2004;110:2150–6.

27. Philips B, de Lemos JA, Patel MJ, et al. Relation of family history of myocardial infarction and the presence of coronary arterial calcium in various age and risk factor groups. Am J Cardiol 2007;99:825–9.

28. Parikh NI, Hwang SJ, Larson MG, et al. Parental occurrence of premature cardiovascular disease predicts increased coronary artery and abdominal aortic calcification in the Framingham Offspring and Third Generation cohorts. Circulation 2007;116: 1473–81.

29. Sheridan SL, Viera AJ, Krantz MJ, et al. The effect of giving global coronary risk information to adults: a systematic review. Arch Intern Med 2010;170:230–9.

30. Kalia NK, Miller LG, Nasir K, et al. Visualizing coronary calcium is associated with improvements in adherence to statin therapy. Atherosclerosis 2006; 185:394–9.

31. Rozanski A, Gransar H, Shaw LJ, et al. Impact of coronary artery calcium scanning on coronary risk factors and downstream testing the EISNER (Early Identification of Subclinical Atherosclerosis by Noninvasive Imaging Research) prospective randomized trial. J Am Coll Cardiol 2011;57:1622–32.

32. Schwartz J, Allison M, Wright CM. Health behavior modification after electron beam computed tomography and physician consultation. J Behav Med 2011;34:148–55.

33. Brenner DJ, Doll R, Goodhead DT, et al. Cancer risks attributable to low doses of ionizing radiation: assessing what we really know. Proc Natl Acad Sci U S A 2003;100:13761–6.

34. Morin RL, Gerber TC, McCollough CH. Radiation dose in computed tomography of the heart. Circulation 2003;107:917–22.

35. Kim KP, Einstein AJ, Berrington de Gonzalez A. Coronary artery calcification screening: estimated radiation dose and cancer risk. Arch Intern Med 2009;169:1188–94.

36. Rumberger JA, Simons DB, Fitzpatrick LA, et al. Coronary artery calcium area by electron-beam computed tomography and coronary atherosclerotic plaque area. A histopathologic correlative study. Circulation 1995;92:2157–62.

37. Gottlieb I, Miller JM, Arbab-Zadeh A, et al. The absence of coronary calcification does not exclude obstructive coronary artery disease or the need for revascularization in patients referred for conventional coronary angiography. J Am Coll Cardiol 2010;55:627–34.

38. Min JK, Lin FY, Gidseg DS, et al. Determinants of coronary calcium conversion among patients with a normal coronary calcium scan: what is the "warranty period" for remaining normal? J Am Coll Cardiol 2010;55:1110–7.

39. Kronmal RA, McClelland RL, Detrano R, et al. Risk factors for the progression of coronary artery calcification in asymptomatic subjects: results from the Multi-Ethnic Study of Atherosclerosis (MESA). Circulation 2007;115:2722–30.

40. Raggi P, Callister TQ, Shaw LJ. Progression of coronary artery calcium and risk of first myocardial infarction in patients receiving cholesterol-lowering therapy. Arterioscler Thromb Vasc Biol 2004;24: 1272–7.

41. Arad Y, Spadaro LA, Roth M, et al. Treatment of asymptomatic adults with elevated coronary calcium scores with atorvastatin, vitamin C, and vitamin E: the St. Francis Heart Study randomized clinical trial. J Am Coll Cardiol 2005;46:166–72.

42. Raggi P, Davidson M, Callister TQ, et al. Aggressive versus moderate lipid-lowering therapy in hypercholesterolemic postmenopausal women: Beyond Endorsed Lipid Lowering with EBT Scanning (BELLES). Circulation 2005;112:563–71.

43. Machaalany J, Yam Y, Ruddy TD, et al. Potential clinical and economic consequences of noncardiac incidental findings on cardiac computed tomography. J Am Coll Cardiol 2009;54:1533–41.

44. Iribarren C, Hlatky MA, Chandra M, et al. Incidental pulmonary nodules on cardiac computed tomography: prognosis and use. Am J Med 2008;121: 989–96.

Identifying and Redefining Stenosis by CT Angiography

Minisha Kochar, MD[a], Reza Arsanjani, MD[d],
Subha V. Raman, MD[b], Leslee J. Shaw, PhD[c],
Daniel S. Berman, MD[d,e], James K. Min, MD, FSCCT[d,e,*]

KEYWORDS

- Coronary artery disease • Coronary angiography • Stenosis
- Computed tomography

Coronary artery disease (CAD) remains the leading cause of morbidity and mortality in the world.[1] Among the 14 million Americans with CAD, the estimated direct and indirect costs exceed $150 billion annually, with cardiovascular costs higher than for any other diagnostic group. Clinical detection of CAD is difficult for many patients, given the absence or minimal nature of symptoms in most, and the initial diagnosis of CAD often occurs at the time of the presentation of acute myocardial infarction or sudden cardiac death.[2]

Coronary atherosclerosis is a complex pathophysiologic process that is initiated by endothelial cell injury, typically occurring at areas of geometric irregularity where sudden changes in the velocity and direction of blood flow occur. Endothelial cells play a vital role in the regulation of coronary blood flow by advancing an antithrombotic and antiinflammatory surface[3–5] as well as by preventing smooth muscle cell proliferation and generating vasoactive substances necessary for regulating coronary vascular tone.[6,7] Insult to endothelial cells precipitates dysfunction and increased permeability, inhibition of vasomotor regulatory systems, and abnormal response to stressors; these processes lead to increased deposition of oxidized low density lipoprotein (LDL).[8] The accumulation of oxidized LDL subsequently triggers overexpression of cell adhesion molecules, which fosters recruitment of inflammatory cells.[9] These intricate processes initially lead to subendothelial accumulation of lipid-laden foam cells and the formation of fatty streaks, which are asymptomatic and nonobstructive.

A dynamic cascade subsequently ensues, including increased inflammation (caused by further monocyte and macrophage recruitment and migration); platelet activation; and smooth muscle cell proliferation, which, along with increased proteolysis and apoptosis, leads to vascular remodeling and procoagulant and complement activation.[4,8] The combination of these processes forms the basis of coronary atheroma progression. As the atheroma increases in size, a compensatory outward expansion of the arterial wall occurs, known as the Glagov phenomenon, in

Disclosures: GE Healthcare (research support).

[a] Department of Cardiology, Kaiser Permanente, 13652 Cantara Street, Panorama City, CA 91402, USA

[b] Division of Cardiology, Department of Medicine, The Ohio State University School of Medicine, 473 West 12th Avenue, Suite 200, Columbus, OH 43210, USA

[c] Division of Cardiology, Department of Medicine, Emory Clinical Cardiovascular Research Institute, Emory University School of Medicine, 1462 Clifton Road NE, Room 530, Atlanta, GA 30306, USA

[d] Cedars-Sinai Heart Institute, Cedars-Sinai Medical Center, 8700 Beverly Boulevard, Room 1253, Los Angeles, CA 90048, USA

[e] Department of Imaging, Cedars-Sinai Medical Center, 8700 Beverly Boulevard, Room 1253, Los Angeles, CA 90048, USA

* Corresponding author. Cedars-Sinai Heart Institute, Cedars-Sinai Medical Center, 8700 Beverly Boulevard, Room 1253, Los Angeles, CA 90048.

E-mail address: James.Min@cshs.org

Cardiol Clin 30 (2012) 57–67

doi:10.1016/j.ccl.2011.11.001

which the luminal integrity is preserved in an effort to maintain coronary flow.[10,11] However, as the atherosclerotic process continues to its late stages, coronary flow is ultimately compromised as the lumen size becomes progressively narrowed.

Traditionally, it has been the significant luminal stenosis for which noninvasive imaging techniques have been focused. Prior seminal studies have revealed a coronary stenosis threshold at approximately 50% at which point coronary blood flow reserve begins to decrease.[12] Critical coronary stenosis has been identified at an 80% stenosis threshold, given a decrease in resting coronary flow at this level.[13] These findings have supported a clinical ceiling for coronary lesions when a greater than or equal to 70% visual luminal stenosis is identified, and this level is routinely used to guide intervention. Although therapeutic paradigms based on measures of high-grade anatomic stenosis severity have been highly effective at reducing symptoms and ischemia, several caveats must be noted. First, not all high-grade stenosis cause ischemia. Indeed, among 70% to 90% stenosis, approximately 1 in 5 lesions do not cause ischemia, and prior multicenter data endorse a conservative noninvasive approach to such lesions.[14] Second, the prognosis of patients with less than 70% stenosis is not entirely benign. Although coronary lesions considered angiographically mild (eg, <50%) are rarely associated with hemodynamically significant reductions in coronary flow, they, nevertheless, confer to affected patients, significantly higher rates of cardiovascular events than those with normal coronaries.[15] Presumably owing to the higher prevalence of angiographically mild coronary artery lesions, angiographically nonobstructive lesions comprise most plaques causal of acute myocardial infarction, with prior data indicating that upwards of two-thirds of acute myocardial infarctions occur at the site of previously observed mild coronary stenoses.[16] Therefore, the importance of identifying these patients cannot be understated, especially if it leads to effective preventative measures.[17]

DIAGNOSTIC EVALUATION FOR HIGH-GRADE CORONARY STENOSIS

For measures of coronary stenosis, invasive coronary angiography is the gold standard for identifying obstructive coronary artery disease. However, because of its invasive nature and non-negligible risk, it is not ideal for widespread diagnostic application for low- to intermediate-risk patients. Instead, traditional methods of coronary evaluation have used noninvasive methods, such as stress testing.[18] By assessing differences between rest and stress-induced images, stress testing has relied on measures of myocardial perfusion or wall motion as surrogate markers of high-grade stenosis that are hemodynamically significant.

Traditionally, myocardial perfusion imaging (MPI) has been the most commonly used noninvasive imaging technique in this population for identifying ischemia as a surrogate measure of high-grade anatomic coronary artery stenosis and for determining prognosis.[18] Although single-photon emission computed tomography (SPECT) has experienced the greatest use, positron emission tomography (PET) offers a noninvasive standard for assessing physiologic stenosis severity both by perfusion assessment and absolute myocardial blood flow and coronary flow reserve.[19] Although neither SPECT nor PET offer the ability to directly visualize coronary stenosis, which is often present despite the absence of perfusion deficits or reduction in flow, a normal MPI scan is, nevertheless, associated with an excellent prognosis.[20,21] However, significant limitations are present with MPI imaging, including the underestimation of the extent of ischemia in patients with left main or 3-vessel coronary artery disease who are at the highest risk for adverse cardiac events.[22,23] In addition, MPI depends on the detection of relative perfusion to indirectly identify flow-limiting lesions; hence, MPI is unable to identify most individuals whose acute coronary events are caused by non–flow-limiting lesions.[16]

Recently, coronary computed tomographic angiography (CCTA) using computed tomography (CT) scanners of 64-detector rows or greater has emerged as an attractive noninvasive alternative to invasive coronary angiography for providing detailed images of the coronary anatomy (**Fig. 1**).[24] Significant advances in CT technology in temporal resolution and volume coverage now allow for the acquisition of virtual motion-free images of the heart and coronary tree in 1 to 8 seconds. Concomitant improvements in spatial resolution have achieved isotropic resolution between 500 to 750 microns. Early studies examining the diagnostic performance of CCTA against an invasive coronary angiographic reference standard were uniformly positive, with a recent meta-analysis reporting sensitivity, specificity, positive predictive value (PPV), and negative predictive value (NPV) of 97%, 90%, 93%, and 96%, respectively (**Fig. 2**).[25] After these single-center studies, which were limited by referral bias (ie, patients already being clinically referred to intracoronary angiography [ICA]) and spectrum bias (patients

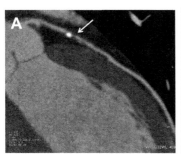
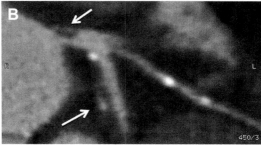

Fig. 1. Curved multiplanar reformat of a coronary CT angiogram demonstrated a high-grade stenosis in the proximal portion of the left anterior descending artery (A) and moderate-severe stenoses of the left main and left circumflex arteries (arrows) (B).

had high pretest CAD likelihood and did not represent those for whom noninvasive imaging is generally performed), prospective multicenter studies were reported.

The first of these studies was the Assessment by Coronary Computed Tomographic Angiography of Individuals UndeRgoing InvAsive Coronary AngiographY (ACCURACY) trial. This prospective 15-center trial evaluated stable patients without known CAD who underwent CCTA before clinically indicated ICA.[26] In 230 patients undergoing CCTA before ICA, with a 25% prevalence of obstructive CAD, CCTA had a diagnostic sensitivity, specificity, PPV, and NPV of 94%, 83%, 48%, and 99%, respectively. NPVs to exclude obstructive CAD at per-patient, per-vessel, and per-segment levels were 99%. Importantly, this study examined consecutive patients regardless of baseline coronary artery calcium score, body mass index, or heart rate. A subsequent multicenter multivendor study by Meijboom and colleagues[27] examined a combination of stable and acute chest pain patients without known CAD. As compared with the 25% prevalence of CAD in the ACCURACY

study, the study by Meijboom observed a 68% prevalence. Despite these large differences in disease prevalence, the sensitivity to detect and NPV to exclude obstructive CAD was 99% and 97%, respectively. These data confirm the high reliability of CCTA to detect and exclude high-grade stenosis across a wide disease prevalence and suggest its usefulness in patients without known CAD.

DIAGNOSTIC PERFORMANCE OF CCTA FOR ADDITIONAL CAD MEASURES BEYOND STENOSIS

One potential benefit of CCTA compared with ICA is its ability to not only assess high-grade coronary stenosis but also atherosclerotic plaque and coronary arterial wall features in a manner akin to intravascular ultrasound (IVUS).[24] One recent study evaluating 100 patients who underwent CCTA, ICA, and IVUS revealed perfect diagnostic performance of CCTA for the identification and exclusion of any atherosclerosis compared with IVUS.[28] In a recent meta-analysis of 33 studies that comprised 946 patients, CCTA was

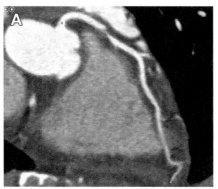
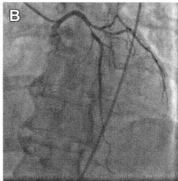

Fig. 2. A 63-year-old woman with history of hypertension and hyperlipidemia referred for coronary CT angiography for evaluation of atypical chest pain. (A) CCTA demonstrated high-grade proximal left anterior artery lesion, which was confirmed (B) by invasive coronary angiography.

noted to demonstrate a high correlation to IVUS for other atherosclerotic measures. Weighted mean differences between CCTA and IVUS were small for cross-sectional area (0.46 mm^2, 95% confidence interval [CI] 0.14–0.79), plaque area (0.09, 95% CI -1.00 to 1.18), area stenosis (-1.81%, 95% CI -4.10 to 0.49), and plaque volume (5.30 mm^3, 95% CI -3.01 to 13.60).[29]

INCREMENTAL PROGNOSTIC VALUE OF CCTA

In addition to its high diagnostic performance against an invasive reference standard, CCTA findings of CAD have been evaluated for their ability to accurately prognosticate events.[30] The first large-scale prognostic study of CCTA evaluated 1127 stable patients with suspected CAD who were followed for an average of 15 months.[31] In a manner comparable to catheter-based angiography, coronary diameter stenosis by CCTA was graded as none or minimal (<30%), mild (30%–49%), moderate (50%–69%), or severe (≥70%) on a per-segment, per-vessel, and per-patient basis. CCTA stenoses were also scored applying a modified Duke prognostic CAD index adapted from an ICA jeopardy score and paralleling its ability to predict 5-year survival by extent and severity of angiographic CAD. Mortality was assessed after 15 months, at which point 39 (3.5%) deaths had occurred.

CCTA measures of CAD predicted risk of all-cause death. Moderate and severe luminal diameter stenoses were associated with higher mortality compared with milder stenosis, and risk of death increased with the number of vessels affected. CT findings predicting higher risk of death by the Duke prognostic CAD index (listed in increasing risk) included the following: (1) 2 segments with moderate stenosis or 1 segment with severe stenosis ($P = .013$); (2) 3 segments with moderate stenosis, 2 segments with severe stenosis, or severe stenosis in the proximal left anterior descending artery (LAD) ($P = .002$); (3) 3 segments with severe stenosis or 2 segments with severe stenosis that included the proximal LAD ($P = .001$); and (4) moderate or severe left main artery stenosis ($P<.001$), with a 15% 1.5-year mortality. Within this cohort, gender-specific differences in prognosis were noted. Specifically, women were more likely to have normal coronary arteries (54% vs 28%, $P<.001$), and the presence of nonobstructive CAD less than 50% stenosis conferred a 1.3-fold higher mortality per nonobstructive lesion ($P = .003$) for women that was not observed for men, with mortality ranging from 2.9% to 10.9% for 0 to 4 or more nonobstructive lesions for women.[32]

Although several subsequent studies affirmed the findings of this initial investigation, they were, nevertheless, uniformly limited to single centers and generally small numbers of patients. In this regard, a recent publication reported the prognostic findings from the dynamic COronary CT Angiography EvaluatioN For Clinical Outcomes: An InteRnational Multicenter (CONFIRM) registry.[33] At present, the CONFIRM registry is comprised of 2 phases. Phase I CONFIRM is a derivation cohort that details demographic, clinical, and CT findings for 27,125 consecutive patients at 12 sites in 6 countries (United States, Canada, Germany, Switzerland, Italy, South Korea), with patients followed for 2.3 ± 1.1 years for a primary endpoint of all-cause death. Phase II CONFIRM is a distinct nonoverlapping validation cohort, detailing identical elements to phase I and with event follow-up for 4682 patients at 6 sites in 4 countries (United States, Canada, Austria, South Korea).

In a 2.3-year follow-up of 23,854 patients without known CAD within CONFIRM, compared with those aged 65 years or older, younger patients experienced a higher risk of death for obstructive 2-vessel (hazard ration [HR] 4.00, $P<.0001$ vs HR 2.46, $P = .0003$) and 3-vessel (HR 6.19, $P<.0001$ vs HR 3.10, $P<.0001$) CAD.[34] For women, the hazards for 3-vessel CAD (HR 4.21, $P<.0001$) were higher compared with men (HR 3.27, $P<.0001$),[34] with similar relationships observed for major adverse cardiovascular events (MACE). Importantly, individuals with nonobstructive CAD, less than 50% experienced a 60% increase in death relative to individuals without CAD ($P = .002$).[34] Importantly, for more than 1000 patients within this study with greater than or equal to a 4-year follow-up, only 1 death occurred, suggesting an NPV for mortality of 99.9% and a warranty period of at least 4 years.

The CONFIRM data support those of Ostrum and colleagues[35] who, to date, have reported the longest follow-up for any CT-based measure of angiography. For 2538 patients followed for nearly 7 years, the risk-adjusted HRs for CCTA-diagnosed CAD were 1.7-, 1.8-, 2.3-, and 2.6-fold for 3-vessel nonobstructive, 1-vessel obstructive, 2-vessel obstructive, and 3-vessel obstructive CAD, respectively. Importantly, at the cessation of 6.8-year follow-up, the annualized death rate for patients with no evident CAD by CCTA was 0.3%, suggesting a warranty period of a normal CCTA that extends to at least 7 years.

Given the ability of CCTA to identify angiographically nonobstructive CAD, recent investigations have examined the prognostic significance of mild CAD by CCTA. In a 2-center study, 2583 patients undergoing CT with a maximal per-patient less than 50% stenosis were followed for 3.1 years, with 54 deaths occurring. Compared with individuals with no CAD, those with nonobstructive CAD experienced higher rates of death (HR 1.98, P = .03).[36] A dose-response relationship was noted for increasing the extent of nonobstructive CAD, with higher mortality for individuals with nonobstructive CAD in 3 vessels (HR 4.75, P = .0002) or greater than or equal to 5 segments (HR 5.12, P = .0002). Importantly, patients with greater than or equal to 5 coronary segments with plaque had a higher percentage of coronary segments with calcified plaque (52% vs 25%, $P<.001$) or mixed plaque (24% vs 13%, P = .002), relative to those with less than 5 coronary segments with plaque, with no differences noted for noncalcified plaque. Notably, the adverse prognosis of nonobstructive CAD was observed even for patients with no medically treatable CAD risk factors and low Framingham risk scores.

This graded increase in adverse prognosis based on none, mild, and severe CAD by CCTA has been observed in numerous additional studies. A study by Schmermund and colleagues followed 706 consecutive patients who had undergone CTA but had no high-grade stenosis.[37] The patients' CCTAs were then categorized as either completely normal (group 1), showing minor plaque (group 2), or showing intermediate stenoses (group 3).[37] In group 1, the probability of event-free survival at 3 years was 100%, whereas it was 96% and 91% in group 2 and 3, respectively, indicating that events were related to the extent of disease. Another study by Russo and colleagues[38] followed 441 patients with suspected CAD who had undergone CCTA to evaluate for the presence and severity of the disease. During the 31.9-month follow-up period, the patients with normal coronary arteries had an annual event rate of 0.88%, whereas those with mild and significant CAD had a 3.89% and 8.09% annual event rate, respectively. Similar findings were noted in studies by Sozzi and colleagues[39] (222 patients with a mean follow-up of 5 years with a 0% event rate for normal coronaries, 1.2% in nonobstructive CAD, and 4.2% in patients with significant stenosis).

COMPARATIVE PROGNOSTIC VALUE OF CCTA AND STRESS TESTING

Prior studies comparing CCTA with myocardial perfusion stress (MPS) testing have found only modest relation between MPI measures of myocardial ischemia and CCTA measures of obstructive CAD, prompting concerns that anatomic-based detection of CAD may be inadequate to identify functionally significant CAD. In a pooled analysis of 4 studies of 231 patients, although agreement between nonobstructive CCTAs and MPS was high (122/143; 85%), agreement was poor when CCTAs demonstrated obstructive CAD (46/88; 52%).[40]

One recent study has examined the relationship of CCTA-identified plaque to MPS-identified ischemia beyond the yes/no dichotomization of obstructive versus nonobstructive CAD. Other measures of plaque severity have been studied and quantified by the authors' group, including summed plaque severity (segment stenosis score), plaque severity accounting for the extent of myocardium subtended by plaques (segments-at-risk score), plaque distribution (segment involvement score), plaque composition (noncalcified, mixed, and calcified plaque scores), and plaque severity in relation to location (prognostic CAD index).

Using these methods to comprehensively compare CCTA anatomic measures of coronary artery plaque extent, distribution, location, and composition with MPI measures of myocardial ischemia, one recent investigation examined 163 intermediate-risk patients without known CAD who underwent both CCTA and MPI.[41] The presence or absence of obstructive CAD by CCTA did not correlate with perfusion defects by MPI; however, segment stenosis scores (odds ratio [OR] 2.0) and segments-at-risk scores (OR 1.7, both $P<.01$) were significantly associated with abnormal MPI scans. Also, increasing numbers of coronary segments with mixed plaque, as compared with calcified or noncalcified plaque, predicted abnormal MPI. Individuals with higher mixed plaque scores (OR 1.64, $P<.01$) had more abnormal MPI scans. Thus, these data demonstrate that CCTA plaque characteristics beyond obstructive versus nonobstructive plaque (of extent, location, and composition) predict functional ischemia by MPI and that the comprehensive assessment of anatomic plaque characteristics may improve the detection of CAD lesions with functional significance.

Also germane for examination is whether the findings of CAD by CCTA and perfusion deficits by MPI are complementary or overlapping. In a study of 1132 outpatients aged 45 years or older compared with 7849 propensity score-matched outpatients undergoing MPI, prognosis was measured for a 2-year outcome of all-cause mortality.[42] In a comparison of the CCTA results by the Duke prognostic CAD index versus the percent ischemic myocardium by SPECT imaging, the annual mortality rates that were predicted by the prognostic CAD index for CCTA were directly proportional to the percent ischemic myocardium by MPS, ranging from 0.2% to 11.0% for CCTA and from 0% to 12% for MPS. Although the range of values for low to high risk was similar, a more gradual increase in risk was noted for CCTA in patients with less extensive CAD. These data identify similar prognostic values of CCTA and MPS and are in accord with the aforementioned prognostic value of milder nonobstructive plaques by CCTA. The aforementioned data are supported by a recent study by van Werkhoven and colleagues,[43] which demonstrated that CCTA findings of high-grade stenosis were independent and incremental predictors of events in 541 patients referred for both CCTA and MPI by supplementing functional assessment with an anatomic one.

PROGNOSIS AND PLAQUE COMPOSITION

Prior studies have demonstrated that certain atherosclerotic plaque features by CCTA, such as plaque burden, positive remodeling, and non-calcified plaque, are associated with higher adverse event rates (**Fig. 3**).[31,44–46] In a 27-month follow-up of 1059 initially stable patients undergoing CCTA, patients who later developed acute coronary syndromes (ACS) had higher rates of plaques with low attenuation plaques (LAP) *and* positive arterial remodeling (PR) compared with those possessing either LAP or PR, or neither LAP nor PR (22.2% vs 3.7% vs 0.5%). Compared with plaques not resulting in ACS, plaques implicated in future ACS demonstrated higher segmental plaque volume (134.9 mm^3 vs 57.8 mm^3) and LAP volume (20.4 mm^3 vs 1.1 mm^3, P<.001).[47] Importantly, all events observed in this study were for patients with less than 75% stenosis. These data are consistent with a study by Kristensen[48] of

patients with non-ST elevation myocardial infarction who underwent a concurrent CT at the time of acute myocardial infarction (AMI). At a 16-month follow-up, 23 out of 312 individuals who experienced a subsequent event had a higher baseline CT total nonobstructive plaque volume (HR 1.06/100 mm^3, P = .01), largely caused by non-calcified plaque volume (HR 1.18/100 mm^3, P = .01).

The mechanisms underlying these findings may be related to arterial injury that may manifest in not only worsened outcome but also heightened ischemia. Cheng[49] examined the relationship of other APCs to myocardial ischemia in 49 patients undergoing CT and MPS. The adverse plaque characteristics (APCs) evaluated included LAP, PR, and spotty intraplaque calcifications (SC).[49] Controlling for stenosis severity, reversible ischemia was more often noted for plaques with LAP (70% vs 14%, P<.001) and PR (70% vs 24%, P = .001) but not SC (55% vs 34%, P = .154). Plaques manifesting both LAP and PR were greater than or equal to 6-fold more likely to be associated with ischemia, as compared with plaques without LAP or PR.[49] These data support the utility of APCs beyond stenosis to identify patients with ischemia, a known risk marker for future AMI.

PROGNOSIS AND VENTRICULAR FUNCTION

CCTA also provides important information about left ventricular function and volumes above and beyond providing information about plaque composition and coronary anatomy (**Fig. 4**). The ability of CCTA to evaluate left ventricular function has been previously validated against echocardiography and other imaging modalities.[50,51] In a 2-center study of 5330 consecutive patients without

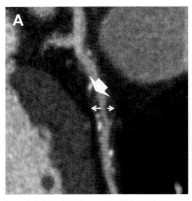 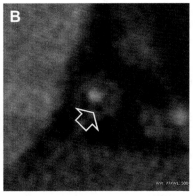

Fig. 3. (*A*) Curved multiplanar reconstruction of a coronary CT angiogram demonstrating partially calcified plaque with high plaque burden. Areas of low attenuation plaque (LAP) (*white thick arrow*) and positive arterial remodeling (*thin arrows*) are noted. (*B*) Cross-sectional arterial analysis again demonstrating area of LAP (*open thick arrow*).

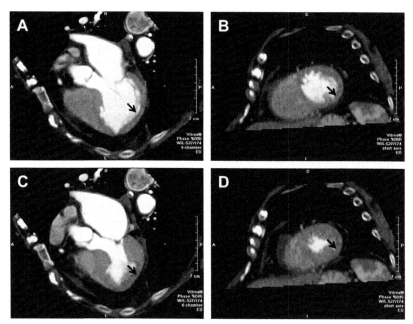

Fig. 4. Left ventricular functional study by CT in an 84-year-old woman. Representative end-diastolic (*A, B*) and systolic (*C, D*) images demonstrate significant hypoattenuation and segmental akinesis (*arrows*) noted in the inferolateral wall suggestive of a prior myocardial infarction. Coronary CT angiography confirmed a high-grade lesion in the obtuse marginal branch of the left circumflex artery.

known CAD undergoing CCTA, left ventricular ejection fraction (LVEF) by CT was judged as normal (>50%) or reduced (≤50%).[52] At a 2.3-year follow-up for all-cause mortality, 100 deaths occurred, with detection of obstructive CAD correlated with mortality (HR 2.44, 95% CI 1.61–3.72, $P<.001$). As compared with those with LVEF greater than 50%, those with LVEF less than or equal to 50% experienced higher rates of death (HR 1.56, 95% CI 1.04–2.36, $P = .03$). Annualized mortality rates in those with nonobstructive CAD and LVEF greater than 50% were very low (0.51%) and increased linearly for nonobstructive CAD and LVEF less than or equal to 50% (0.74%), obstructive CAD and LVEF greater than 50% (1.76%), and obstructive CAD and LVEF less than or equal to 50% (3.97%) (log-rank test $P<.001$).

A similar study by de Graaf and colleagues[53] evaluated 728 patients, with known or suspected CAD, for the presence of significant stenosis (defined as >50%) and left ventricular function. During a 765-day median follow-up period, 45 events were identified. A multivariate analysis, after correcting for risk factors and degree of stenosis, identified LVEF less than 49% and left ventricular end-systolic volume (LVESV) of greater than 90 mL as independent predictors of events. Both LVEF and LVESV were prognostically incremental to high-grade stenosis by CCTA. Finally, in one recent study, 333 patients presenting to

the emergency department with acute chest pain followed for 23 months also noted incremental prognostic information provided by regional wall motion abnormality above and beyond those provided by degree of stenosis.[54]

FUTURE DIRECTIONS

Prior data suggest an important diagnostic impact to ischemia detection for the guidance of decisions related to medical therapy versus revascularization. Although CCTA has been definitively shown to accurately identify and exclude high-grade anatomic coronary artery stenosis, which offers important prognostic findings, it has been less reliable for the diagnosis of hemodynamically significant CAD.[55,56] At present, fractional flow reserve (FFR)[57] is widely considered the gold standard for assessing the functional significance of discrete coronary lesions. At states of maximal hyperemia, the pressure ratio within the coronary artery distal to a lesion compared with the pressure within the aorta indicates ischemia at ratio values less than or equal to 0.80. FFR effectively guides the management of patients with multivessel disease, with coronary intervention decisions based on FFR rather than angiography alone associated with a reduced MACE event rate.[58,59]

Recently, a novel noninvasive approach addresses the functional severity of a coronary stenosis by using computational fluid dynamics (CFD) to evaluate FFR by CCTA. CFD uses mathematical algorithms using a fluid model to predict blood flow and pressure fields in coronary arteries as well as calculating the lesion-specific FFR.[60–62] The first prospective, multicenter study to evaluate the diagnostic accuracy of FFR utilizing CT to determine lesion-specific ischemia as compared with invasive FFR at the time of ICA has recently been completed.[63] In the diagnosis of ischemia-causing stenoses obtained via non-invasive fractional flow reserve study, 103 stable patients with known or suspected CAD underwent both CCTA and coronary angiography with FFR. In 159 vessels, the diagnostic accuracy, sensitivity, specificity, PPV, and NPV for FFR_{CT} less than 0.80 and CCTA stenosis greater than 50% were 84%, 88%, 82%, 74%, and 92% and 59%, 91%, 40%, 47%, and 89%, respectively. The area under the receiver operator characteristics curve was 0.90 for FFR_{CT} and 0.75 for CCTA stenosis ($P = .001$), with very good correlation between FFR_{CT} and invasive FFR ($r = 0.717$, $P<.001$). A larger parallel trial designed to evaluate the per-patient diagnostic performance of FFR_{CT} is ongoing, with enrollment recently completed.

SUMMARY

CCTA has emerged as a novel noninvasive method for the evaluation of not only coronary artery stenosis but also arterial wall and plaque features. The diagnostic performance of CCTA for these characteristics is high, with concordant prognostic utility. Recent developments in CCTA technology enable the simultaneous assessment of coronary stenosis, atherosclerotic plaque characteristics, and physiologic significance of lesion-specific ischemia. Future studies are needed to establish the totality of coronary artery plaque measures that offer clinical usefulness.

REFERENCES

1. Lloyd-Jones D, Adams RJ, Brown TM, et al. Heart disease and stroke statistics–2010 update: a report from the American Heart Association. Circulation 2010;121(7):e46–215.
2. Lerner DJ, Kannel WB. Patterns of coronary heart disease morbidity and mortality in the sexes: a 26-year follow-up of the Framingham population. Am Heart J 1986;111(2):383–90.
3. Ross R. Atherosclerosis–an inflammatory disease. N Engl J Med 1999;340(2):115–26.
4. Libby P, Ridker PM, Hansson GK. Inflammation in atherosclerosis: from pathophysiology to practice. J Am Coll Cardiol 2009;54(23):2129–38 PMCID: 2834169.
5. Gauthier TW, Scalia R, Murohara T, et al. Nitric oxide protects against leukocyte-endothelium interactions in the early stages of hypercholesterolemia. Arterioscler Thromb Vasc Biol 1995;15(10):1652–9.
6. Furchgott RF, Zawadzki JV. The obligatory role of endothelial cells in the relaxation of arterial smooth muscle by acetylcholine. Nature 1980;288(5789): 373–6.
7. Bian K, Doursout MF, Murad F. Vascular system: role of nitric oxide in cardiovascular diseases. J Clin Hypertens (Greenwich) 2008;10(4):304–10.
8. Borissoff JI, Spronk HM, ten Cate H. The hemostatic system as a modulator of atherosclerosis. N Engl J Med 2011;364(18):1746–60.
9. Crowther MA. Pathogenesis of atherosclerosis. Hematology Am Soc Hematol Educ Program 2005; 1:436–41.
10. Glagov S, Bassiouny HS, Sakaguchi Y, et al. Mechanical determinants of plaque modeling, remodeling and disruption. Atherosclerosis 1997; 131(Suppl):S13–4.
11. Glagov S, Weisenberg E, Zarins CK, et al. Compensatory enlargement of human atherosclerotic coronary arteries. N Engl J Med 1987;316(22):1371–5.
12. Gould KL, Lipscomb K, Hamilton GW. Physiologic basis for assessing critical coronary stenosis. Instantaneous flow response and regional distribution during coronary hyperemia as measures of coronary flow reserve. Am J Cardiol 1974;33(1): 87–94.
13. Uren NG, Melin JA, De Bruyne B, et al. Relation between myocardial blood flow and the severity of coronary-artery stenosis. N Engl J Med 1994; 330(25):1782–8.
14. Tonino PA, Fearon WF, De Bruyne B, et al. Angiographic versus functional severity of coronary artery stenoses in the FAME study fractional flow reserve versus angiography in multivessel evaluation. J Am Coll Cardiol 2010;55(25):2816–21.
15. Emond M, Mock MB, Davis KB, et al. Long-term survival of medically treated patients in the Coronary Artery Surgery Study (CASS) registry. Circulation 1994;90(6):2645–57.
16. Falk E, Shah PK, Fuster V. Coronary plaque disruption. Circulation 1995;92(3):657–71.
17. Shah PK. Screening asymptomatic subjects for subclinical atherosclerosis: can we, does it matter, and should we? J Am Coll Cardiol 2010;56(2): 98–105.
18. Klocke FJ, Baird MG, Lorell BH, et al. ACC/AHA/ ASNC guidelines for the clinical use of cardiac radionuclide imaging–executive summary: a report of the American College of Cardiology/American

Heart Association Task Force on Practice Guidelines (ACC/AHA/ASNC Committee to Revise the 1995 Guidelines for the Clinical Use of Cardiac Radionuclide Imaging). J Am Coll Cardiol 2003;42(7): 1318–33.

19. Gould KL. Does coronary flow trump coronary anatomy? JACC Cardiovasc Imaging 2009;2(8): 1009–23.

20. Shaw LJ, Hendel R, Borges-Neto S, et al. Prognostic value of normal exercise and adenosine (99m) Tc-tetrofosmin SPECT imaging: results from the multicenter registry of 4,728 patients. J Nucl Med 2003; 44(2):134–9.

21. Hachamovitch R, Hayes S, Friedman JD, et al. Determinants of risk and its temporal variation in patients with normal stress myocardial perfusion scans: what is the warranty period of a normal scan? J Am Coll Cardiol 2003;41(8):1329–40.

22. Berman DS, Kang X, Slomka PJ, et al. Underestimation of extent of ischemia by gated SPECT myocardial perfusion imaging in patients with left main coronary artery disease. J Nucl Cardiol 2007;14(4): 521–8.

23. Martin W, Tweddel AC, Hutton I. Balanced triple-vessel disease: enhanced detection by estimated myocardial thallium uptake. Nucl Med Commun 1992;13(3):149–53.

24. Min JK, Shaw LJ, Berman DS. The present state of coronary computed tomography angiography a process in evolution. J Am Coll Cardiol 2010; 55(10):957–65.

25. Hamon M, Biondi-Zoccai GG, Malagutti P, et al. Diagnostic performance of multislice spiral computed tomography of coronary arteries as compared with conventional invasive coronary angiography: a meta-analysis. J Am Coll Cardiol 2006;48(9): 1896–910.

26. Budoff MJ, Dowe D, Jollis JG, et al. Diagnostic performance of 64-multidetector row coronary computed tomographic angiography for evaluation of coronary artery stenosis in individuals without known coronary artery disease: results from the prospective multicenter ACCURACY (Assessment by Coronary Computed Tomographic Angiography of Individuals Undergoing Invasive Coronary Angiography) trial. J Am Coll Cardiol 2008;52(21): 1724–32.

27. Meijboom WB, Meijs MF, Schuijf JD, et al. Diagnostic accuracy of 64-slice computed tomography coronary angiography: a prospective, multicenter, multivendor study. J Am Coll Cardiol 2008;52(25):2135–44.

28. Pundziute G, Schuijf JD, Jukema JW, et al. Evaluation of plaque characteristics in acute coronary syndromes: non-invasive assessment with multislice computed tomography and invasive evaluation with intravascular ultrasound radiofrequency data analysis. Eur Heart J 2008;29(19):2373–81.

29. Voros S, Rinehart S, Qian Z, et al. Coronary atherosclerosis imaging by coronary CT angiography: current status, correlation with intravascular interrogation and meta-analysis. JACC Cardiovasc Imaging 2011;4(5):537–48.

30. Hulten EA, Carbonaro S, Petrillo SP, et al. Prognostic value of cardiac computed tomography angiography: a systematic review and meta-analysis. J Am Coll Cardiol 2011;57(10):1237–47.

31. Min JK, Shaw LJ, Devereux RB, et al. Prognostic value of multidetector coronary computed tomographic angiography for prediction of all-cause mortality. J Am Coll Cardiol 2007;50(12):1161–70.

32. Shaw LJ, Min JK, Narula J, et al. Sex differences in mortality associated with computed tomographic angiographic measurements of obstructive and non-obstructive coronary artery disease: an exploratory analysis. Circ Cardiovasc Imaging 2010;3(4): 473–81.

33. Min JK, Dunning A, Lin FY, et al. Rationale and design of the CONFIRM (COronary CT Angiography EvaluatioN For Clinical Outcomes: an InteRnational Multicenter) registry. J Cardiovasc Comput Tomogr 2011;5(2):84–92.

34. Min JK, Dunning A, Lin FY, et al. Age- and sex-related differences in all-cause mortality risk based on coronary computed tomography angiography findings results from the International Multicenter CONFIRM (Coronary CT Angiography Evaluation for Clinical Outcomes: an International Multicenter Registry) of 23,854 patients without known coronary artery disease. J Am Coll Cardiol 2011;58(8): 849–60.

35. Ostrom MP, Gopal A, Ahmadi N, et al. Mortality incidence and the severity of coronary atherosclerosis assessed by computed tomography angiography. J Am Coll Cardiol 2008;52(16):1335–43.

36. Lin FY, Shaw LJ, Dunning AM, et al. Mortality risk in symptomatic patients with nonobstructive coronary artery disease: a prospective 2-center study of 2,583 patients undergoing 64-detector row coronary computed tomographic angiography. J Am Coll Cardiol 2011;58(5):510–9.

37. Schmermund A, Elsasser A, Behl M, et al. Comparison of prognostic usefulness (three years) of computed tomographic angiography versus 64-slice computed tomographic calcium scanner in subjects without significant coronary artery disease. Am J Cardiol 2010;106(11):1574–9.

38. Russo V, Zavalloni A, Bacchi Reggiani ML, et al. Incremental prognostic value of coronary CT angiography in patients with suspected coronary artery disease. Circ Cardiovasc Imaging 2010;3(4):351–9.

39. Sozzi FB, Civaia F, Rossi P, et al. Long-term follow-up of patients with first-time chest pain having 64-slice computed tomography. Am J Cardiol 2011; 107(4):516–21.

40. Schuijf JD, Bax JJ. CT angiography: an alternative to nuclear perfusion imaging? Heart 2008;94(3): 255–7.

41. Lin F, Shaw LJ, Berman DS, et al. Multidetector computed tomography coronary artery plaque predictors of stress-induced myocardial ischemia by SPECT. Atherosclerosis 2008;197(2):700–9.

42. Shaw LJ, Berman DS, Hendel RC, et al. Prognosis by coronary computed tomographic angiography: matched comparison with myocardial perfusion single-photon emission computed tomography. J Cardiovasc Comput Tomogr 2008;2(2):93–101.

43. van Werkhoven JM, Schuijf JD, Gaemperli O, et al. Prognostic value of multislice computed tomography and gated single-photon emission computed tomography in patients with suspected coronary artery disease. J Am Coll Cardiol 2009;53(7): 623–32.

44. Hammer-Hansen S, Kofoed KF, Kelbaek H, et al. Volumetric evaluation of coronary plaque in patients presenting with acute myocardial infarction or stable angina pectoris-a multislice computerized tomography study. Am Heart J 2009;157(3):481–7.

45. Hoffmann U, Moselewski F, Nieman K, et al. Noninvasive assessment of plaque morphology and composition in culprit and stable lesions in acute coronary syndrome and stable lesions in stable angina by multidetector computed tomography. J Am Coll Cardiol 2006;47(8):1655–62.

46. Imazeki T, Sato Y, Inoue F, et al. Evaluation of coronary artery remodeling in patients with acute coronary syndrome and stable angina by multislice computed tomography. Circ J 2004;68(11):1045–50.

47. Motoyama S, Sarai M, Harigaya H, et al. Computed tomographic angiography characteristics of atherosclerotic plaques subsequently resulting in acute coronary syndrome. J Am Coll Cardiol 2009;54(1): 49–57.

48. Kristensen TS, Kofoed KF, Kühl JT, et al. Prognostic implications of nonobstructive coronary plaques in patients with non-ST-segment elevation myocardial infarction: a multidetector computed tomography study. J Am Coll Cardiol 2011;58(5):502–9.

49. Shmilovich H, Cheng VY, Tamarappoo BK, et al. Vulnerable plaque features on coronary CT angiography as markers of inducible regional myocardial hypoperfusion from severe coronary artery stenoses. Atherosclerosis 2011. [Epub ahead of print].

50. Yamamuro M, Tadamura E, Kubo S, et al. Cardiac functional analysis with multi-detector row CT and segmental reconstruction algorithm: comparison with echocardiography, SPECT, and MR imaging. Radiology 2005;234(2):381–90.

51. Henneman MM, Schuijf JD, Jukema JW, et al. Assessment of global and regional left ventricular function and volumes with 64-slice MSCT: a comparison with 2D echocardiography. J Nucl Cardiol 2006;13(4):480–7.

52. Min JK, Lin FY, Dunning AM, et al. Incremental prognostic significance of left ventricular dysfunction to coronary artery disease detection by 64-detector row coronary computed tomographic angiography for the prediction of all-cause mortality: results from a two-centre study of 5330 patients. Eur Heart J 2010;31(10):1212–9.

53. de Graaf FR, van Werkhoven JM, van Velzen JE, et al. Incremental prognostic value of left ventricular function analysis over non-invasive coronary angiography with multidetector computed tomography. J Nucl Cardiol 2010;17(6):1034–40 PMCID: 2990018.

54. Schlett CL, Banerji D, Siegel E, et al. Prognostic value of CT angiography for major adverse cardiac events in patients with acute chest pain from the emergency department: 2-year outcomes of the RO-MICAT trial. JACC Cardiovasc Imaging 2011;4(5): 481–91.

55. Di Carli MF, Dorbala S, Curillova Z, et al. Relationship between CT coronary angiography and stress perfusion imaging in patients with suspected ischemic heart disease assessed by integrated PET-CT imaging. J Nucl Cardiol 2007;14(6):799–809.

56. Hacker M, Jakobs T, Hack N, et al. Sixty-four slice spiral CT angiography does not predict the functional relevance of coronary artery stenoses in patients with stable angina. Eur J Nucl Med Mol Imaging 2007;34(1):4–10.

57. Wu CK, Lin JW, Caffrey JL, et al. Cystatin C and long-term mortality among subjects with normal creatinine-based estimated glomerular filtration rates: NHANES III (Third National Health and Nutrition Examination Survey). J Am Coll Cardiol 2010; 56(23):1930–6.

58. Pijls NH, Fearon WF, Tonino PA, et al. Fractional flow reserve versus angiography for guiding percutaneous coronary intervention in patients with multivessel coronary artery disease: 2-year follow-up of the FAME (Fractional Flow Reserve Versus Angiography for Multivessel Evaluation) study. J Am Coll Cardiol 2010;56(3):177–84.

59. Tonino PA, De Bruyne B, Pijls NH, et al. Fractional flow reserve versus angiography for guiding percutaneous coronary intervention. N Engl J Med 2009; 360(3):213–24.

60. Kim HJ, Jansen KE, Taylor CA. Incorporating autoregulatory mechanisms of the cardiovascular system in three-dimensional finite element models of arterial blood flow. Ann Biomed Eng 2010;38(7):2314–30.

61. Kim HJ, Vignon-Clementel IE, Coogan JS, et al. Patient-specific modeling of blood flow and pressure in human coronary arteries. Ann Biomed Eng 2010;38(10):3195–209.

62. Kim HJ, Vignon-Clementel IE, Figueroa CA, et al. On coupling a lumped parameter heart model and a three-dimensional finite element aorta model. Ann Biomed Eng 2009;37(11):2153–69.

63. Koo BK, Erglis A, Doh JH, et al. Diagnosis of ischemia-causing coronary stenoses by noninvasive fractional flow reserve computed from coronary computed tomographic angiograms results from the prospective multicenter DISCOVER-FLOW (Diagnosis of Ischemia-Causing Stenoses Obtained Via Noninvasive Fractional Flow Reserve) study. J Am Coll Cardiol 2011;58(19):1989–97.

Evaluation of Plaque Morphology by Coronary CT Angiography

Shinichiro Fujimoto, MD, PhD[a],*, Takeshi Kondo, MD, PhD[a],
Jagat Narula, MD, PhD, FRCP[b]

KEYWORDS

- Vulnerable plaque • Positive remodeling
- Low-attenuation plaque • Napkin ring sign
- No-reflow phenomenon
- Circumferential plaque calcification

Coronary computed tomographic angiography (CTA) is a promising noninvasive tool that allows the visualization of plaque morphology. Plaques characterized by positive remodeling, low attenuation, and napkin ring circular enhancement on contrast-enhanced coronary CTA have been regarded as rupture-prone vulnerable plaques, which account for about 60% of all vulnerable lesions and may be precursors of plaque rupture. Recently, we demonstrated that the distribution and prevalence of computed tomography (CT)-verified vulnerable plaques were approximately similar to that of thin-cap fibroatheroma (TCFA) reported in autopsy cases, and that coronary artery calcium score (CACS) alone may not be as useful for exclusion of a risk of acute coronary syndrome (ACS). If a more widespread use of coronary CTA is considered in the future, coronary CTA needs to demonstrate incremental prognostic value beyond the Framingham Risk Score (FRS) and other prognostic markers. The clinical usefulness of CT-based detection of vulnerable plaque remains to be demonstrated. In a somewhat different setting, CT-derived plaque features were demonstrated to predict the occurrence of slow-flow complications during percutaneous coronary interventions (PCIs), which opens a further potential field for coronary CTA.

DIAGNOSIS OF THE VULNERABLE PLAQUE

In pathology studies, ACSs are caused by plaque rupture in up to 60% of cases, plaque erosion in 30% to 35% of cases, and calcified nodules in 3% to 7% of cases.[1,2] Narula and colleagues[3] reported that the characteristics of rupture-prone vulnerable plaques include positive remodeling (so that the plaque accounts for more than 25–50% of the entire cross section of the artery), the presence of a large necrotic core (more than 25% of plaque volume), the presence of vasa vasorum within the plaque, macrophage infiltrates in the fibrous cap, a fibrous cap less than 65 μm thick, as well as increased matrix metalloproteinase expression.

ACS may occur without precursory symptoms, and its prediction remains both important and difficult to achieve. A meta-analysis of coronary angiography during a 5-year period before the onset of ACS reported that 68% of culprit lesions showed no significant luminal stenosis.[4] It has been proposed noted that the traditional FRS may be supported by the noninvasive diagnostic imaging tool that allows the detection of a truly high-risk group with a more than 15% risk of developing ACS per year.[5]

Based on comparisons with intravascular ultrasound (IVUS),[6] it was established that CT has the

a Department of Cardiology, Takase Clinic, 885-2 Minami-orui, Takasaki 370-0036, Japan
b Mount Sinai School of Medicine, One Gustave L. Levy Place, Box 1030, New York, NY 10029-6574, USA
* Corresponding author.
E-mail address: s-fujimo@tj8.so-net.ne.jp

Cardiol Clin 30 (2012) 69–75
doi:10.1016/j.ccl.2011.10.002
0733-8651/12/$ – see front matter © 2012 Elsevier Inc. All rights reserved.

ability to visualize and characterize coronary atherosclerotic plaque. With further progress in technology and the increasing accumulation of clinical data, coronary CTA has developed into a most promising noninvasive tool for the identification of vulnerable plaques.

CT-VERIFIED VULNERABLE PLAQUE

Motoyama and colleagues[6] reported that the average CT densities of soft, fibrous, and calcified plaques as determined by IVUS echogenicity were 11 ± 12 HU, 78 ± 21 HU, and 516 ± 198 HU, respectively. They concluded that a threshold of 30 HU was a reasonable cutoff value to define lipid-rich plaque in coronary CTA. Moreover, Motoyama and colleagues[7] reported that, compared with the culprit lesions of patients with stable angina pectoris, the culprit lesions in ACS were significantly more frequently characterized by spotty calcification, positive remodeling (remodeling index >1.1), and the presence of low-attenuation plaque (CT <30 HU). Prospectively, the investigators were able to demonstrate that plaques positive for 2 features with positive remodeling and low CT attenuation had a probability of 22.2% of an ACS within 2 years (Fig. 1).[8] Recently, Kashiwagi and colleagues[9] compared coronary CTA with optical coherence tomography for the detection of TCFA. Again, findings on coronary CTA that were predictive of TCFA were positive remodeling, the presence of a low–CT attenuation plaque (35 ± 32 HU) and ringlike attenuation. The presence of ringlike attenuation in CT was 11-fold higher in the TCFA group compared with the non-TCFA group. However, the background to the phenomenon remains unclear, and speculation includes the presence of deep microcalcification, intraplaque enhancement due to the presence of neovascularization and/or intraplaque

hemorrhage, the presence of a large central lipid core surrounded by fibrous plaque tissue, or even completed rupture with thrombotic material and surrounding contrast agent. It is presently assumed that high-risk plaques in CT should demonstrate positive remodeling, low-attenuation plaque, and ringlike attenuation (sometimes referred to as the napkin ring sign) (Fig. 2).

SPATIAL DISTRIBUTION OF CT-VERIFIED VULNERABLE PLAQUE AND THE RELATIONSHIP WITH SIGNIFICANT STENOSIS

Most TCFAs are localized in the proximal portion of the 3 major coronary arteries. Kolodgie and colleagues[10] reported that the proximal portion of the left anterior descending coronary artery was the most frequent location; the proximal right and left circumflex coronary arteries were about half as common. Moreover, Virmani and colleagues[11] reported that 74% of TCFAs demonstrated less than 75% narrowing of their cross-sectional area. We examined the distribution of plaques positive for 2 features with positive remodeling and low CT attenuation and their relationship with significant stenosis. The study included 4870 patients (male/female = 2418/2452, 65 ± 12 years) who underwent coronary CTA for suspected coronary artery disease (CAD). Four hundred seventy-four lesions with both characteristics were observed in 342 patients (7.0%). Most of these lesions were localized in the proximal portion of the 3 major coronary arteries. About half of the plaques positive for 2 features (52.5%) occurred in the proximal portion and/or midportion of the left anterior descending artery: 18% in the proximal portion of the right coronary artery, 5% in the proximal portion of the left circumflex coronary artery, and 8% in the left main trunk. Of the 474 high-risk

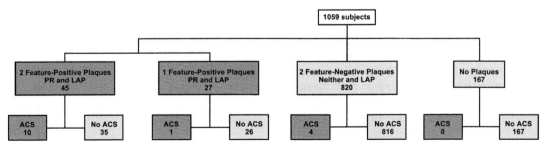

Fig. 1. Relationship between acute coronary events and plaque characteristics based on coronary CTA. The plaque characteristics of lesions developing ACS during 27 ± 10 months of follow-up were evaluated. Of the 45 patients showing plaques positive for 2 features (positive remodeling [PR] and low-attenuation plaque [LAP]), ACS developed in 10 (22.2%), compared with 1 (3.7%) of the 27 patients with plaques positive for 1 feature (either PR or LAP). ACS developed in only 4 (0.5%) of the 820 patients with neither PR nor LAP. (From Motoyama S, Sarai M, Harigaya H, et al. Computed tomographic angiography characteristics of atherosclerotic plaques subsequently resulting in acute coronary syndrome. J Am Coll Cardiol 2009;54:52; with permission.)

A   **B**

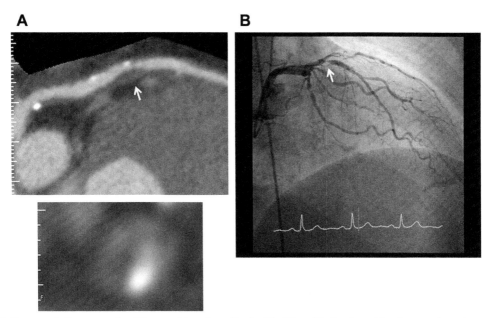

Fig. 2. Representative case of a 57-year-old male patient with CT-verified vulnerable plaque who subsequently developed ACS. Coronary risk factors included hypertension and dyslipidemia. The patient underwent coronary CT angiography, which revealed a 50% stenotic lesion with positive remodeling, low-attenuation plaque, napkin ring sign, and spotty calcification within the proximal left anterior descending artery (*A*). He was treated medically. After 177 days, the patient experienced ACS with negative T waves in V2 to V4. Emergency coronary angiography revealed a 90% stenotic lesion at the site corresponding to the CT-verified vulnerable plaque in the proximal left anterior descending artery (*B*).

lesions, 310 (65.4%) were not associated with significant luminal stenosis. Hence, the distribution and prevalence of high-risk coronary plaques as demonstrated by CT were approximately similar to that of TCFA reported in autopsy cases (**Fig. 3**).

THE RELATIONSHIP WITH CALCIFICATION IN CT-VERIFIED VULNERABLE PLAQUE

The CACS is closely associated with the presence of coronary atherosclerosis. It has been well established that increasing calcium scores are associated with an increased likelihood of cardiac events.[12] On the other hand, most vulnerable plaques have no or only very small calcifications.[1] Noncalcified plaques are more prevalent in patients with ACS than in those with stable angina pectoris.[13] We examined the relationship of high-risk plaques in coronary CTA with the presence and extent of coronary calcium in the patient group mentioned earlier. No calcification was present in 260 lesions (54.9%), spotty calcium in 101 lesions (21.3%), moderate calcification in 107 lesions (22.6%), and severe calcification in only 6 lesions (1.3%). The frequency of plaques with high-risk morphology increased as calcium scores increased from 0 to 499, but it decreased when calcium scores exceeded 500 (**Fig. 4**). Spotty

calcification, one of the characteristics for vulnerable plaque, might not be detectable in traditional coronary calcium scans because their slice thickness is often limited to 3 mm. High-risk plaques could be found in individuals with a calcium score of 0. Of the 2160 patients with unknown CAD, 1019 individuals had a calcium score of 0 (male/female = 455/564, 60.5 ± 12.0 years). In 47 of these individuals (4.6%), plaques positive for 2 features were found in coronary CTA. One hundred and four patients (10.2%) had spotty calcification, and 10 (9.6%) of these 104 patients had high-risk plaques in coronary CTA. Of 915 patients (89.8%) with calcification patterns that were not spotty, 37 (4.0%) had plaques positive for 2 features (**Fig. 5**).[14] These results suggest that the calcium score alone may not be useful for the reliable exclusion of vulnerable plaques.

THE RELATIONSHIP BETWEEN CT-VERIFIED VULNERABLE PLAQUE AND THE FRS

Recent CT hardware developments have led to a reduction in the dose of contrast medium and radiation exposure, which facilitates more widespread use of coronary CTA. The international multicenter CONFIRM (Coronary CT Angiography Evaluation For Clinical Outcomes International Multicenter)

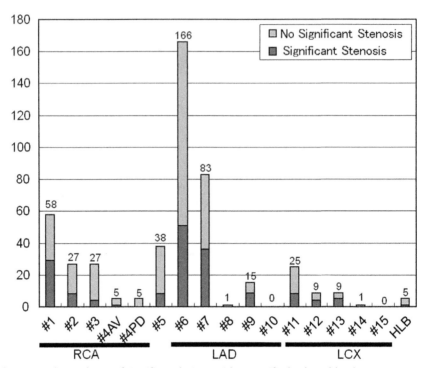

Fig. 3. Distribution and prevalence of significant lesions with CT-verified vulnerable plaque. Coronary atherosclerotic plaques with positive remodeling and low CT attenuation occur predominantly in the proximal portion of the 3 major coronary arteries, and only 34.6% of such lesions are associated with significant luminal stenosis. LAD, left anterior descending artery; LCX, left circumflex coronary artery; RCA, right coronary artery.

registry, which includes 23,854 patients without known CAD who underwent coronary CTA, demonstrated convincingly that nonobstructive plaque detected by CT was positively associated with all-cause mortality.[15] Hence, the detection of vulnerable plaque in coronary CTA might be clinically useful for risk stratification of individuals even if obstructive CAD was not detected. We examined

the relationship between CT-verified vulnerable plaque and the FRS in 1458 patients (male/female = 798/660, 61.6 ± 9.2 years [30–74]) without known CAD. Plaques positive for 2 features were observed in 104 cases (7.1%). In relation to the FRS, plaques positive for 2 features were observed in 1 of 122 individuals (0.8%) in the low Framingham risk group (<5%), in 55 of 1018 patients (5.4%) in the

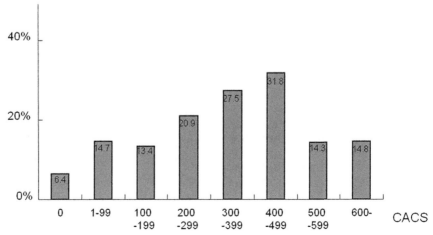

Fig. 4. Relationship between CACS and CT-verified vulnerable plaque. Frequency of patients with plaques positive for 2 features increased from CACS 0 to 499 but decreased adversely when CACS exceeded 500.

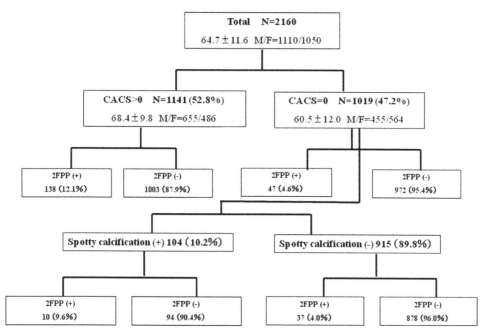

Fig. 5. Prevalence of plaques positive for 2 features (2FPP) in patients with a CACS of 0 with or without spotty calcification.

intermediate Framingham risk group (5%–20%), and in 48 of 318 patients (15.1%) in the high Framingham risk group (>20%) **(Fig. 6)**. The CACS was not a significant predictor. These results suggest that coronary CTA would be most useful for risk restratification in individuals with intermediate and high risk according to the FRS.

PLANNING CORONARY INTERVENTION

The slow-flow (also referred to as no-reflow) phenomenon has been frequently reported in the

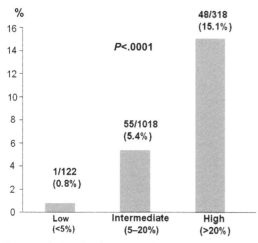

Fig. 6. Relationship between the FRS and CT-verified vulnerable plaque.

context of PCIs. The phenomenon is associated with myocardial damage and prolonged hospitalization.[16,17] Some previous reports have shown that plaque assessment by IVUS was useful for predicting the development of slow flow.[18,19] Similarly, CT has been shown to permit prediction of slow-flow and procedural complications. Nakazawa and colleagues[20] reported significant differences concerning the prevalence of low-attenuation plaque and napkin ring–like appearance of culprit plaques between patients with slow flow and those without it. We compared pre-PCI CT plaque characteristics of patients with stable angina who developed slow flow with those who did not develop slow flow during PCI. Multivariate logistic regression analyses revealed that low-attenuation plaque, dyslipidemia, and circumferential plaque calcification were significant predictors of the development of slow flow. Circumferential plaque calcification was the strongest predictor. The presence of such characteristics should alert the operator to potential complications.

LIMITATION AND FUTURE PERSPECTIVE FOR ASSESSMENT OF PLAQUE MORPHOLOGY IN CORONARY CTA

In coronary CTA, lesions with positive remodeling, low CT attenuation, and ringlike attenuation are widely regarded as rupture-prone vulnerable plaques. However, CT density values are influenced by factors such as the concentration of contrast

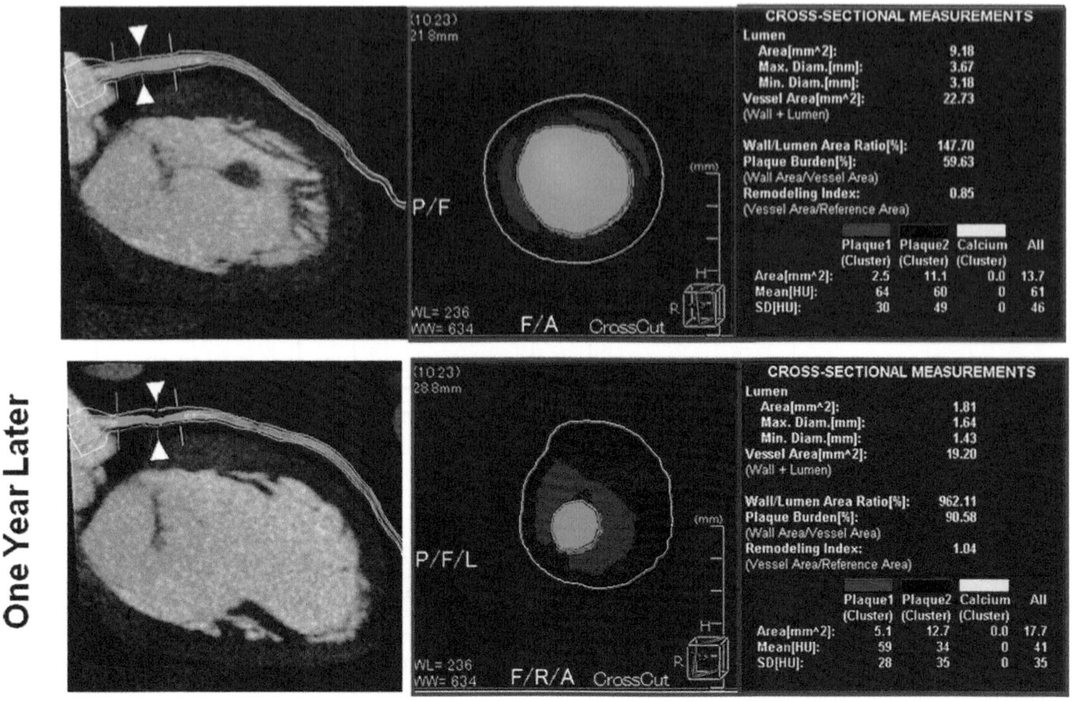

Fig. 7. Evaluation of plaque characteristics using new plaque analyzing software (Plaque Labeling Method). The patient, a 60-year-old man with atypical chest pain, underwent coronary CTA at our hospital, which revealed 25% stenotic lesion at the left main trunk. One year later, he suffered typical chest pain frequently. The patient underwent coronary CTA again, which revealed a progressive 75% stenotic lesion at the left main trunk. Plaque characteristics in this lesion were also evaluated by new plaque analyzing software. Quantitative analysis for vessel area and plaque area and plaque characteristics (*red*, necrotic core; *blue*, fibrous and/or fibrofatty; *yellow*, calcification) could be evaluated. The results showed that the necrotic core area (*red area*) progressed remarkably after 1 year.

medium in the coronary artery lumen, the degree of stenosis of coronary lesions, tube voltage, and reconstruction kernel.[21] In some studies, CT attenuations as high as 58 ± 43 HU for lipid-rich plaque have been reported.[22] Dedicated plaque analysis software to automatically determine plaque area and to classify lesions as lipid rich, fibrous, and calcified now use not only on CT values but also on their three-dimensional continuity, position, and shape (**Fig. 7**).[23]

As a further and important limitation, approximately 30% of coronary events are caused by plaque erosion. Such lesions may escape detection by CT.[24]

Although inflammation plays an important role in atherosclerotic plaque rupture,[25] coronary CTA cannot evaluate the presence or activity of inflammatory cells in atherosclerotic plaques. Recently, Hyafil and colleagues[26] showed that CT contrast agent, composed of iodinated nanoparticles dispersed with surfactant given intravenously to rabbits, accumulates in macrophages within atherosclerotic plaque 2 hours after injection, allowing for identification of macrophage cells with

coronary CTA. Hence, the development of specific contrast agents may be of value.[27]

More and larger clinical trials, optimally designed as intervention trials, will need to demonstrate clinical usefulness and improved outcome through CT-based plaque analysis.

REFERENCES

1. Naghavi M, Libby P, Falk E, et al. From vulnerable plaque to vulnerable patient: a call for new definitions and risk assessment strategies; part I. Circulation 2003;108:1664–72.
2. Virmani A, Burke AP, Farb A, et al. Pathology of the vulnerable plaque. J Am Coll Cardiol 2006;47: C13–8.
3. Narula J, Finn AV, Demaria AN. Picking plaques that pop. J Am Coll Cardiol 2005;45:1970–3.
4. Falk E, Shah PK, Fuster V. Coronary plaque disruption. Circulation 1995;92:657–71.
5. Braunwald E. Epilogue: what do clinicians expect from imagers? J Am Coll Cardiol 2006;47(Suppl 8): C101–3.

6. Motoyama S, Kondo T, Anno H, et al. Atherosclerotic plaque characterization by 0.5-mm-slice multislice computed tomographic imaging. Circ J 2007;71: 363–6.

7. Motoyama S, Kondo T, Sarai M, et al. Multislice computed tomographic characteristics of coronary lesions in acute coronary syndromes. J Am Coll Cardiol 2007;50:319–26.

8. Motoyama S, Sarai M, Harigaya H, et al. Computed tomographic angiography characteristics of atherosclerotic plaques subsequently resulting in acute coronary syndrome. J Am Coll Cardiol 2009;54: 49–57.

9. Kashiwagi M, Tanaka A, Kitabata H, et al. Feasibility of noninvasive assessment of thin-cap fibroatheroma by multidetector computed tomography. JACC Cardiovasc Imaging 2009;2:1412–9.

10. Kolodgie FD, Burke AP, Farb A, et al. The thin-cap fibroatheroma: a type of vulnerable plaque: the major precursor lesion to acute coronary syndromes. Curr Opin Cardiol 2001;16:285–92.

11. Virmani R, Burke AP, Kolodgie FD, et al. Vulnerable plaque: the pathology of unstable coronary lesions. J Interv Cardiol 2002;15:439–46.

12. Greenland P, Bonow RO, Brundage BH, et al. ACCF/ AHA 2007 clinical expert consensus document on coronary artery calcium scoring by computed tomography in global cardiovascular risk assessment and in evaluation of patients with chest pain: a report of the American College of Cardiology Foundation Clinical Expert Consensus Task Force (ACCF/AHA Writing Committee to Update the 2000 Expert Consensus Document on Electron Beam Computed Tomography). J Am Coll Cardiol 2007; 49:378–402.

13. Henneman MM, Schuijf JD, Pundziute G, et al. Noninvasive evaluation with multislice computed tomography in suspected acute coronary syndrome: plaque morphology on multislice computed tomography versus coronary calcium score. J Am Coll Cardiol 2008;52:216–22.

14. Morita H, Fujimoto S, Kondo T, et al. Prevalence of computed tomographic angiography-verified high risk plaques and significant luminal stenosis in patients with zero coronary calcium score. Int J Cardiol, in press.

15. Min JK, Dunning A, Lin FY, et al. Age- and sex-related differences in all cause mortality risk based on coronary computed tomography angiography findings. J Am Coll Cardiol 2011;58:849–60.

16. Ramirez-Moreno A, Cardenal R, Pera C, et al. Predictors and prognostic value of myocardial injury following stent implantation. Int J Cardiol 2004;97: 193–8.

17. Mehta RH, Harjai KJ, Boura J, et al. Prognostic significance of transient no-reflow during primary percutaneous coronary intervention for ST-elevation acute myocardial infarction. Am J Cardiol 2003;92:1445–7.

18. Okura H, Taguchi H, Kubo T, et al. Atherosclerotic plaque with ultrasonic attenuation affects coronary reflow and infarct size in patients with acute coronary syndrome: an intravascular ultrasound study. Circ J 2007;71:648–53.

19. Hong YJ, Jeong MH, Choi YH, et al. Impact of plaque components on no-reflow phenomenon after stent deployment in patients with acute coronary syndrome: a virtual histology-intravascular ultrasound analysis. Eur Heart J 2011;32:2059–66.

20. Nakazawa G, Tanabe K, Onuma Y, et al. Efficacy of culprit assessment by 64-slice multidetector computed tomography to predict transient no-reflow phenomenon during percutaneous coronary intervention. Am Heart J 2008;155:1150–7.

21. Cademartiri F, Mollet NR, Runza G, et al. Influence of intracoronary attenuation on coronary plaque measurements using multislice computed tomography: observations in an ex vivo model of coronary computed tomography angiography. Eur Radiol 2005;15:1426–31.

22. Pohlea K, Achenbach S, Macneill B, et al. Characterization of non-calcified coronary atherosclerotic plaque by multi-detector row CT: comparison to IVUS. Atherosclerosis 2007;190:174–80.

23. Kodama T, Kondo T, Orihara T, et al. Comparison between new labeling method of MDCT and virtual histology of IVUS for non-calcified plaque analysis. Circ J 2009;73(Suppl 1):228(OE-156).

24. Ozaki Y, Okumura M, Ismail TF, et al. Coronary CT angiographic characteristics of culprit lesions in acute coronary syndromes not related to plaque rupture as defined by optical coherence tomography and angioscopy. Eur Heart J 2011;32:2814–23.

25. Libby P. Inflammation in atherosclerosis. Nature 2001;420:868–74.

26. Hyafil F, Cornily JC, Feig JE, et al. Noninvasive detection of macrophages using a nanoparticulate contrast agent for computed tomography. Nat Med 2007;13:636–41.

27. Narula J, Strauss HW. The popcord plaques [editorial]. Nature Med 2007;13:532–4.

Prognostic Value of Coronary CT Angiography

Michael K. Cheezum, MD[a],
Edward A. Hulten, MD, MPH[b,c,d], Collin Fischer, MD[a],
Ryan M. Smith, DO[a], Ahmad M. Slim, MD[e],
Todd C. Villines, MD, FSCCT[a,f],*

KEYWORDS

- Coronary computed tomography angiography
- Computed tomography • Prognosis
- Coronary artery disease • Agatston score
- Coronary artery calcification

Over the past decade, coronary computed tomography angiography (CTA) has rapidly advanced. At present, the clinical performance of coronary CTA is guided by detailed consensus Appropriate Use Criteria regarding patient selection,[1] and guidelines on its performance,[2–4] scan interpretation and results reporting,[5,6] and coronary CTA provider training and competency.[2,7] Owing to newer scanner technologies and acquisition protocols that have resulted in improved spatial and temporal resolution of coronary CTA, image quality has been significantly augmented while patient radiation exposure has been dramatically reduced. The result is a highly accurate noninvasive method for the diagnosis of coronary artery disease (CAD), and a reasonable alternative to invasive coronary angiography (ICA) in appropriately selected patients.[8–11] Indeed, increased scrutiny regarding health care use and the reported low yield of ICA for obstructive CAD, especially among patients without known prior CAD, has opened the door for coronary CTA as a potential noninvasive gatekeeper to invasive coronary catheterization in low- to intermediate-risk patients.[12,13] While this role is shared with other noninvasive cardiac testing modalities, coronary CTA possesses the unique ability to accurately assess coronary arterial plaque for its presence, distribution, lesion severity, morphology, and composition. Recent data have convincingly demonstrated that coronary CTA provides robust prognostic information related to the extent and severity of both obstructive and nonobstructive coronary atherosclerosis. Furthermore, the prognostic implications derived

The authors have no disclosures. The views expressed here are those of the authors only, and are not to be construed as those of the Department of the Army or Department of Defense.

[a] Cardiology Service, Walter Reed National Military Medical Center, 8901 Rockville Pike, Bethesda, MD 20889, USA

[b] Non-invasive Cardiovascular Imaging Program, Brigham and Women's Hospital, Harvard Medical School, 75 Francis Street, Boston, MA 02115, USA

[c] Department of Medicine, Brigham and Women's Hospital, Harvard Medical School, 75 Francis Street, Boston, MA 02115, USA

[d] Department of Radiology, Brigham and Women's Hospital, Harvard Medical School, 75 Francis Street, Boston, MA 02115, USA

[e] Cardiology Service, San Antonio Military Medical Center, 3551 Roger Brooke Drive, Fort Sam Houston, TX, USA

[f] Cardiac CT Program, Cardiovascular Research, Walter Reed National Military Medical Center, Uniformed Services University, 8901 Rockville Pike, Bethesda, MD 20889, USA

* Corresponding author. Cardiac CT Program, Cardiovascular Research, Walter Reed National Military Medical Center, Uniformed Services University, 8901 Rockville Pike, Bethesda, MD 20889.

E-mail address: todd.villines@us.army.mil

Cardiol Clin 30 (2012) 77–91
doi:10.1016/j.ccl.2011.11.005
0733-8651/12/$ – see front matter Published by Elsevier Inc.

from novel measures of plaque composition and morphology, as well as the potential refinement of computed tomography (CT) myocardial perfusion, seem likely to further enhance the prognostic yield of coronary CTA and are active areas of research. Here the full potential of coronary CTA remains to be seen, and subsequent image-based treatment strategies have awaited mature data regarding the prognostic value of coronary CTA to identify patients at higher risk. Armed with recent evidence clearly demonstrating the prognostic value of coronary CTA, studies prospectively examining the clinical and cost outcomes of therapeutics tailored to coronary CTA-based measures of cardiovascular risk are needed.[14]

PROGNOSTIC VALUE OF CORONARY CTA IN SYMPTOMATIC PATIENTS

Significant prognostic data have emerged across diverse patient populations with a range of clinical presentations undergoing coronary CTA, varying from symptoms of stable chest pain to possible acute coronary syndromes. Relative to other non-invasive modalities, data demonstrate the independent predictive significance of coronary CTA for future major adverse cardiac events (MACE), and confirm the incremental prognostic value of CAD burden visualized on coronary CTA, beyond traditional risk factors.

Stable Chest Pain

Recently, two large meta-analyses summarized numerous single-center data regarding the prognostic value of coronary CTA findings in patients with primarily stable symptoms concerning obstructive CAD.[15,16] In the first, the authors' group performed an analysis of 18 trials published through March 2010 (**Table 1**) that included 9592 symptomatic patients followed for a median of 20 months following coronary CTA.[15] Among patients included in this analysis, the mean age was 59 years, 58% were men, and fewer than 2% of patients previously had known CAD. There were 449 MACE including 180 deaths, 56

Table 1
Eighteen studies included in a meta-analysis on prognosis following coronary CT angiography

Author	Year	Design	Population: Known or Suspected CAD	Scanner	n	Follow-up (mo)	Age (y)	% Male
Gopal[17]	2009	PCO	Known or suspected	EBCT	454	40	58	70
Ostrom[18]	2008	RetCO	Suspected	EBCT	2538	78	59	70
Min[19]	2007	PCO	Suspected	16-Slice	1127	15.3	62	43
Noda[20]	2008	PCO	Suspected	16-Slice	30	9.9	65	43
Pundziute[21]	2007	PCO	Known or suspected	16-Slice	100	13	59	73
Shaw[22]	2008	PCO	Suspected	16-Slice	693	15.6	62	52
Abidov[23]	2009	PCO	Suspected	64-Slice	199	27.6	54	54
Aldrovandi[24]	2009	PCO	Suspected	64-Slice	187	24	63	64
Barros[25]	2009	RetCO	Suspected	64-Slice	31	21	58	70
Cademartiri[26]	2008	PCO	Known or suspected	64-Slice	98	20	67	32
Carrigan[27]	2009	RetCO	Suspected	64-Slice	227	27.6	54	61
Chow[28]	2010	PCO	Suspected	64-Slice	2076	16.8	58	52
Danciu[29]	2007	PCO	Suspected	64-Slice	421	15	64	63
Fazel[30]	2009	RetCO	Suspected	64-Slice	436	36	55	45
Gaemperli[31]	2008	PCO	Known or suspected	64-Slice	220	14.4	63	65
Hay[32]	2009	RetCO	Suspected	64-Slice	138	19.9	57	73
Rubinshtein[33]	2006	RetCO	Suspected	64-Slice	100	12	56	57
van Werkhoven[34]	2009	PCO	Suspected	64-Slice	517	22.4	59	59
Total					9592	429		
Mean/median					224	20	59	58

Abbreviations: CAD, coronary artery disease; EBCT, electron-beam computed tomography; PCO, prospective cohort; RetCO, retrospective cohort.

Reproduced from Hulten EA, Carbonaro S, Petrillo SP, et al. Prognostic value of cardiac computed tomography angiography: a systematic review and meta-analysis. J Am Coll Cardiol 2011;57(10):1239; with permission.

myocardial infarctions (MIs), and 213 coronary revascularizations, for an annualized event rate of 4.5% for combined MACE and 2.4% for death and nonfatal MI (excluding revascularizations). The pooled, weighted annualized event rate for patients with obstructive (any stenosis ≥50%) versus nonobstructive (<50% stenosis) and normal coronary CTA was 8.8% versus 1.4% and 0.17% for all MACE (P<.05), and 2.2% versus 0.7% and 0.15% for death (P<.05), respectively (**Fig. 1**). These results demonstrate that patients with no appreciable CAD on coronary CTA have a very low annualized risk of MACE (<1%) that is similar to rates seen in healthy, low-risk populations and slightly lower than that reported for patients with normal exercise myocardial perfusion imaging or exercise echocardiography.[35,36] Conversely, patients with nonobstructive and obstructive CAD had combined event rates of 1.4% and 8.8% per year, respectively. Although revascularizations accounted for a large proportion of subsequent events reported across multiple studies, and notwithstanding potential biases inherent to following patients prospectively after coronary angiography, patients with obstructive disease on coronary CTA nevertheless experienced a significantly increased number of hard events, including death and MI, which are less subjective outcome measures than is revascularization.

More recently, Bamberg and colleagues[16] reported their meta-analysis of 7335 symptomatic patients undergoing coronary CTA for suspected CAD. Similar to the authors' findings, after a mean follow-up of 20 months they demonstrated increased annualized MACE with and without revascularization (11.9% and 6.4%) among patients with any significant stenosis (≥50%), and a very low combined event rate (0.4%) in patients with no CAD. Of note, they performed the first expanded analysis of MACE associated with various subgroups of plaque burden (**Table 2**), whereby each significant coronary stenosis (maximum of 17) and the presence of left main coronary artery stenosis conferred a 35% (hazard ratio [HR] 1.35; P<.001) and a more than 500% (HR 6.64; P = .009) increased relative risk, respectively. Of interest, the association between the

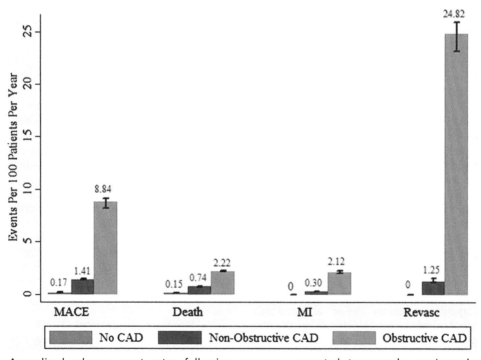

Fig. 1. Annualized adverse event rates following coronary computed tomography angiography (CTA). Percentage of annualized event rates for combined major adverse cardiac events (MACE), death (all-cause), myocardial infarction (MI), and revascularization (Revasc), stratified by cardiac CTA diagnosis of no coronary artery disease (CAD), nonobstructive CAD (50% stenosis), and obstructive CAD (50% stenosis). All groups were significantly different by analysis of variance (P<.05). (*Reproduced from* Hulten EA, Carbonaro S, Petrillo SP, et al. Prognostic value of cardiac computed tomography angiography: a systematic review and meta-analysis. J Am Coll Cardiol 2011;57(10):1240; with permission.)

Table 2
Summary estimates of relative risks associated with secondary coronary CTA findings

CTA Finding	$n_{Studies}$	$n_{Participants}$	Events	Hazard Ratio[a] (95% CI)	I^2 (%)	P Value	Z	P Value
Significant coronary stenosis	9	3670	252	10.74 (6.4–18.1)	85	<.001	1.34	.18
Left main coronary artery stenosis	4	1674	142	6.64 (2.6–17.3)	71.9	.009	0.49	.62
Each significant coronary stenosis	4	1879	145	1.35 (1.1–1.7)	95.1	<.001	0.41	.52
3-vessel disease	2	3665	125	2.50 (1.9–3.3)	0	.55	0.32	.87
Any atherosclerotic plaque	6	4733	244	4.51 (2.2–9.3)	26.7	.33	0.96	.32
Each coronary segment containing plaque	5	2106	163	1.23 (1.17–1.29)	7.6	.35	−0.7	.50
Each coronary segment containing noncalcified plaque	4	979	124	1.29 (1.2–1.4)	0	.13	0.27	.91

Abbreviations: CI, confidence interval; $n_{Participants}$, number of subjects included in analysis; $n_{Studies}$, number of studies included in analysis.

[a] As derived from meta-regression analysis for mortality, acute coronary syndrome, and coronary revascularization.

Reproduced from Bamberg F, Sommer WH, Hoffmann V, et al. Meta-analysis and systematic review of the long-term predictive value of assessment of coronary atherosclerosis by contrast-enhanced coronary computed tomography angiography. J Am Coll Cardiol 2011;57(24):2430; with permission.

presence of significant coronary stenosis or any plaque and adverse outcomes remained highly significant even after adjustment for coronary calcium scores (HR 11.24 vs 10.42 after adjustment; $P = .79$). In conclusion, they summarize significant limitations of current research to include population differences (age primarily), study quality, and the importance of excluding revascularization in outcomes to limit heterogeneity. Indeed, future comparative research on image-based treatment strategies versus traditional management would ideally exclude coronary revascularization (and unstable angina), and/or report this separately, to limit bias related to differences in practice patterns regarding revascularization, and to remain consistent with common definitions of "hard" cardiovascular events, such as that used by current National Cholesterol Education Panel guidelines.[37]

Recently, results from the CONFIRM (Coronary CT Angiography Evaluation For Clinical Outcomes) international registry were reported, providing the first large-scale, prospective, multicenter data on prognosis following coronary CTA.[38] The investigators evaluated 24,775 symptomatic patients without known CAD who were clinically referred for at least 64-slice coronary CTA at 12 sites. Coronary disease was evaluated on a per-patient, per-vessel, and per-segment basis and graded as no disease, mild (1%–49%), moderate (50%–70%), or severe (≥70%) stenosis. The primary end point was all-cause mortality, occurring in 404 patients. Patients without CAD had excellent survival (99.7%) during the mean reported follow-up duration of 2.3 years; the risk of mortality increased in a statistically significant manner for nonobstructive, 1-vessel, 2-vessel, and 3-vessel obstructive (≥50% stenosis) disease (adjusted HR 1.62, 2.00, 2.92, and 3.70, respectively) (**Fig. 2**). The investigators further demonstrated that the extent and severity of CAD measured on a per-segment level, and especially when the left main artery and proximal left anterior descending artery are involved, are important to most accurately assess post-CTA mortality risk (**Table 3**). Within the CONFIRM registry, consistent with prior single-center studies,[19,28,39] several semiquantitative scores of CAD burden have been described that may refine risk prediction by coronary CTA:

- Segment Involvement Score (SIS). The number of segments with any atherosclerosis that confers risk-adjusted HR = 1.10 (95% confidence interval [CI]: 1.06–1.13) per segment involved (maximum of 16 segments)[38]
- Segment Stenosis Score (SSS). Each segment is scored as 1 (mild stenosis), 2 (moderate stenosis), or 3 (severe stenosis),

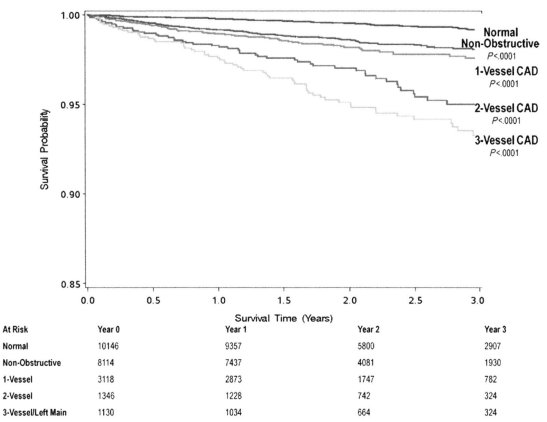

At Risk	Year 0	Year 1	Year 2	Year 3
Normal	10146	9357	5800	2907
Non-Obstructive	8114	7437	4081	1930
1-Vessel	3118	2873	1747	782
2-Vessel	1346	1228	742	324
3-Vessel/Left Main	1130	1034	664	324

Fig. 2. Unadjusted, all-cause 3-year Kaplan-Meier analysis of survival according to presence, extent, and severity of coronary artery disease by coronary CTA. Note the dose relationship of mortality to increasing numbers of vessels with obstructive CAD. (*Reproduced from* Min JK, Dunning A, Lin FY, et al. Age- and sex-related differences in all-cause mortality risk based on coronary computed tomography angiography findings. Results from the international multicenter CONFIRM (Coronary CT Angiography Evaluation for Clinical Outcomes: An International Multicenter Registry) of 23,854 patients without known coronary artery disease. J Am Coll Cardiol 2011;58(8):854; with permission.)

where per-segment severity confers risk-adjusted HR = 1.06 (95% CI: 1.05–1.08)[38]
- Modified Duke Prognostic Index. An angiographic 5-year prognostic index integrating proximal CAD, plaque extent, and left main disease, whereby survival worsens with higher-risk Duke scores, ranging from 96% survival for 1 stenosis ≥70% or 2 stenoses ≥50% (P = .013) to 85% survival for ≥50% left main artery stenosis (P<.0001)[19]

In an important subgroup analysis from the CONFIRM registry of patients with recorded left ventricular systolic function, the severity of CAD and left ventricular ejection fraction were each independently predictive of all-cause mortality, beyond standard cardiovascular risk factors.[40]

Nonobstructive CAD

When coronary CTA is clinically used according to current Appropriate Use Criteria,[1] the majority of

patients studied will ultimately demonstrate no obstructive CAD (74% of patients in the CONFIRM registry) while the identification of nonobstructive, subclinical CAD is common. Given evidence that most MIs result from plaque disruption involving a previously nonobstructive lesion and the known prognostic value of subclinical CAD, identified on noncontrast CT scans for Agatston calcium scoring,[41,42] the prognostic value of nonobstructive CAD on coronary CTA has come under considerable focus.

Expanding on prior studies, Lin and colleagues[43] evaluated 2583 primarily symptomatic (85%) adults (mean age 52.7 years; 58% women) without known CAD or obstructive disease (≥50% stenosis) on 64-slice coronary CTA. Over a mean follow-up period of 3.1 years, the investigators demonstrated clear strata in the risk for all-cause mortality according to the extent of nonobstructive CAD (**Fig. 3**). The visualization of any plaque increased the risk factor–adjusted

Table 3
Univariable and adjusted hazard ratios for all-cause mortality by per-patient, per-vessel, and per-segment analysis based on obstructive CAD at the 50% and 70% stenosis level

CCTA Result	Obstructive CAD (Defined at 50% Level)				Obstructive CAD (Defined at 70% Level)			
	Univariable HR (95% CI)	P Value	Risk-Adjusted HR (95% CI)	P Value	Univariable HR (95% CI)	P Value	Risk-Adjusted HR (95% CI)	P Value
Per-patient analysis								
Normal	1.00	Reference	1.00	Reference	1.00	Reference	1.00	Reference
Nonobstructive CAD	2.88 (2.15–3.86)	<.0001	1.60 (1.18–2.16)	.0023	3.29 (2.50–4.34)	<.0001	1.76 (1.32–2.34)	.0001
Obstructive CAD	6.05 (4.58–7.99)	<.0001	2.60 (1.94–3.49)	<.0001	8.11 (6.00–11.0)	<.0001	3.13 (2.27–4.31)	<.0001
Per-vessel analysis								
Normal	1.00	Reference	1.00	Reference	1.00	Reference	1.00	Reference
Nonobstructive	2.88 (2.15–3.86)	<.0001	1.62 (1.20–2.19)	.0018	3.30 (2.50–4.34)	<.0001	1.77 (1.33–2.36)	<.0001
1-vessel obstructive	4.12 (2.96–5.72)	<.0001	2.00 (1.43–2.82)	<.0001	5.67 (3.97–8.10)	<.0001	2.35 (1.62–3.42)	<.0001
2-vessel obstructive	6.93 (4.82–9.96)	<.0001	2.92 (2.00–4.25)	<.0001	11.40 (7.56–17.2)	<.0001	3.94 (2.57–6.04)	<.0001
3-vessel or left main obstructive	10.52 (7.50–14.7)	<.0001	3.70 (2.58–5.29)	<.0001	15.52 (10.1–23.9)	<.0001	5.27 (3.36–8.27)	<.0001
Per-segment analysis								
Segment involvement score (per segment involved)	1.22 (1.18–1.25)	<.0001	1.10 (1.06–1.13)	<.0001	NA	NA	NA	NA
Segment stenosis score (per segment severity)	1.12 (1.11–1.14)	<.0001	1.06 (1.05–1.08)	<.0001	NA	NA	NA	NA
Any severe proximal stenosis	4.01 (3.12–5.17)	<.0001	2.15 (1.66–2.78)	<.0001	NA	NA	NA	NA
Any left main stenosis	2.51 (2.01–3.13)	<.0001	1.45 (1.15–1.82)	.0015	NA	NA	NA	NA

Abbreviations: CCTA, coronary CTA; CI, confidence interval; HR, hazard ratio; NA, not applicable.
Reproduced from Min JK, Dunning A, Lin FY, et al. Age- and sex-related differences in all-cause mortality risk based on coronary computed tomography angiography findings. Results from the international multicenter CONFIRM (Coronary CT Angiography Evaluation for Clinical Outcomes: An International Multicenter Registry) of 23,854 patients without known coronary artery disease. J Am Coll Cardiol 2011;58(8):854; with permission.

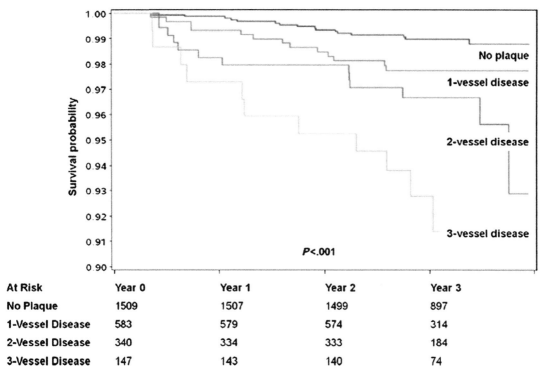

At Risk	Year 0	Year 1	Year 2	Year 3
No Plaque	1509	1507	1499	897
1-Vessel Disease	583	579	574	314
2-Vessel Disease	340	334	333	184
3-Vessel Disease	147	143	140	74

Fig. 3. Prognosis of nonobstructive coronary artery disease burden. Unadjusted all-cause 3-year Kaplan-Meier analysis of survival according to absence of CAD versus nonobstructive CAD in 1, 2, or 3 major epicardial coronary arteries. (*Reproduced from* Lin FY, Shaw LJ, Dunning AM, et al. Mortality risk in symptomatic patients with non-obstructive coronary artery disease: a prospective 2-center study of 2,583 patients undergoing 64-detector row coronary computed tomographic angiography. J Am Coll Cardiol 2011;58(5):515; with permission.)

mortality risk (HR 1.98), but risk was particularly higher with multivessel nonobstructive disease (HR 4.75 for 3-vessel nonobstructive disease) or if 5 segments or more were involved (HR 5.12). Of importance, the increased risk from nonobstructive CAD was also seen in patients with low Framingham Risk Scores (FRS), a patient subset that does not typically qualify for aggressive primary cardiovascular preventive therapies. Similarly, the presence of any plaque demonstrated an improvement in the net reclassification index when compared with risk estimates using the FRS alone.

Ahmadi and colleagues[44] similarly followed 1102 consecutive symptomatic patients with nonobstructive (<50%) CAD on coronary CTA for a mean of 78 months, the primary outcome being all-cause mortality. Again, the number of coronary vessels with nonobstructive disease independently predicted all-cause mortality. However, of additional interest was the finding that mortality incrementally increased according to the type of nonobstructive disease present: purely calcified plaque (1.4%), to partially calcified plaque (3.3%), to noncalcified plaque (9.6%) (*P*<.001).

Whereas prognostic data regarding nonobstructive CAD on coronary CTA has been derived primarily from low- to intermediate-risk patients, Kristensen and colleagues[45] recently provided an interesting look at the prognostic implications of nonobstructive CAD in high-risk patients presenting with suspected non–ST-segment MIs (NSTEMI). The investigators evaluated 312 consecutive patients presenting with acute chest pain, elevated troponin T, and the absence of ST-segment elevation, and performed 64-slice coronary CTA followed by invasive angiography. Total plaque volume for all nonobstructive lesions on coronary CTA and plaque composition (noncalcified, partially calcified, and calcified) was assessed. The primary outcome was combined MACE (cardiovascular death, MI, unstable angina, or symptom-driven revascularization) over a median follow-up of 16 months. It was demonstrated that increasing noncalcified plaque volume on coronary CTA is independently associated with increased rates of recurrent events, and is superior to Agatston calcium scoring and traditional risk factors in this high-risk cohort.

Prognostic Comparison with Agatston Calcium Scoring

A noncontrast CT scan to calculate Agatston coronary artery calcium scores (CACS) and to assist in coronary CTA planning is often performed before coronary CTA. Because of the increase in radiation from this additional scan, some have questioned the routine performance of CACS at the time of CTA, due to its unclear prognostic value relative to the information obtained from coronary angiography.

Kwon and colleagues[46] assessed the comparative prognostic value of coronary CTA versus CACS and risk factors in 4388 patients clinically referred for coronary CTA at a single center. Patients were of a mean age of 60 years, 52% were men, 29% had low pretest probability of obstructive CAD, and the mean Agatston CACS was relatively low (76 units). After a mean follow-up of 838 days there were 105 MACE (only 2 among 2073 patients with no CAD). Similar to the aforementioned studies, event rates increased according to the presence and severity of obstructive and nonobstructive CAD. There was no significant incremental value of CACS beyond coronary CTA measures of CAD when assessing prognosis. The investigators questioned the further use of CAC scoring for purely prognostic reasons. In a study of both symptomatic and asymptomatic patients, Russo and colleagues[47] demonstrated similar findings. However, it must be noted that the performance of CACS at the time of coronary CTA may be done in select patients for reasons unrelated to prognostic considerations. For example, the identification of significant coronary calcification on the pre-CTA noncontrast scan may allow providers to appropriately adjust coronary CTA acquisition variables to optimize coronary CTA study quality.

Acute Chest Pain

While significant prognostic data exist for coronary CTA in stable, symptomatic patients, data extending these findings to patients presenting with acute cardiovascular symptoms is limited. Chest pain is a common complaint among patients presenting for emergency care, accounting for approximately 8 to 10 million visits at a cost of approximately $10 to $12 billion in the United States annually.[48–50] Here, the potential for coronary CTA to accurately and efficiently triage low- to intermediate-risk patients and to reduce costs relative to other noninvasive evaluation strategies is of great interest.[51–53] To this end, findings from the ROMI-CAT (Rule Out Myocardial Infarction Using Computer Assisted Tomography) trial provide the longest follow-up to date among patients undergoing coronary CTA as an initial diagnostic strategy in the emergency department (ED).[54] This single-center, prospective, blinded, observational analysis enrolled 368 patients presenting with acute chest pain, normal initial troponin levels, and no ischemic electrocardiographic findings, to undergo 64-slice coronary CTA before evaluation according to the usual standard of care. Both caregivers and patients were blinded to the results of coronary CTA, and patients were followed for the primary end point of combined MACE (cardiac death, nonfatal MI, or coronary revascularization). Reassuringly, a normal coronary CTA was associated with the complete absence of MACE at 2-year follow-up, similar to prior data.[55] Further, patients with nonobstructive CAD (<50%) and obstructive CAD (≥50% stenosis) had significantly increased MACE (4.6% and 30.3%, respectively) at 2-year follow-up (P<.0001), driven primarily by coronary revascularization (23 of 35 total events).

The CT-STAT (Coronary Computed Tomographic Angiography for Systematic Triage of Acute Chest Pain Patients to Treatment) trial provided the first multicenter, randomized analysis of coronary CTA in the ED setting.[53] Across 16 centers, low- to intermediate-risk patients (Thrombolysis in Myocardial Infarction risk score ≤4) presenting with acute chest pain were randomized to either early, at least 64-slice, coronary CTA (n = 361) or rest-stress myocardial perfusion imaging (MPI) (n = 338), and followed for the time to diagnosis (primary outcome), as well as costs of care (total billed ED charges) and safety, defined as combined MACE (cardiac death, acute coronary syndrome [ACS], or revascularization). At 6-month follow-up, patients with a normal index coronary CTA had no difference in their low rates of combined MACE when compared with a normal MPI (0.8% vs 0.4%; P = .29), demonstrating excellent short-term prognosis in these patients. Although patients undergoing coronary CTA relative to rest-stress MPI were shown to have 38% lower costs and a 54% reduction in their time to diagnosis, the investigators acknowledge several limitations to this study and existing data to include limited follow-up in a small sample size (not powered for safety outcomes), inherent limitations in cost estimation with lack of formal cost-effectiveness data, and the absence of other comparative strategies (eg, stress-only MPI, exercise stress echo, and treadmill testing alone). In this regard, future research is awaited (such as ROMICAT II)[56] to build on current understanding of the long-term prognosis and comparative effectiveness in the ED setting.

PROGNOSTIC VALUE OF CORONARY CTA IN UNIQUE POPULATIONS

Inconclusive Stress Tests

In a cohort of 529 low- to intermediate-risk patients with inconclusive functional stress testing, de Azevedo and colleagues[57] found a majority (69%) to demonstrate no significant CAD (≤50% stenosis) by coronary CTA. The presence of obstructive (≥50% stenosis) CAD and CAD burden as calculated by the modified Duke prognostic index were each independently shown to predict the primary composite outcome of all-cause mortality and nonfatal MIs over a mean 30-month follow-up period. Of interest, the pretest likelihood of obstructive CAD by Diamond-Forrester risk analysis was not significantly associated with an increase in adverse events (HR 1.31, 95% CI 0.86–2.00; P = .2), similar to findings in the ROMICAT trial.[54] Of importance is that the prognostic value of coronary CTA findings was superior to both clinical risk factors and Agatston CACS.

Prior Coronary Artery Bypass Graft

Coronary CTA is highly accurate for the assessment of coronary artery bypass graft (CABG) stenosis,[58] and its use for this purpose is endorsed by current Appropriate Use Criteria.[1] However, the assessment of native coronary arteries in patients with prior CABG may be less accurate compared with coronary CTA in patients without prior CABG, owing primarily to increased prevalence of dense coronary calcification.[59] Recently, Chow and colleagues[60] described the prognostic value of coronary CTA among 250 consecutively referred post-CABG patients undergoing retrospective electrocardiogram-gated 64-slice coronary CTA. Patients were followed for 20.8 months for the combined (MACE) end point of cardiac death and nonfatal MI. The investigators stratified patients by the number of unprotected coronary territories (UCTs), defined as: (1) ungrafted native coronary artery with 70% or more stenosis (≥50% stenosis if left main); (2) 70% or more stenosis distal to the graft insertion; or (3) 70% or more stenosis in the native artery and its graft. The investigators demonstrated that the absence of UCTs was associated with a significantly lower annualized rate of MACE (2.4%), compared with 1 (5.8%), 2 (11.1%), or 3 UCTs (21.7%), respectively (P<.001). Furthermore, the number of UCTs significantly improved the prediction of adverse events beyond clinical variables alone (area under the curve [AUC] 0.76 vs 0.61; P = .001), demonstrating for the first time the potential for coronary CTA to provide prognostic information in post-CABG patients.

PROGNOSTIC IMPLICATIONS OF PLAQUE MORPHOLOGY

Beyond the prognostic value of CAD severity and the type of calcification pattern (in patients with nonobstructive CAD), coronary CTA can identify additional characteristics in plaque morphology and composition that may provide important prognostic information. Of particular interest is the potential for coronary CTA to identify coronary lesions most prone to disruption and the resultant adverse coronary events. Based on pathology specimens and intracoronary imaging studies, the precursor lesion to plaque rupture or erosion is the thin cap fibrous atheroma (TCFA), which is typified by a large necrotic, macrophage-rich, lipid-rich core and an overlying thin (<65 μm) cap.[42,61] Although modern coronary CTA, with an isotropic spatial resolution of approximately 0.4 mm (400 μm), cannot image cap thickness, TCFA lesions typically have associated features that can be reliably visualized in high-quality coronary CTA data sets, and have been correlated to unstable coronary lesions on intravascular ultrasonography (IVUS) and optical coherence tomography (OCT).[62]

Several investigators have identified characteristics of culprit lesions imaged during an ACS, and have proposed that these may identify high-risk lesions when present in clinically stable patients. Specifically, studies have consistently demonstrated that culprit lesions in ACS are more likely than stable plaques to possess a higher plaque volume,[63,64] higher degree of positive remodeling,[64–67] lower-attenuation plaque,[64,67,68] less overall calcification,[63–65,67–70] a pattern of spotty calcification,[64,67] and a peripheral contrast rim (also termed ringlike enhancement).[64]

In an effort to prospectively validate these observations, Motoyama and colleagues[71] prospectively examining 1059 consecutive patients who underwent 64-slice coronary CTA for suspected or known CAD, measured the degree of positive remodeling (PR) and looked for the presence of low-attenuation plaque (LAP: <30 HU). Over a mean of 27 months, the presence of both PR and LAP was associated with a nearly 23-fold increased likelihood of the occurrence of ACS (HR 22.8, 95% CI 6.9–75.2; P<.001). In addition, coronary lesions that resulted in ACS had an increased remodeling index (1.27 vs 1.13; P = .003), total plaque volume (134.9 vs 57.8 mm^3; P<.001), and LAP volume (20.4 vs 1.1 mm^3; P<.001) (**Fig. 4**).

At present the clinical use of the aforementioned plaque characteristics is limited, due to the dependence of these measurements on very high-quality coronary CTA data sets, the need for

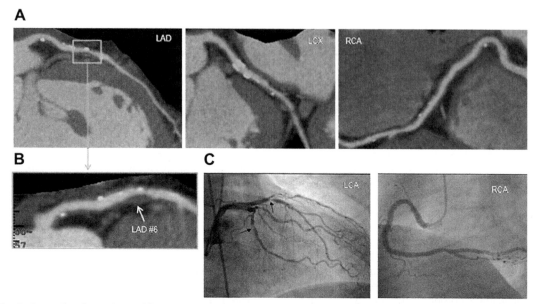

Fig. 4. Example of a patient with acute coronary syndrome 6 months after coronary CTA. (*A*) Curved multiplanar reformation images of left anterior descending artery (LAD), left circumflex artery (LCX), and right coronary artery (RCA). (*B*) Positive remodeling, low-attenuation plaque, and spotty calcification were detected in LAD #6 on coronary CTA. (*C*) Acute coronary syndrome occurred 6 months after coronary CTA. LAD #6 was determined as the culprit lesion, based on invasive angiography findings. LCA, left coronary artery. (*Reproduced from Motoyama S, Sarai M, Harigaya H, et al. Computed tomographic angiography characteristics of atherosclerotic plaques subsequently resulting in acute coronary syndrome. J Am Coll Cardiol 2009;54(1):52; with permission.*)

precise measurements with unclear interobserver reproducibility, and the lack of outcomes data that define the optimal treatment of patients with potentially high-risk nonobstructive plaque characteristics. It is also important that the measurement of intraplaque density can be significantly influenced by study noise as well as the density and proximity of contrast and calcium, due to volume averaging, thereby limiting this technique in many patients. Further studies are warranted to better standardize the measurements of potentially high-risk plaque morphology. Significant efforts are under way to develop semiautomated and automated tools for the quantification of plaque composition, degree of remodeling and, potentially, plaque composition.[62]

CORONARY CTA AND PROGNOSIS IN ASYMPTOMATIC PATIENTS?

Despite declining mortality rates, cardiovascular diseases remain the most common cause of death in the United States, with a substantial proportion of cardiac events occurring suddenly in previously asymptomatic patients, many of whom are considered to be at low to intermediate risk by standard global cardiovascular risk scores.[72,73] The performance of CACS using noncontrast CT scanning

has been shown to be superior to standard risk-score approaches,[41] including the measurement of highly sensitive C-reactive protein,[74,75] for the prediction of future cardiovascular risk. Hence, with the goal of refining risk prediction and guiding preventive treatments and despite a lack of data demonstrating improved outcomes with its use, CACS is now endorsed in clinical guidelines for use as a screening test in select populations.[76,77] Of interest is whether coronary CTA could add incremental prognostic information in asymptomatic screening patients, beyond CACS, a technology that quantifies only calcified atherosclerosis. A recent consideration that has arisen in this debate is the markedly reduced radiation exposure from modern coronary CTA that is comparable with effective radiation doses from multidetector CACS in many patients.[78] However, the use of coronary CTA as a screening test is not currently recommended[1,76,77] because of the relatively low prevalence of future adverse events associated with obstructive CAD in an asymptomatic population[79,80]; moreover, CACS is currently cheaper, logistically simpler, faster, free of iodinated contrast, and easier to interpret.

Studies evaluating the prognostic value of coronary CTA in asymptomatic patients are currently limited to single-center, retrospective analyses of select ethnicities with relatively short follow-up durations. In the largest analysis to date, Choi and colleagues[81] retrospectively identified 1000 asymptomatic, self-referred, predominantly middle-aged Korean adults (mean age 50 years) with low to intermediate 10-year FRS (mean 5.2%) who underwent 64-slice coronary CTA as part of a general health evaluation. In this lower-risk cohort the investigators found a relatively low percentage of patients with any coronary athero-sclerosis (22%), with 4% of patients having purely noncalcified plaque (4%), and a 5% prevalence of at least one significant ($\geq$50%) stenosis. After a relatively limited follow-up duration of 17 months, there were 15 cardiac events of which 14 were from revascularizations occurring early (<90 days) following coronary CTA. In a subse-quent analysis, the investigators noted that patients with any CAD had significantly higher rates of statin and aspirin use at 90 days and 18 months compared with patients without CAD or nonscreened matched controls.[80] However, significantly higher rates of additional cardiovas-cular testing were observed in patients who underwent coronary CTA relative to matched nonscreened patients with no difference in hard cardiovascular events at 18 months.

By contrast, Hadamitzky and colleagues[79] retro-spectively evaluated 451 asymptomatic patients referred for coronary CTA based on "elevated CAD risk" (not a true screening population). Conse-quently, relative to those studied by Choi and colleagues, these patients were older (mean age 59 years) with higher baseline FRS (mean 10.6%), and were found to have very high rates of non-obstructive (54%) and obstructive CAD (24% with $\geq$50% stenosis). On follow-up (median 27.5 months), there were 2 cases of unstable angina and 8 revascularizations among patients with obstructive CAD. Hence, excluding revasculariza-tions, rates of hard events were low. However, the investigators identified 19% of patients with purely noncalcified plaque who were not identified using CACS, and demonstrated that coronary CTA was superior to CACS in reclassifying patients from intermediate to low or high risk. Of interest, the combination of coronary CTA and FRS significantly improved the ability to predict cardiac events compared with FRS alone ($P = .001$), whereas the combined model of CACS and FRS relative to FRS alone demonstrated a less marked improve-ment ($P = .02$).

SUMMARY

In addition to its role as a highly accurate test for the diagnosis of CAD, coronary CTA provides robust prognostic information that is incremental to cardiovascular risk factors, CACS, and left ventricular ejection fraction. Patients without appreciable coronary atherosclerosis on coronary CTA have a very favorable prognosis for at least the following 3 years, and longer-term follow-up studies are ongoing. Conversely, mortality signifi-cantly increases with both increasing degree and extent of obstructive and nonobstructive CAD. Differences in plaque morphology and composition may further identify patients at higher risk for future cardiovascular events. Ongoing research involving large-scale registries (eg, CONFIRM) and multicenter randomized trials, to include RESCUE (Randomized Evaluation of Patients with Stable Angina Comparing Diagnostic Examinations) and PROMISE (Prospective Multi-center Imaging Study for Evaluation of Chest Pain),[82] may improve our understanding of the prognostic value of coronary CTA and down-stream management of these patients in compar-ison with other noninvasive tests for CAD, while active research in CT perfusion imaging[83] and CT fractional flow reserve[84] may add to the prognostic and diagnostic value of coronary CTA by mea-suring the hemodynamic significance of coronary lesions. Unfortunately, it has not been proved that modifications in medical therapy and patient lifestyle can mitigate the risk predicted by coro-nary CTA. Although the authors typically prescribe standard cardiovascular preventive treatments, such as statins, to patients with nonobstructive CAD on coronary CTA irrespective of cholesterol values and guideline recommendations, data sup-porting this common practice are lacking. To this end, randomized long-term clinical outcomes trials designed to prospectively evaluate preventive therapies that are differentially applied according to coronary CTA risk variables are needed.

REFERENCES

1. Taylor AJ, Cerqueira M, Hodgson JM, et al. ACCF/SCCT/ACR/AHA/ASE/ASNC/NASCI/SCAI/SCMR 2010 appropriate use criteria for cardiac computed tomography. A report of the American College of Cardiology Foundation Appropriate Use Criteria Task Force, the Society of Cardiovascular Computed Tomography, the American College of Radiology, the American Heart Association, the American Society of Echocardiography, the American Society of Nuclear Cardiology, the North American Society for Cardiovascular Imaging, the Society for Cardio-vascular Angiography and Interventions, and the Society for Cardiovascular Magnetic Resonance. J Am Coll Cardiol 2010;56(22):1864–94.
2. ACR-NASCI-SPR practice guideline for the per-formance and interpretation of cardiac computed

tomography (CT). Available at: http://www.acr.org/SecondaryMainMenuCategories/quality_safety/guidelines/dx/cardio/ct_cardiac.aspx. Accessed September 15, 2011.

3. Abbara S, Arbab-Zadeh A, Callister TQ, et al. SCCT guidelines for performance of coronary computed tomographic angiography: a report of the Society of Cardiovascular Computed Tomography Guidelines Committee. J Cardiovasc Comput Tomogr 2009; 3(3):190–204.

4. Halliburton SS, Abbara S, Chen MY, et al. SCCT guidelines on radiation dose and dose-optimization strategies in cardiovascular CT. J Cardiovasc Comput Tomogr 2011;5(4):198–224.

5. Raff GL, Abidov A, Achenbach S, et al. SCCT guidelines for the interpretation and reporting of coronary computed tomographic angiography. J Cardiovasc Comput Tomogr 2009;3(2):122–36.

6. Weigold WG, Abbara S, Achenbach S, et al. Standardized medical terminology for cardiac computed tomography: a report of the Society of Cardiovascular Computed Tomography. J Cardiovasc Comput Tomogr 2011;5(3):136–44.

7. Budoff MJ, Achenbach S, Berman DS, et al. Task force 13: training in advanced cardiovascular imaging (computed tomography) endorsed by the American Society of Nuclear Cardiology, Society of Atherosclerosis Imaging and Prevention, Society for Cardiovascular Angiography and Interventions, and Society of Cardiovascular Computed Tomography. J Am Coll Cardiol 2008;51(3):409–14.

8. Meijboom WB, Meijs MF, Schuijf JD, et al. Diagnostic accuracy of 64-slice computed tomography coronary angiography: a prospective, multicenter, multivendor study. J Am Coll Cardiol 2008;52(25): 2135–44.

9. Miller JM, Rochitte CE, Dewey M, et al. Diagnostic performance of coronary angiography by 64-row CT. N Engl J Med 2008;359(22):2324–36.

10. Budoff MJ, Dowe D, Jollis JG, et al. Diagnostic performance of 64-multidetector row coronary computed tomographic angiography for evaluation of coronary artery stenosis in individuals without known coronary artery disease: results from the prospective multicenter ACCURACY (Assessment by Coronary Computed Tomographic Angiography of Individuals Undergoing Invasive Coronary Angiography) trial. J Am Coll Cardiol 2008;52(21): 1724–32.

11. Schuetz GM, Zacharopoulou NM, Schlattmann P, et al. Meta-analysis: noninvasive coronary angiography using computed tomography versus magnetic resonance imaging. Ann Intern Med 2010;152(3): 167–77.

12. Cheezum MK, Hulten EA, Taylor AJ, et al. Cardiac CT angiography compared with myocardial perfusion stress testing on downstream resource utilization. J Cardiovasc Comput Tomogr 2011; 5(2):101–9.

13. Patel MR, Peterson ED, Dai D, et al. Low diagnostic yield of elective coronary angiography. N Engl J Med 2010;362(10):886–95.

14. Shaw LJ, Min JK, Hachamovitch R, et al. Cardiovascular imaging research at the crossroads. JACC Cardiovasc Imaging 2010;3(3):316–24.

15. Hulten EA, Carbonaro S, Petrillo SP, et al. Prognostic value of cardiac computed tomography angiography: a systematic review and meta-analysis. J Am Coll Cardiol 2011;57(10):1237–47.

16. Bamberg F, Sommer WH, Hoffmann V, et al. Meta-analysis and systematic review of the long-term predictive value of assessment of coronary atherosclerosis by contrast-enhanced coronary computed tomography angiography. J Am Coll Cardiol 2011; 57(24):2426–36.

17. Gopal A, Nasir K, Ahmadi N, et al. Cardiac computed tomographic angiography in an outpatient setting: an analysis of clinical outcomes over a 40-month period. J Cardiovasc Comput Tomogr 2009;3(2):90–5.

18. Ostrom MP, Gopal A, Ahmadi N, et al. Mortality incidence and the severity of coronary atherosclerosis assessed by computed tomography angiography. J Am Coll Cardiol 2008;52(16):1335–43.

19. Min JK, Shaw LJ, Devereux RB, et al. Prognostic value of multidetector coronary computed tomographic angiography for prediction of all-cause mortality. J Am Coll Cardiol 2007;50(12):1161–70.

20. Noda M, Takagi A, Kuwatsuru R, et al. Prognostic significance of multiple-detector computed tomography in conjunction with TIMI risk score for patients with non-ST elevation acute coronary syndrome. Heart Vessels 2008;23(3):161–6.

21. Pundziute G, Schuijf JD, Jukema JW, et al. Prognostic value of multislice computed tomography coronary angiography in patients with known or suspected coronary artery disease. J Am Coll Cardiol 2007;49(1):62–70.

22. Shaw LJ, Berman DS, Hendel RC, et al. Prognosis by coronary computed tomographic angiography; matched comparison with myocardial perfusion single-photon emission computed tomography. J Cardiovasc Comput Tomogr 2008;2(2):93–101.

23. Abidov A, Gallagher MJ, Chinnaiyan KM, et al. Clinical effectiveness of coronary computed tomographic angiography in the triage of patients to cardiac catheterization and revascularization after inconclusive stress testing: results of a 2-year prospective trial. J Nucl Cardiol 2009;16(5):701–13.

24. Aldrovandi A, Maffei E, Palumbo A, et al. Prognostic value of computed tomography coronary angiography in patients with suspected coronary artery disease: a 24-month follow-up study. Eur Radiol 2009;19(7):1653–60.

25. Barros AJ, Blazquez MA, Leta R, et al. Noninvasive coronary angiography using multidetector computed tomography in patients with suspected coronary artery disease and a non-diagnostic exercise treadmill test result. Med Clin (Barc) 2009;132(17): 661–4.

26. Cademartiri F, Seitun S, Romano M, et al. Prognostic value of 64-slice coronary angiography in diabetes mellitus patients with known or suspected coronary artery disease compared with a nondiabetic population. Radiol Med 2008;113(5):627–43.

27. Carrigan TP, Nair D, Schoenhagen P, et al. Prognostic utility of 64-slice computed tomography in patients with suspected but no documented coronary artery disease. Eur Heart J 2009;30(3):362–71.

28. Chow BJ, Wells GA, Chen L, et al. Prognostic value of 64-slice cardiac computed tomography severity of coronary artery disease, coronary atherosclerosis, and left ventricular ejection fraction. J Am Coll Cardiol 2010;55(10):1017–28.

29. Danciu SC, Herrera CJ, Stecy PJ, et al. Usefulness of multislice computed tomographic coronary angiography to identify patients with abnormal myocardial perfusion stress in whom diagnostic catheterization may be safely avoided. Am J Cardiol 2007;100(11):1605–8.

30. Fazel P, Peterman MA, Schussler JM. Three-year outcomes and cost analysis in patients receiving 64-slice computed tomographic coronary angiography for chest pain. Am J Cardiol 2009;104(4): 498–500.

31. Gaeperli O, Valenta I, Schepis T, et al. Coronary 64-slice CT angiography predicts outcome in patients with known or suspected coronary artery disease. Eur Radiol 2008;18(6):1162–73.

32. Hay CS, Morse RJ, Morgan-Hughes GJ, et al. Prognostic value of coronary multidetector CT angiography in patients with an intermediate probability of significant coronary heart disease. Br J Radiol 2010;83(988):327–30.

33. Rubinshtein R, Halon DA, Gaspar T, et al. Usefulness of 64-slice cardiac computed tomographic angiography for diagnosing acute coronary syndromes and predicting clinical outcome in emergency department patients with chest pain of uncertain origin. Circulation 2007;115(13):1762–8.

34. van Werkhoven JM, Schuijf JD, Gaemperli O, et al. Prognostic value of multislice computed tomography and gated single-photon emission computed tomography in patients with suspected coronary artery disease. J Am Coll Cardiol 2009;53(7): 623–32.

35. Wilson PW, D'Agostino RB, Levy D, et al. Prediction of coronary heart disease using risk factor categories. Circulation 1998;97(18):1837–47.

36. Metz LD, Beattie M, Hom R, et al. The prognostic value of normal exercise myocardial perfusion imaging and exercise echocardiography: a meta-analysis. J Am Coll Cardiol 2007;49(2):227–37.

37. Expert Panel on Detection, Evaluation, and Treatment of High Blood Cholesterol in Adults. Executive Summary of The Third Report of The National Cholesterol Education Program (NCEP) Expert Panel on Detection, Evaluation, and Treatment of High Blood Cholesterol in Adults (Adult Treatment Panel III). JAMA 2001;285(19):2486–97.

38. Min JK, Dunning A, Lin FY, et al. Age- and sex-related differences in all-cause mortality risk based on coronary computed tomography angiography findings. Results from the international multicenter CONFIRM (Coronary CT Angiography Evaluation for Clinical Outcomes: An International Multicenter Registry) of 23,854 patients without known coronary artery disease. J Am Coll Cardiol 2011; 58(8):849–60.

39. Lin F, Shaw LJ, Berman DS, et al. Multidetector computed tomography coronary artery plaque predictors of stress-induced myocardial ischemia by SPECT. Atherosclerosis 2008;197(2):700–9.

40. Chow BJ, Small G, Yam Y, et al. The incremental prognostic value of cardiac CT in CAD using CONFIRM (COroNary computed tomography angiography evaluation For clinical outcomes: an InteRnational Multicenter registry). Circ Cardiovasc Imaging 2011;4(5):463–72.

41. Polonsky TS, McClelland RL, Jorgensen NW, et al. Coronary artery calcium score and risk classification for coronary heart disease prediction. JAMA 2010; 303(16):1610–6.

42. Stone GW, Maehara A, Lansky AJ, et al. A prospective natural-history study of coronary atherosclerosis. N Engl J Med 2011;364(3):226–35.

43. Lin FY, Shaw LJ, Dunning AM, et al. Mortality risk in symptomatic patients with nonobstructive coronary artery disease: a prospective 2-center study of 2,583 patients undergoing 64-detector row coronary computed tomographic angiography. J Am Coll Cardiol 2011;58(5):510–9.

44. Ahmadi N, Nabavi V, Hajsadeghi F, et al. Mortality incidence of patients with non-obstructive coronary artery disease diagnosed by computed tomography angiography. Am J Cardiol 2011;107(1):10–6.

45. Kristensen TS, Kofoed KF, Kuhl JT, et al. Prognostic implications of nonobstructive coronary plaques in patients with non-ST-segment elevation myocardial infarction: a multidetector computed tomography study. J Am Coll Cardiol 2011;58(5):502–9.

46. Kwon SW, Kim YJ, Shim J, et al. Coronary artery calcium scoring does not add prognostic value to standard 64-section CT angiography protocol in low-risk patients suspected of having coronary artery disease. Radiology 2011;259(1):92–9.

47. Russo V, Zavalloni A, Bacchi Reggiani ML, et al. Incremental prognostic value of coronary CT

angiography in patients with suspected coronary artery disease. Circ Cardiovasc Imaging 2010;3(4): 351–9.

48. Owens PL, Barrett ML, Gibson TB, et al. Emergency department care in the United States: a profile of national data sources. Ann Emerg Med 2010;56(2): 150–65.

49. Tatum JL, Jesse RL, Kontos MC, et al. Comprehensive strategy for the evaluation and triage of the chest pain patient. Ann Emerg Med 1997;29(1):116–25.

50. Heller GV, Stowers SA, Hendel RC, et al. Clinical value of acute rest technetium-99m tetrofosmin tomographic myocardial perfusion imaging in patients with acute chest pain and nondiagnostic electrocardiograms. J Am Coll Cardiol 1998;31(5):1011–7.

51. Goldstein JA, Gallagher MJ, O'Neill WW, et al. A randomized controlled trial of multi-slice coronary computed tomography for evaluation of acute chest pain. J Am Coll Cardiol 2007;49(8):863–71.

52. Khare RK, Courtney DM, Powell ES, et al. Sixty-four-slice computed tomography of the coronary arteries: cost-effectiveness analysis of patients presenting to the emergency department with low-risk chest pain. Acad Emerg Med 2008;15(7):623–32.

53. Goldstein JA, Chinnaiyan KM, Abidov A, et al. The CT-STAT (Coronary Computed Tomographic Angiography for Systematic Triage of Acute Chest Pain Patients to Treatment) trial. J Am Coll Cardiol 2011; 58(14):1414–22.

54. Schlett CL, Banerji D, Siegel E, et al. Prognostic value of CT angiography for major adverse cardiac events in patients with acute chest pain from the emergency department: 2-year outcomes of the ROMICAT trial. JACC Cardiovasc Imaging 2011;4(5):481–91.

55. Hollander JE, Chang AM, Shofer FS, et al. One-year outcomes following coronary computerized tomographic angiography for evaluation of emergency department patients with potential acute coronary syndrome. Acad Emerg Med 2009;16(8):693–8.

56. ClinicalTrials.gov. Multicenter Study to Rule Out Myocardial Infarction by Cardiac Computed Tomography (ROMICAT-II). Available at: http://www. clinicaltrials.gov/ct2/show/NCT01084239. Accessed September 9, 2011.

57. de Azevedo CF, Hadlich MS, Bezerra SG, et al. Prognostic value of CT angiography in patients with inconclusive functional stress tests. JACC Cardiovasc Imaging 2011;4(7):740–51.

58. Nieman K, Pattynama PM, Rensing BJ, et al. Evaluation of patients after coronary artery bypass surgery: CT angiographic assessment of grafts and coronary arteries. Radiology 2003;229(3): 749–56.

59. Romagnoli A, Patrei A, Mancini A, et al. Diagnostic accuracy of 64-slice CT in evaluating coronary artery bypass grafts and of the native coronary arteries. Radiol Med 2010;115(8):1167–78.

60. Chow BJ, Ahmed O, Small G, et al. Prognostic value of CT angiography in coronary bypass patients. JACC Cardiovasc Imaging 2011;4(5):496–502.

61. Virmani R, Burke AP, Farb A, et al. Pathology of the vulnerable plaque. J Am Coll Cardiol 2006; 47(Suppl 8):C13–8.

62. Voros S, Rinehart S, Qian Z, et al. Coronary atherosclerosis imaging by coronary CT angiography: current status, correlation with intravascular interrogation and meta-analysis. JACC Cardiovasc Imaging 2011; 4(5):537–48.

63. Hammer-Hansen S, Kofoed KF, Kelbaek H, et al. Volumetric evaluation of coronary plaque in patients presenting with acute myocardial infarction or stable angina pectoris-a multislice computerized tomography study. Am Heart J 2009;157(3):481–7.

64. Pflederer T, Marwan M, Schepis T, et al. Characterization of culprit lesions in acute coronary syndromes using coronary dual-source CT angiography. Atherosclerosis 2010;211(2):437–44.

65. Hoffmann U, Moselewski F, Nieman K, et al. Noninvasive assessment of plaque morphology and composition in culprit and stable lesions in acute coronary syndrome and stable lesions in stable angina by multidetector computed tomography. J Am Coll Cardiol 2006;47(8):1655–62.

66. Imazeki T, Sato Y, Inoue F, et al. Evaluation of coronary artery remodeling in patients with acute coronary syndrome and stable angina by multislice computed tomography. Circ J 2004;68(11):1045–50.

67. Motoyama S, Kondo T, Sarai M, et al. Multislice computed tomographic characteristics of coronary lesions in acute coronary syndromes. J Am Coll Cardiol 2007;50(4):319–26.

68. Schuijf JD, Beck T, Burgstahler C, et al. Differences in plaque composition and distribution in stable coronary artery disease versus acute coronary syndromes; non-invasive evaluation with multi-slice computed tomography. Acute Card Care 2007; 9(1):48–53.

69. Henneman MM, Schuijf JD, Pundziute G, et al. Noninvasive evaluation with multislice computed tomography in suspected acute coronary syndrome: plaque morphology on multislice computed tomography versus coronary calcium score. J Am Coll Cardiol 2008;52(3):216–22.

70. Pundziute G, Schuijf JD, Jukema JW, et al. Evaluation of plaque characteristics in acute coronary syndromes: non-invasive assessment with multi-slice computed tomography and invasive evaluation with intravascular ultrasound radiofrequency data analysis. Eur Heart J 2008;29(19):2373–81.

71. Motoyama S, Sarai M, Harigaya H, et al. Computed tomographic angiography characteristics of atherosclerotic plaques subsequently resulting in acute coronary syndrome. J Am Coll Cardiol 2009;54(1): 49–57.

72. Lloyd-Jones D, Adams RJ, Brown TM, et al. Heart disease and stroke statistics—2010 update: a report from the American Heart Association. Circulation 2010;121(7):e46–215.

73. Murabito JM, Evans JC, Larson MG, et al. Prognosis after the onset of coronary heart disease. An investigation of differences in outcome between the sexes according to initial coronary disease presentation. Circulation 1993;88(6):2548–55.

74. Arad Y, Goodman KJ, Roth M, et al. Coronary calcification, coronary disease risk factors, C-reactive protein, and atherosclerotic cardiovascular disease events: the St. Francis Heart Study. J Am Coll Cardiol 2005;46(1):158–65.

75. Blaha MJ, Budoff MJ, DeFilippis AP, et al. Associations between C-reactive protein, coronary artery calcium, and cardiovascular events: implications for the JUPITER population from MESA, a population-based cohort study. Lancet 2011;378(9792):684–92.

76. Greenland P, Alpert JS, Beller GA, et al. 2010 ACCF/AHA guideline for assessment of cardiovascular risk in asymptomatic adults: a report of the American College of Cardiology Foundation/American Heart Association Task Force on Practice Guidelines. J Am Coll Cardiol 2010;56(25):e50–103.

77. Perrone-Filardi P, Achenbach S, Mohlenkamp S, et al. Cardiac computed tomography and myocardial perfusion scintigraphy for risk stratification in asymptomatic individuals without known cardiovascular disease: a position statement of the Working Group on Nuclear Cardiology and Cardiac CT of the European Society of Cardiology. Eur Heart J 2011; 32(16):1986–93.

78. Achenbach S, Goroll T, Seltmann M, et al. Detection of coronary artery stenoses by low-dose, prospectively ECG-triggered, high-pitch spiral coronary CT angiography. JACC Cardiovasc Imaging 2011;4(4): 328–37.

79. Hadamitzky M, Meyer T, Hein F, et al. Prognostic value of coronary computed tomographic angiography in asymptomatic patients. Am J Cardiol 2010;105(12):1746–51.

80. McEvoy JW, Blaha MJ, Nasir K, et al. Impact of coronary computed tomographic angiography results on patient and physician behavior in a low-risk population. Arch Intern Med 2011;171(14): 1260–8.

81. Choi EK, Choi SI, Rivera JJ, et al. Coronary computed tomography angiography as a screening tool for the detection of occult coronary artery disease in asymptomatic individuals. J Am Coll Cardiol 2008;52(5):357–65.

82. ClinicalTrials.gov. Prospective multicenter imaging study for evaluation of chest pain (PROMISE). Available at: http://clinicaltrials.gov/ct2/show/NCT01174550. Accessed September 9, 2011.

83. Bamberg F, Becker A, Schwarz F, et al. Detection of hemodynamically significant coronary artery stenosis: incremental diagnostic value of dynamic CT-based myocardial perfusion imaging. Radiology 2011;260(3):689–98.

84. Min JK, Berman DS, Budoff MJ, et al. Rationale and design of the DeFACTO (Determination of Fractional Flow Reserve by Anatomic Computed Tomographic AngiOgraphy) study. J Cardiovasc Comput Tomogr 2011;5(5):301–9.

Subtraction Coronary CT Angiography for Calcified Lesions

Kunihiro Yoshioka, MD, PhD[a],*, Ryoichi Tanaka, MD, PhD[a],
Kenta Muranaka, RT[b]

KEYWORDS

- Coronary artery • Computed tomography • Angiography
- Subtraction

Several studies have demonstrated that assessment of the coronary arteries using 64-row computed tomography (CT) provides high diagnostic accuracy in the depiction of stenotic lesions.[1–9] CT coronary angiography is now widely accepted as a noninvasive method for assessing the coronary arteries in patients with ischemic heart disease. On the other hand, the results of these studies have also shown that CT coronary angiography techniques suffer from several limitations and problems.[10] One of the most serious problems is that the presence of severe calcification in the coronary arteries reduces diagnostic accuracy, and it may even be impossible to assess some coronary segments if extremely severe calcification is present.

New higher-row CT scanners, have been introduced as the next generation after 64-row scanners. For instance, 320-row CT scanners incorporate an extremely wide detector composed of 320 rows of 0.5-mm detector elements, to permit a range of 16 cm in the z-axis direction to be scanned in a single rotation. This means that the entire heart can be scanned in a single rotation without moving the patient table. Specifically, 320-row CT permits data for the entire heart to be acquired by a simple snapshot (sequential) scan in a single rotation, whereas 64-row CT requires a helical scan (which involves continuous table movement and tube rotation) to acquire data over the same range. Consequently, the image data obtained for the heart using 320-row CT have the advantage of uniform temporal phase (cardiac phase) in all parts of the image. In addition, 320-row CT uses the half reconstruction technique as the image reconstruction method, which is much simpler than the complex techniques such as the multisegmental (multisector) reconstruction method used in helical CT systems, in which a single slice is generated from data acquired in multiple cardiac phases.

We considered that these features of the 320-row CT scanner might be useful in overcoming the problems related to severe calcification in the coronary arteries. Specifically, we attempted to eliminate calcification by using a subtraction method in which noncontrast CT (precontrast CT) image data are subtracted from contrast-enhanced CT (postcontrast CT) image data. The ability to perform such subtraction examinations was anticipated from the earliest stages in the development of 320-row CT, and the usefulness of subtraction in the central nervous system has been reported.[11,12] However, it has generally been believed that the subtraction method would be difficult to apply to the cardiovascular system because of cardiac motion.[13] Nevertheless, we expected that the positional shift between 2 scans could be minimized in

This work was supported by a Grant-in-Aid for Scientific Research (C) from the Ministry of Education, Culture, Sports, Science and Technology of Japan (grant 21591576).

The authors have nothing to disclose.

[a] Division of Cardiovascular Radiology, Department of Radiology, Iwate Medical University Hospital, 19-1 Uchimaru, Morioka 020-8505, Japan

[b] Center for Radiological Science, Iwate Medical University Hospital, 19-1 Uchimaru, Morioka 020-8505, Japan

* Corresponding author.

E-mail address: kyoshi@iwate-med.ac.jp

doi:10.1016/j.ccl.2011.10.004

320-row CT because image data in the same temporal phase can be obtained in a single rotation by the simple sequential scan method and half reconstruction technique. Moreover, even if positional shift was to occur, we considered that it would be possible to compensate for reasonably small amounts of positional shift by using suitable image postprocessing techniques.

This article describes the current status, limitations, and future prospects of subtraction coronary CT angiography and also presents some clinical cases.

CT IMAGING METHODS

The CT scanner used in this study was a 320-row CT system (Aquilion ONE, Toshiba Medical Systems, Otawara, Japan). Data over a range of up to 16 cm in the z-axis direction were acquired to cover the entire heart by performing a snapshot scan with a slice thickness of 0.5 mm and a gantry rotation speed of 350 milliseconds without moving the patient couch. Although examination of the coronary arteries usually requires electrocardiography (ECG)-gated scanning, Prospective CTA scan mode (Toshiba Medical Systems, Otawara, Japan) was used to image the coronary arteries.

The Prospective CTA method is a scanning method in which x-rays are generated only in a preset cardiac phase in accordance with ECG-gating signals. This is the most commonly used method for imaging the coronary arteries with 320-row CT.[14–16] The scanning is performed during a diastolic phase in which cardiac motion is small. With the R-R interval on the ECG tracing corresponding to the entire cardiac cycle (100%), a time point at about 65% to 85% of the cardiac cycle (which is during the diastolic phase) is selected usually. We set the system so that image data are acquired in the cardiac phases from 70% to 80%, corresponding to 10% of the cardiac cycle. To use the Prospective CTA method, the patient's heart rate must be 65 beats per minute or less. Therefore, patients in whom control of the heart rate is required are given an oral β-blocker (metoprolol, 20 mg) therapy 1 to 2 hours before the examination.

The same method was also used for calcium scoring, but in the calcium scoring method used with our CT scanner, the cardiac phase is set to 75%. The coronary artery images were acquired with a tube voltage of 120 kV and a tube current of 300 to 580 mA for the Prospective CTA method. For calcium scoring, the tube voltage was 120 kV and the tube current was 300 mA.

High-osmolarity iodine contrast medium (370 mg iodine/mL; iopamidol 370, Bayer AG, Germany)

was injected via a right antecubital vein at a rate of body weight × 0.07 mL/s over a period of 7 to 10 seconds. The total amount injected was therefore body weight × 0.49 to 0.7 mL. The injection of contrast medium was immediately followed by normal saline solution flush of 35 mL injected at the same rate. A dual-cylinder–type power injector (Dual Shot GX, Nemoto Kyorindo, Tokyo, Japan) was used for injection.

The optimal scan start timing was determined using the bolus-tracking method or the test-injection method. In the bolus-tracking method, a region of interest (ROI) was set in the ascending aorta, and scanning was started when the CT number in the ROI reached 150 HU. In the test-injection method, the injection rate was determined as described earlier, with injection over 3 seconds. An ROI was set in the ascending aorta, and a time-density curve was generated to identify the time to peak density of the contrast medium.

IMAGE ACQUISITION METHODS USED IN SUBTRACTION CORONARY CT

In subtraction coronary CT examinations performed at our institution, 2 acquisition protocols are used to obtain the precontrast CT image data.

Single Breath-Hold Method

During a single breath-hold of 20 to 40 seconds, scanning is performed twice to acquire both precontrast CT image data and postcontrast CT image data using the Prospective CTA method. The optimal scan start timing is determined using the test-injection method. The main advantage of this method is that misregistration artifacts due to differences in the breath-holding position are minimized. The main disadvantage is that the radiation dose is increased because of the additional dose for the precontrast CT scan.

Two Breath-Hold Method

This is a method in which the image data acquired for calcium scoring are used as the precontrast CT image data. Calcium scoring and postcontrast CT are performed separately. This means that patients must hold their breath twice, and we therefore refer to this method as the 2 breath-hold method. In this method, patients first undergo a calcium scoring examination. After scanning is completed, the operator waits for the patient to return to normal respiration at rest and prepares the CT system for calcium score measurement and postcontrast CT scanning. After several minutes, the postcontrast CT image data are acquired using the bolus-tracking method. The main advantage of this method is that it can be performed by following exactly the same procedures as for conventional CT coronary angiography. The main disadvantage is that there is a high likelihood of misregistration artifacts because the 2 breath-holding positions do not match exactly. If misregistration artifacts are severe, subtraction may be impossible.

At our institution, a calcium scoring examination is performed for all patients who undergo CT coronary angiography. The 2 breath-hold method allows us to perform subtraction CT coronary angiography without any additional radiation exposure for the entire examination, compared with conventional CT coronary angiography performed at our institution.

In general, we prefer to use the single breath-hold method, in which there is a low likelihood of misregistration artifacts. The 2 breath-hold method is selected only if the single breath-hold method is judged to be unsuitable because the breath holding for the required period is impossible or because the radiation dose must be minimized.

SUBTRACTION METHOD

Using a function provided in the CT system, subtraction images are obtained by subtracting precontrast CT data from postcontrast CT data. Specifically, volume datasets of all parts of the images obtained by precontrast CT and postcontrast CT are used to create the subtraction image by subtracting the CT value of each pixel in the precontrast CT image from the CT value of the corresponding pixel in the postcontrast CT image.

If misregistration artifacts due to positional shift are observed, they are corrected manually based on visual assessment using the Volume Position Matching function (Toshiba Medical Systems, Otawara, Japan) that is also provided in the CT

system. This is a manual method for correcting positional shift by adjusting the positions of the images in 3 dimensions, similar to the pixel-shift function in digital subtraction angiography.[17] This technique has been used in 64-row CT systems to perform subtraction CT angiography in the arteries of the central nervous system as well as peripheral arteries.

IMAGE ANALYSIS

The volume dataset obtained using the subtraction method is transferred to a workstation (Zio M900, Ziosoft, Tokyo, Japan) for image analysis. At this time, the postcontrast CT volume dataset is also sent to the same workstation.

Image analysis is performed for the postcontrast CT volume dataset. From the postcontrast CT volume dataset, we generate a volume-rendered image, an angiographic view[18] (maximum intensity projection image), a curved planar reformation (CPR) image, and a cross-sectional image, all of which are generated in routine coronary CT examinations performed at our institution.

From the volume dataset obtained using the subtraction method, we generate a CPR image of the region in which severe calcification was observed in postcontrast CT. This CPR image is created at a position as close as possible to that of the postcontrast CT scan (**Fig. 1**).

When generating the subtraction image, misregistration artifacts must be corrected manually using the Volume Position Matching function, in which a long processing time is needed to create even a single CPR image. For example, it takes approximately 1 hour to create a CPR image of a single artery or segment with severe calcification. The creation of cross-sectional images takes even longer because such images require the

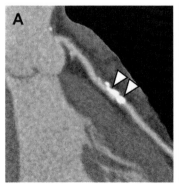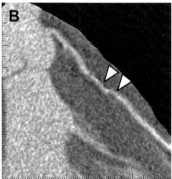

Fig. 1. Demonstration of the coronary arteries by postcontrast CT and subtraction coronary CT. (*A*) Postcontrast CT. A CPR image of the left anterior descending branch shows a dense calcification (*arrowheads*). (*B*) Subtraction coronary CT. The CPR image was created at a position as close as possible to that of the postcontrast CT scan. The calcification is eliminated (*arrowheads*).

correction of more complicated and finer misregistration artifacts than CPR images. It is therefore not practical to create cross-sectional images in routine examinations, and such images are created only when they are judged to be essential for assessing a specific lesion (**Fig. 2**).

USEFULNESS OF THE CORONARY CALCIUM SCORE IN DECIDING WHETHER CONVENTIONAL CORONARY CT SHOULD BE PERFORMED

At present, there is no consensus regarding the highest calcium score at which conventional coronary CT can be performed with an acceptable level of diagnostic accuracy.[10] However, one multicenter study, called the ACCURACY (Assessment by Coronary Computed Tomographic Angiography of Individuals Undergoing Invasive Coronary Angiography) study, using 64-row CT has reported that the specificity is significantly reduced when the calcium score is higher than 400.[8] In another international multicenter study using 64-row CT, the CorE 64 (Coronary Artery Evaluation Using 64-Row Multidetector Computed Tomography Angiography) study, patients with calcium scores higher than 600 were excluded from the study group.[7] Furthermore, the guidelines published in 2009 by the Society of Cardiovascular Computed Tomography suggest that several hospitals do not proceed to coronary CT if the calcium score

is higher than 600 to 1000.[19] The appropriate use criteria announced jointly by many societies in 2010 specify a threshold level, with a calcium score of 400 or less considered appropriate and a calcium score of more than 400 considered uncertain.[20]

Based on the reports mentioned earlier, we have tentatively decided that, at our institution, patients with a calcium score of 600 or more should be classified as clinical cases with severe calcification in whom conventional coronary CT would be difficult and that such patients should be examined using subtraction coronary CT instead.

A CASE REPORT

An 83-year-old woman who was receiving medical treatment for diabetes and hypertension presented with suspected effort angina pectoris. A stress ECG test was recommended for suspected angina pectoris, but the test could not be completed because the patient had lumbar spinal canal stenosis, and assessment was impossible. Coronary CT was therefore performed.

Calcium scoring was performed first, and the patient was found to have a high calcium score of 1315.32 (**Fig. 3**A). Because the calcium score was greater than 600, it was judged that subtraction coronary CT was indicated. In addition, because the patient was able to hold her breath for approximately 40 seconds, subtraction coronary CT using

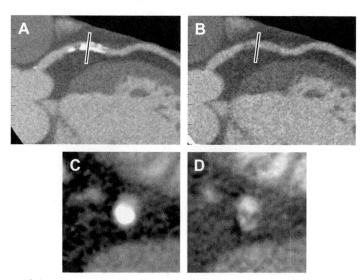

Fig. 2. Demonstration of the coronary arteries by postcontrast CT and subtraction coronary CT. (*A*) Postcontrast CT. A CPR image of the left anterior descending branch shows some calcifications. (*B*) Subtraction coronary CT. A CPR image at the same position as in (*A*). The calcifications are eliminated. (*C*) Postcontrast CT. A cross-sectional image of the left anterior descending branch at the line indicated in (*A*) shows a nodular calcification. (*D*) Subtraction coronary CT. A cross-sectional image at the line indicated in (*B*). The calcification is eliminated. For cross-sectional images in subtraction CT coronary angiography, there is a high likelihood of misregistration artifacts. Image processing therefore often takes a long time.

A

Calcium Score

Region	# Lesion	Agatston
RCA	4	440.58
LM	2	213.35
LAD	4	609.46
LCx	2	51.92
Aorta	0	0.00
Other	0	0.00
Total*	12	1315.32

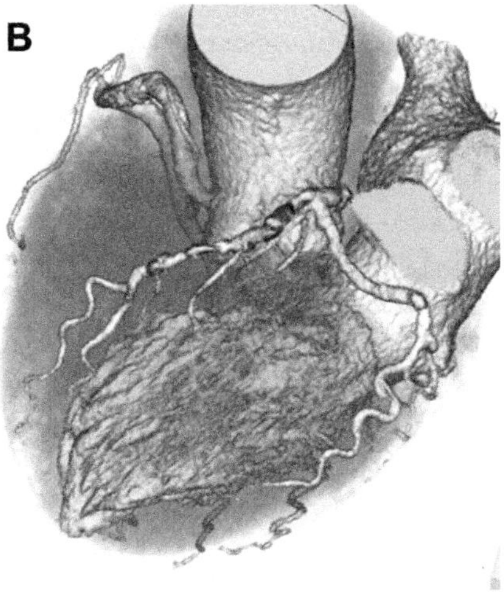

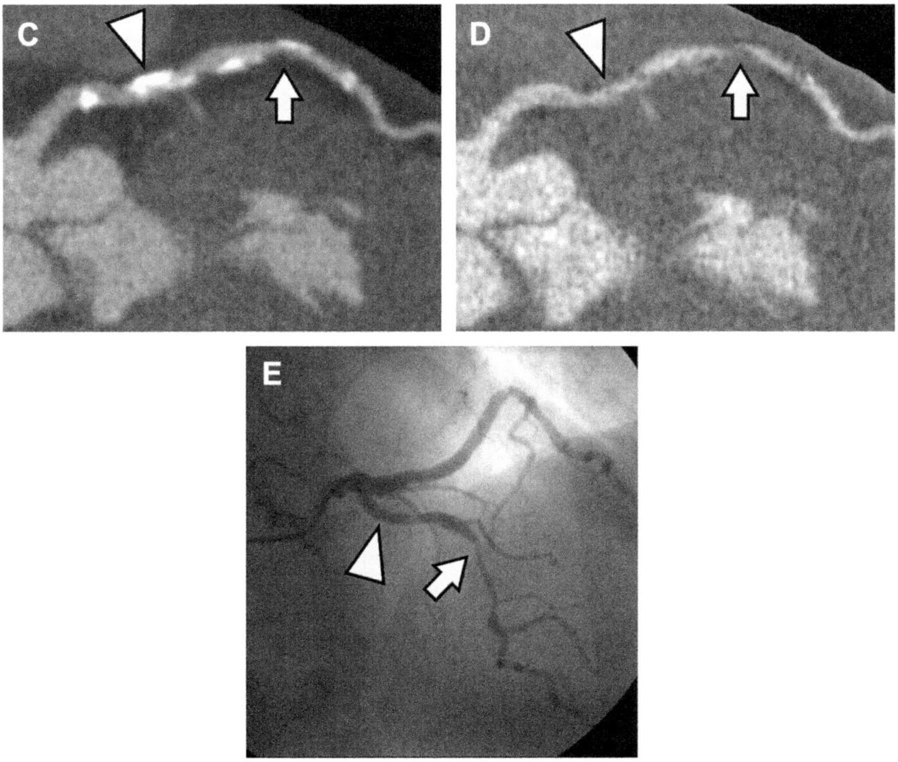

Fig. 3. An 83-year-old woman with suspected effort angina pectoris. (A) Calcium score. The patient's total calcium score was 1315.32. LAD, left anterior descending; LCx, left circumflex; LM, left main; RCA, right coronary artery. (B) A volume-rendered image created from the postcontrast CT volume dataset. Severe calcifications are observed in the proximal segments of the LAD branch. (C) A CPR image of the LAD generated from the postcontrast CT volume dataset. A severe calcification that makes it difficult to assess the lumen is observed in the proximal segment (arrowhead). A severe stenotic lesion with mild calcification is seen in a more distal segment (arrow). (D) A CPR image of the LAD generated from the subtraction coronary CT data, adjusted to show the same position as in (C). The severe calcification seen in the proximal segment is eliminated, making it possible to observe the lumen. No severe stenosis is seen (arrowhead). The mild calcification in the distal segment is also eliminated (arrow). (E) Invasive coronary angiography. No severe stenosis is observed in the region in which severe calcification is seen in CT images (arrowhead). A severe stenosis is observed in the distal segment (arrow).

the single breath-hold method was selected. **Fig. 3**B shows a volume-rendered image generated from the postcontrast CT volume dataset, and **Fig. 3**C shows a CPR image of the left anterior descending branch. The CPR image shows several severe nodular calcifications in this branch that make it impossible to assess a part of the lumen (arrowhead in **Fig. 3**C). These calcifications are eliminated in the subtraction coronary CT image (see **Fig. 3**D), and the postcontrast CT image clearly depicts even the part of the lumen that was difficult to assess because of calcification, making it possible to rule out the presence of a significant stenotic lesion (arrowhead in **Fig. 3**D). The patient subsequently underwent invasive coronary angiography, which also confirmed that no significant stenosis was present in the region where severe calcification was seen (arrowhead in **Fig. 3**E). In addition, a severe stenotic lesion with mild calcification was observed in a segment of the left anterior descending branch distal to this calcified lesion (arrows in **Fig. 3**C–E).

PRELIMINARY RESULTS FOR SUBTRACTION CORONARY CT

At an early stage of our study, we evaluated the image quality of subtraction coronary CT images in terms of the severity of misregistration artifacts.[21] Specifically, the following 4-grade scale was used for evaluation: score 4, no misregistration artifacts; score 3, minor misregistration artifacts; score 2, moderate misregistration artifacts but not so severe as to make diagnosis impossible; and score 1, severe misregistration artifacts making diagnosis impossible. The subjects were 10 patients with calcium scores of 600 or more. A total of 61 segments that contained severe calcification were evaluated. The scan method used was the 2 breath-hold method. This method was used because this evaluation was conducted during the early period of our research into subtraction coronary CT and only the 2 breath-hold method with a low radiation dose was used at that time.

The results showed that the average score was 2.4, with 6 segments (9.8%) showing a score of 1. We concluded that subtraction coronary CT, given its level of technological development at that time, was not suitable for use in the clinical setting and that further reduction in misregistration artifacts was required. We therefore decided to aggressively introduce the single breath-hold method, in which there is a low likelihood of misregistration artifacts, although the radiation dose is increased. Further evaluation of image quality in terms of misregistration artifacts in the single breath-hold method is currently being conducted.

USEFULNESS OF SUBTRACTION CORONARY CT FOR THE ASSESSMENT OF CORONARY ARTERY STENTS

It is possible to use subtraction coronary CT to assess not only calcified lesions but also coronary artery stents. The scan method, contrast enhancement method, and image processing method for the assessment of stents are the same as those for the assessment of calcified lesions.

Generally, it is considered that coronary CT is suitable for the evaluation of coronary artery stents with a diameter of 3 mm or more, whereas evaluation is difficult for stents with a diameter of less than 3 mm.[10] It is therefore expected that subtraction coronary CT should be able to depict the lumen of coronary artery stents with a diameter less than 3 mm (**Fig. 4**). Subtraction coronary CT is also expected to be useful for examining cases

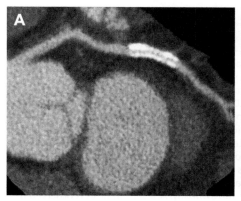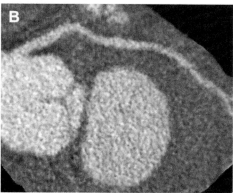

Fig. 4. Evaluation of a coronary artery stent by subtraction coronary CT. Patient with a stent 2.5 mm in diameter (S660, Johnson & Johnson Interventional Systems, New Brunswick, NJ, USA) placed in the left anterior descending branch (LAD). (*A*) Postcontrast CT. A CPR image of the LAD shows the stent. (*B*) Subtraction coronary CT. A CPR image created at the same position as in (*A*). The stent is completely eliminated.

in which evaluation of the lumen is difficult, such as when a stent is placed in a stenotic lesion with severe calcification or when another stent is placed over an existing stent. **Fig. 5** shows a clinical case in which a thin stent measuring 2.5 mm in diameter was placed in a stenotic lesion with severe calcification.

In our research to date, we have been selecting patients with severe calcification in the coronary arteries as the primary candidates for subtraction coronary CT, and we therefore have limited experience in the evaluation of coronary artery stents using this method. Consequently, we do not have much data demonstrating the usefulness of subtraction coronary CT for the evaluation of coronary artery stents at this time. It should be noted, however, that we have recently been receiving an increasing number of requests for such examinations from cardiologists, and, as a result, research focusing on coronary artery stents is currently underway.

RADIATION DOSE IN SUBTRACTION CORONARY CT

This section focuses on the estimated effective radiation dose in subtraction coronary CT. The effective radiation dose can be estimated based on the dose-length product (DLP, mGy × cm) using the formula effective radiation dose = DLP × k, where k = 0.014 mSv × mGy^{-1} × cm^{-1}, which is recommended by the European Working Group for Guidelines on Quality Criteria in CT and the American Association of Physicists in Medicine.[22,23]

When Prospective CTA was used for subtraction CT coronary angiography, the estimated effective radiation doses were 2.6 mSv minimum and 5.0 mSv maximum at a heart rate of 60 beats per minute, and the estimated effective radiation dose for calcium scoring was 2.3 mSv. Therefore, the effective radiation dose for the single breath-hold method was 5.2 to 10 mSv for subtraction coronary CT alone or 7.5 to 12.3 mSv with calcium scoring included. For the 2 breath-hold method, the calcium scoring images were used as the pre-contrast CT images, and the effective radiation dose was therefore 4.9 to 7.3 mSv.

The results mentioned earlier are based on the assumption that all the 320 rows of detector elements in the CT scanner are used (ie, when a scan range of 16 cm is set). However, in 320-row CT, the scan range in the z-axis direction can be reduced according to the size of the heart to be scanned.[24] Specifically, 280 rows (14 cm), 256 rows (12.8 cm), 240 rows (12 cm), or 200 rows (10 cm) can be selected, making it possible to reduce the radiation dose to 12.5%, 20%, 25%, or 37.5%, respectively, compared with the radiation dose for 320-row scanning. At present, 240-row or 256-row scanning is used for assessment in more than 60% of cases at our institution; 320-row scanning is used for assessment in less than 10% of cases. For example, the radiation dose in 256-row scanning is 6.0 to 9.8 mSv for the single breath-hold method or 3.9 to 5.8 mSv for the 2 breath-hold method, because the effective radiation dose is 2.1 to 4.0 mSv for Prospective CTA and 1.8 mSv for calcium scoring. This means that subtraction coronary CT can be performed with a total radiation dose of less than 10 mSv.

Setting an x-ray tube voltage lower than 120 kV is another reasonable approach for reducing the radiation dose, and studies on the low-dose assessment of the coronary arteries using 320-row CT have been reported.[25,26] However, because the changes in the volume of calcifications and blooming artifacts caused by changes in the tube voltage have not yet been investigated in detail, we have not used this technique for subtraction coronary CT. Image reconstruction technologies based on iterative methods are also said to be useful for reducing the radiation dose. One study has reported that using an iterative reconstruction method in coronary CT makes it possible to reduce the radiation dose by 44% compared with the commonly used filtered back projection method.[27] It has recently become possible to apply such iterative reconstruction methods to Prospective CTA and calcium scoring even in 320-row CT.

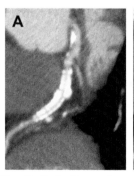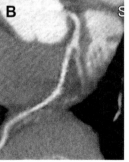

Fig. 5. Evaluation of a coronary artery stent by subtraction coronary CT. Patient with a stent 2.5 mm in diameter (Cypher, Cordis Corp, Miami, FL, USA) placed at a stenotic lesion with severe calcification in the left anterior descending branch (LAD). (*A*) Post-contrast CT. A CPR image of the LAD shows the stent. Severe nodular calcifications are also seen around the stent. It is difficult to assess the lumen of the stent. (*B*) Subtraction coronary CT. A CPR image created at the same position as in **Fig. 4A**. Both the stent and calcification are eliminated, and the lumen can be easily assessed.

We would therefore like to aggressively introduce this method and determine how much further the radiation dose can be reduced.

MISREGISTRATION ARTIFACTS

Subtraction coronary CT requires 2 scans (precontrast and postcontrast CT), but it is nearly impossible to perfectly match the positions of these scans. Misregistration artifacts due to positional shift must therefore be corrected to generate clear subtraction images. However, at present, such positional correction must be performed manually, which requires a great deal of time and effort. This is one of the major limitations of this method. Because misregistration artifacts must be corrected for each calcification, a long time is needed for image processing if multiple severe calcifications are present. Although the time required varies depending on the severity of misregistration and the number of severe calcifications, image processing currently requires at least 1 hour for 1 lesion. The processing time is doubled for 2 lesions, tripled for 3 lesions, and so on. The long time required for processing makes it difficult to use this method in the clinical setting. One of the reasons for the difficulty in image processing is that the position correction method (Volume Position Matching) used is not intended for coronary arteries. Specifically, this method was developed for the examination of regions exhibiting relatively little motion, such as the central nervous system and the peripheral arteries, and it therefore supports only simple position matching. To address this limitation, we are currently involved in the research and development of a software program intended specifically for subtraction coronary CT that supports not only complicated position matching but also semiautomatic subtraction.

FUTURE PROSPECTS

Subtraction coronary CT currently has several limitations, such as misregistration artifacts, long image processing times, and a higher radiation dose when the single breath-hold method is used. Because of these limitations, we currently use subtraction CT coronary angiography only in

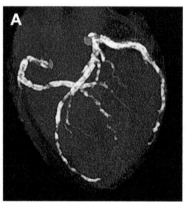

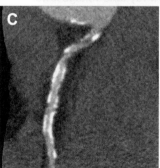
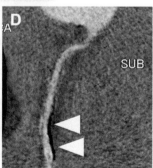
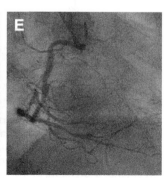

B

Calcium Score

Region	# Lesion	Agatston
RCA	2	1176.26
LM	1	175.31
LAD	8	2457.39
LCx	5	654.70
Aorta	0	0.00
Other	0	0.00
Total*	16	4463.66

Fig. 6. Subtraction coronary CT performed in a patient receiving hemodialysis. (*A*) Angiographic view (maximum intensity projection image). Diffuse extremely severe calcification is seen in all 3 branches of the coronary artery. (*B*) Calcium score. The patient had a calcium score of 4463.66. LAD, left anterior descending; LCx, left circumflex; LM, left main; RCA, right coronary artery. (*C*) Postcontrast CT. CPR image of the proximal RCA. Thick wall calcification is seen. (*D*) Subtraction coronary CT. The calcification is eliminated. Misregistration artifacts at a sufficiently low level that does not interfere with image interpretation are noted (*arrowheads*). No significant stenosis is seen. (*E*) Invasive coronary angiography. No significant stenosis is seen in the RCA.

patients with a calcium score of 600 or more. However, if this method could be applied to other patients with localized severely calcified lesions, it is expected that diagnostic accuracy would be improved. Similarly, this method may prove to be useful for the assessment of coronary artery stents. Moreover, if this method undergoes further development to a sufficiently high level, it may prove to be applicable to patients who are currently not candidates for conventional coronary CT because of extremely severe calcification (**Fig. 6**).

In the meantime, the dual-energy method is attracting a great deal of attention as a method for eliminating calcifications in CT images. The application of this method to peripheral arteries and the central nervous system has already been reported.[28–35] At this time, the dual-energy method cannot be used in combination with ECG-gated scanning, and application to the coronary arteries has therefore not yet been realized. Although application to the coronary arteries is expected in the near future, it will be necessary to evaluate the dual-energy method in comparison with the subtraction method used in the present study. It is considered that each method will prove to have both advantages and disadvantages, but it would be desirable for both of these methods to be available because it would provide greater flexibility in clinical practice.

REFERENCES

1. Vanhoenacker PK, Heijenbrok-Kal MH, Van Heste R, et al. Diagnostic performance of multidetector CT angiography for assessment of coronary artery disease: meta-analysis. Radiology 2007;244:419–28.

2. Hamon M, Morello R, Riddell JW, et al. Coronary arteries: diagnostic performance of 16- versus 64- section spiral CT compared with invasive coronary angiography—meta-analysis. Radiology 2007;245: 720–31.

3. Janne d'Othée B, Siebert U, Cury R, et al. A systematic review on diagnostic accuracy of CT-based detection of significant coronary artery disease. Eur J Radiol 2008;65:449–61.

4. Mowatt G, Cummins E, Waugh N, et al. Systematic review of the clinical effectiveness and cost-effectiveness of 64-slice or higher computed tomography angiography as an alternative to invasive coronary angiography in the investigation of coronary artery disease. Health Technol Assess 2008; 12(17):iii–iiv, ix–143.

5. Stein PD, Yaekoub AY, Matta F, et al. 64-slice CT for diagnosis of coronary artery disease: a systematic review. Am J Med 2008;121:715–25.

6. Sun Z, Lin C, Davidson R, et al. Diagnostic value of 64-slice CT angiography in coronary artery disease: a systematic review. Eur J Radiol 2008; 67:78–84.

7. Miller JM, Rochitte CE, Dewey M, et al. Diagnostic performance of coronary angiography by 64-row CT. N Engl J Med 2008;359:2324–36.

8. Budoff MJ, Dowe D, Jollis JG, et al. Diagnostic performance of 64-multidetector row coronary computed tomographic angiography for evaluation of coronary artery stenosis in individuals without known coronary artery disease: results from the prospective multicenter ACCURACY (Assessment by Coronary Computed Tomographic Angiography of Individuals Undergoing Invasive Coronary Angiography) trial. J Am Coll Cardiol 2008;52:1724–32.

9. Meijboom WB, Meijs MF, Schuijf JD, et al. Diagnostic accuracy of 64-slice computed tomography coronary angiography: a prospective, multicenter, multivendor study. J Am Coll Cardiol 2008;52: 2135–44.

10. Mark DB, Berman DS, Budoff MJ, et al. ACCF/ACR/ AHA/NASCI/SAIP/SCAI/SCCT 2010 expert consensus document on coronary computed tomographic angiography: a report of the American College of Cardiology Foundation Task Force on Expert Consensus Documents. Circulation 2010;121(22): 2509–43.

11. Mori S, Endo M. Candidate image processing for real-time volumetric CT subtraction angiography. Eur J Radiol 2007;61:335–41.

12. Yahyavi-Firouz-Abadi N, Wynn BL, Rybicki FJ, et al. Steroid responsive large vessel vasculitis: application of whole-brain 320-detector row dynamic volume CT angiography and perfusion. AJNR Am J Neuroradiol 2009;30:1409–11.

13. Hsiao EM, Rybicki FJ, Steigner M. CT coronary angiography: 256-slice and 320-detector row scanners. Curr Cardiol Rep 2010;12:68–75.

14. Rybicki FJ, Otero HJ, Steigner ML, et al. Initial evaluation of coronary images from 320-detector row computed tomography. Int J Cardiovasc Imaging 2008;24:535–46.

15. Steinger ML, Otero HJ, Cai T, et al. Narrowing the phase window width in prospectively ECG-gated single heart beat 320-detector row coronary CT angiography. Int J Cardiovasc Imaging 2009;25: 85–90.

16. Dewey M, Zimmermann E, Deissenrieder F, et al. Noninvasive coronary angiography by 320-row computed tomography with lower radiation exposure and maintained diagnostic accuracy: comparison of results with cardiac catheterization in a head-to-head pilot investigation. Circulation 2009;120:867–75.

17. Watanabe Y, Kashiwagi N, Yamada N, et al. Synchronized helical scan technique for the evaluation of postoperative cerebral aneurysms treated with cobalt-alloy clips. AJNR Am J Neuroradiol 2008;29:1071–5.

18. Jinzaki M, Sato K, Tanami, et al. Novel method of displaying coronary CT angiography: Angiographic view. Circ J 2006;70:1661–2.

19. Abbara S, Arbab-Zadeh A, Callister TQ, et al. SCCT guidelines for performance of coronary computed tomographic angiography: a report of the Society of Cardiovascular Computed Tomography Guidelines Committee. J Cardiovasc Comput Tomogr 2009;3:190–204.

20. Taylor AJ, Cerqueira M, Hodgson JM, et al. ACCF/SCCT/ACR/AHA/ASE/ASNC/NASCI/SCAI/SCMR 2010 appropriate use criteria for cardiac computed tomography. A report of the American College of Cardiology Foundation Appropriate Use Criteria Task Force, the Society of Cardiovascular Computed Tomography, the American College of Radiology, the American Heart Association, the American Society of Echocardiography, the American Society of Nuclear Cardiology, the North American Society for Cardiovascular Imaging, the Society for Cardiovascular Angiography and Interventions, and the Society for Cardiovascular Magnetic Resonance. J Cardiovasc Comput Tomogr 2010;4(6):407. e1–33.

21. Yoshioka K, Tanaka R, Muranaka K, et al. Subtraction coronary CTA: evaluation in patients with severe calcification [abstract]. Nippon Act Radiol 2010;(70 Suppl):s262–3 [in Japanese].

22. Bongartz G, Golding SJ, Jurik AG, et al. European guidelines for multislice computed tomography. Available at: http://www.msct.eu/CT_Quality_Criteria.htm#Download%20the%202004%20CT%20Quality%20Criteria. Accessed August 18, 2011.

23. McCollough CH, Primak AN, Braun N, et al. Strategies for reducing radiation dose in CT. Radiol Clin N Am 2009;47:27–40.

24. Khan A, Nasir K, Khosa F, et al. Prospective gating with 320-MDCT angiography: effect of volume scan length on radiation dose. AJR Am J Roentgenol 2011;196:407–11.

25. Hoe J, Toh KH. First experience with 320-row multidetector CT coronary angiography with prospective electrocardiogram gating to reduce radiation dose. J Cardiovasc Comput Tomogr 2009;3:257–61.

26. Einstein AJ, Elliston CD, Arai AE, et al. Radiation dose from single-heartbeat coronary CT angiography performed with a 320-detector row volume scanner. Radiology 2010;254:698–706.

27. Leipsic J, LaBountry TM, Heibron B, et al. Estimated radiation dose reduction using adaptive statistical iterative reconstruction in coronary CT angiography: the ERASIR study. AJR Am J Roentgenol 2010;195:655–60.

28. Meyer BC, Werncke T, Hopfenmuller W, et al. Dual energy CT of peripheral arteries: effect of automatic bone and plaque removal on image quality and grading of stenoses. Eur J Radiol 2008;68:414–22.

29. Brockmann C, Jochum S, Sadick M, et al. Dual-energy CT angiography in peripheral arterial occlusive disease. Cardiovasc Intervent Radiol 2009;32:630–7.

30. Yamamoto S, McWilliams J, Arellano C, et al. Dual-energy CT angiography and lower extremity arteries: dual-energy bone subtraction versus manual bone subtraction. Clin Radiol 2009;64:1088–96.

31. Uotani K, Watanabe Y, Higashi M, et al. Dual-energy CT head bone and plaque removal for quantification of calcified carotid stenosis: utility and comparison with digital subtraction angiography. Eur Radiol 2009;19:2060–5.

32. Deng K, Liu C, Ma R, et al. Clinical evaluation of dual-energy bone removal in CT angiography of the head and neck: comparison with conventional bone-subtraction CT angiography. Clin Radiol 2009;64:534–41.

33. Thomas C, Korn A, Ketelsen D, et al. Automatic lumen segmentation in calcified plaques: dual-energy CT versus standard reconstructions in comparison with digital subtraction angiography. AJR Am J Roentgenol 2010;194:1590–5.

34. Zhang LJ, Wu SY, Niu JB, et al. Dual-energy CT angiography in the evaluation of intracranial aneurysms: image quality, radiation dose, and comparison with 3D rotation digital subtraction angiography. AJR Am J Roentgenol 2010;194:23–30.

35. Zhang LJ, Wu SY, Poon CS, et al. Automatic bone removal dual-energy CT angiography for the evaluation of intracranial aneurysms. J Comput Assist Tomogr 2010;34:816–24.

CT Detection of Pulmonary Embolism and Aortic Dissection

Philipp Blanke, MD[a,b], Paul Apfaltrer, MD[a,c],
Ullrich Ebersberger, MD[a,d], Andreas Schindler, BS[a],
Mathias Langer, MD[b], U. Joseph Schoepf, MD[a,*]

KEYWORDS

- Pulmonary embolism • Aortic dissection
- Acute chest pain • Computed tomography
- Computed tomography angiography

Chest pain accounts for nearly 40% of all emergency department (ED) diagnoses in the United States and is the single most common presenting ED complaint of adults.[1,2] Chest pain is the presenting symptom of various pathologies, making immediate and efficient risk stratification and management challenging. The most clinically relevant conditions causing chest pain that have to be differentiated in this setting are acute coronary syndrome (ACS), pulmonary embolism (PE), and acute aortic syndrome (AAS). Patients with acute chest pain are evaluated by clinical and medical history, risk factors, electrocardiogram (ECG), and serum cardiac enzyme levels. These elements have been combined into the Thrombosis in Myocardial Infarction (TIMI) score.[3] However, most patients will not have definite evidence of ACS and thus pose a significant diagnostic challenge. A variety of different tests are competing for the filling of this diagnostic void. "Chest pain" computed tomography (CT) or "triple rule-out" CT may represent a reasonable approach in this respect. However, dedicated CT imaging strategies for PE and AAS exist, and in certain scenarios might even be more suitable than the rather unselective triple rule-out CT. Although computed tomography angiography (CTA) has been for more than a decade considered the accepted clinical reference standard for evaluation of patients with suspected PE and AAS, new data-acquisition techniques are evolving, enabling reduction of radiation dose, improved image quality, and higher information content.[4–6]

In this article the authors discuss current imaging strategies for PE and AAS, imaging parameters and typical findings, and current issues and recent advances of CT imaging for these disease entities, in particular, radiation-dose reduction and pulmonary CT perfusion imaging.

AORTIC DISSECTION
Epidemiology and Clinical Presentation

Thoracic aortic dissection (TAD) belongs to the category of life-threatening pathologies of the aorta, referred to as AAS, which also includes intramural hematoma (IMH) and penetrating aortic ulcer

Dr Schoepf is a consultant for and receives research support from Bayer, Bracco, GE, Medrad, and Siemens. The other authors have no conflict of interest to disclose.

[a] Department of Radiology and Radiological Science, Medical University of South Carolina, Ashley River Tower, 25 Courtenay Drive, Charleston, SC 29401, USA
[b] Department of Diagnostic Radiology, University Hospital Freiburg, Hugstetter Strasse 55, 79106 Freiburg, Germany
[c] Institute of Clinical Radiology and Nuclear Medicine, University Medical Center Mannheim, Medical Faculty Mannheim - Heidelberg University, Theodor-Kutzer-Ufer 1-3, 68167 Mannheim, Germany
[d] Department of Cardiology and Intensive Care Medicine, Heart Center Munich-Bogenhausen, Englschalkinger Strasse 77, 81925 Munich, Germany
* Corresponding author.
E-mail address: Schoepf@musc.edu

Cardiol Clin 30 (2012) 103–116
doi:10.1016/j.ccl.2011.11.006
0733-8651/12/$ – see front matter © 2012 Elsevier Inc. All rights reserved.

(PAU). AAS is characterized by acute onset of symptoms. TAD is estimated to occur at a rate of 3 to 4 cases per 100,000 persons per year, and is associated with a high mortality.[7–10] Reported rates most likely underestimate the true incidence of TAD because a substantial portion of patients dies before reaching a hospital or before the diagnosis is established.[11] TAD is most common in men and older individuals, with a male-to-female ratio of approximately 2:1 and average age at onset of 63 years.[12,13] Aortic dilatation is a well-established risk factor for TAD but is not a prerequisite; most ascending aortic dissections occur when the aortic diameter is less than 5.5 cm.[14,15] Congenital cardiovascular defects, such as bicuspid aortic valve, and certain genetic syndromes, such as Marfan syndrome, Loeys-Dietz syndrome, and Ehlers-Danlos syndrome, are most commonly associated with TAD.[16] Extent and localization of acute aortic dissection (AAD) is classified using the Stanford or DeBakey classifications.[5] After the initial intimal tear, the dissection may migrate in either an antegrade or retrograde direction. Due to pressure differences, the false lumen may compress or obstruct the true lumen. The false lumen may remain patent, thrombose, or recommunicate with the true lumen through fenestrations (reentry). Worse, thinning of the outer wall of the false lumen can lead to progressive dilatation and finally rupture into pericardial, pleural, or peritoneal cavities.

According to data from The International Registry of Acute Aortic Dissections (IRAD), the most common presenting symptom of AAD is severe pain reported by 96% of patients, with an abrupt onset in approximately 85% of patients.[12] The majority of patients complain of chest pain; anterior chest pain is more typical in patients with type A dissection, whereas interscapular pain or pain in the back and abdomen is more common in patients with type B dissection. However, there is a substantial overlap in presenting symptoms, and most importantly, more than 25% of patients do not present with chest pain.[12,17] The pain is usually described as worst ever or sharp, but also as tearing or ripping.[12,18]

In untreated patients the associated mortality rate of Stanford type A dissection is 1% to 2% per hour immediately after symptom onset.[8,19] Thus timely diagnosis is essential for successful management. However, the relative infrequency of AAD coupled with clinical presentations that may mimic more common clinical situations, such as ACS, can impede immediate establishment of diagnosis. In fact, the median time from arrival at the ED to diagnosis is approximately 4.3 hours and has not changed over the last 2 decades.[20] Variables associated with delayed diagnosis include atypical presentation with lack of typical symptoms such as abrupt onset, chest or back pain, and absence of high-risk physical findings such as hypotension or pulse deficit.[20] Establishing the diagnosis by CTA is associated with the shortest time intervals between admission and time of final diagnosis.[20]

Available Imaging Modalities and Diagnostic Accuracies

Common imaging options include chest radiography and cross-sectional imaging such as CTA, as well as transthoracic echocardiography (TTE) or transesophageal echocardiography (TEE). Selection of the most appropriate imaging modality may depend on patient-related factors (ie, hemodynamic stability, renal function, contrast allergy) and institutional capabilities (ie, rapid availability, state-of-the-art technology, and expertise).

Chest radiography often serves as a part of the initial evaluation of patients with potential AAS, primarily to identify other causes of the patient's symptoms but also as a screening test to identify imaging surrogates of a dilated aorta or bleeding. Of importance is that chest radiography is inadequately sensitive to definitively exclude the presence of AAS. In fact, typical chest radiographic findings of type A dissection, such as mediastinal widening, were not evident in 37% of patients in the IRAD registry, and no chest radiograph abnormalities were noted in 12% of patients.[12]

TEE is superior to TTE for assessment of the thoracic aorta, in particular for the distal aorta.[5] TEE has a sensitivity and specificity for diagnosing AAS of 98% and 95%, respectively.[21] However, TEE may be operator dependent and is limited by blind spots in the distal ascending aorta and proximal aortic arch, as well as by the incapability of visualizing the abdominal aorta.[5]

Advantages of CTA include nearly universal availability, and the ability to rapidly image the entire aorta including lumen, wall, and periaortic regions. Furthermore, CTA allows for assessment of potential involvement of branch vessels as well as the differentiation of other causes of AAS, namely IMH and PAU. ECG-assisted data acquisition techniques allow for motion-free imaging of the aortic root, and conceivably improve sensitivity and specificity of AAS assessment. Reported sensitivity and specificity of CTA is up to 100% and 98% to 99%, respectively.[22–24] In a meta-analysis of magnetic resonance imaging (MRI), TEE, and CTA, patients with a 50% pretest probability of TAD (high risk) had a 96%, 93%, and 93% posttest probability of AAD following a positive result at these 3 modalities, respectively.[21] By contrast, patients with a 5% pretest probability of AAD (low risk) had a 0.3%, 0.2%, and 0.1% post-test probability of AAD following a negative result at MRI, TEE, and CTA, respectively.[21] CTA yielded a sensitivity of 100% and a specificity of 98%, and it was superior to the other 2 modalities for ruling out TAD in patients at low risk for AAD.[21] However, disadvantages of CT are exposure to ionizing radiation and the need for contrast media.

Imaging Strategies with CTA

Because of the broad variety of possible imaging settings for CTA, such as acquisition window, number of contrast phases, scan length, tube current, and voltage, mainly influencing radiation exposure but also potential information content of the CTA study, the examiner should be aware of the pretest probability of AAD and further differentials to exclude. First, it has to be decided whether to perform ECG-assisted or nongated data acquisition and whether data acquisition should be limited to a single arterial phase. ECG-assisted data acquisition has led to a reduction in motion artifacts of the aortic root (**Fig. 1**), but historically at the cost of a significant increase in radiation exposure unless the newest CT technology is used. Second, an additional noncontrast study can be performed preceding the contrast-enhanced data acquisition to detect subtle changes of IMH.[25] The contrast-enhanced study itself is needed to delineate the presence and extent of the dissection flap, and thus to identify organ malperfusion and contrast leaks indicating rupture. Scan range should extend from the thoracic inlet to the pelvis to provide information on involvement of the iliac and femoral arteries, essential for endovascular treatment. Extending the scan range further cranially to include the neck yields valuable information on the extent of

dissection into the carotid arteries, especially in the presence of neurologic symptoms, which is also important for intraoperative strategies.

CTA Imaging Technique

Multidetector CT (MDCT) scanners, with at least 16-slice or 64-slice data acquisition, can be considered as a reasonable standard requirement for aortic imaging. Modern MDCT scanners allow for volumetric data acquisition with isotropic voxel size resolution in the x, y, and z axes, thereby allowing for multiplanar reformations with no limitation to the orientation and angulation. Contrast-enhanced data sets are usually acquired after intravenous injection of 90 to 130 mL of nonionic contrast media at an injection rate of 3 to 4 mL/s followed by a saline bolus chaser. Compared with-nongated data acquisition, ECG-assisted data acquisition has led to a substantial decrease in pulsation and motion artifacts of the thoracic aorta, in particular for the aortic root and ascending aorta.[26] Different ECG-assistance techniques are available: retrospective ECG gating for helical data acquisition, prospective ECG triggering for sequential data acquisition, also referred to as "step-and-shoot," and ECG-triggered high-pitch data acquisition.[27,28] Retrospectively ECG-gated helical data acquisition is characterized by low pitch values of 0.2 to 0.5 in order to cover the full cardiac cycle and to avoid data gaps. This technique allows for cine imaging of the cardiovascular system, and is beneficial for assessment of aortic valve anatomy (**Fig. 2**) and function, as well as for providing sufficient raw data for further image reconstructions throughout the cardiac cycle (eg, end-systole) in addition to standard diastolic reconstructions in cases of irregular and high heart rates. A disadvantage of this technique is the inherent increase in radiation exposure.[27] With

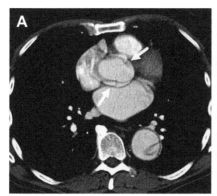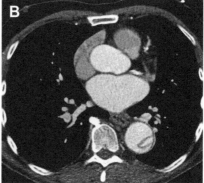

Fig. 1. (*A*) Nongated axial image depicts contour doubling of the aortic root (*arrow*) and an intimal flap in the descending aorta due to motion artifacts. (*B*) ECG-gated axial images of the same patient depict sharp wall delineation of the aortic root, with the dissection confined to the descending aorta (Stanford type B).

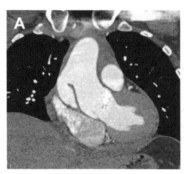
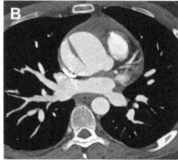
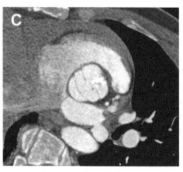

Fig. 2. A 35-year-old male patient with type A dissection. Intimal flap, aneurysmal widening of the ascending aorta, and pericardial effusion are appreciated on the coronal (*A*) and sagittal (*B*) images. (*C*) Multiplanar reconstruction of the aortic valve depicts a bicuspid aortic valve.

prospective ECG triggering, data acquisition is limited to a certain part of the cardiac cycle without any overlapping or redundant data acquisition, usually allowing for reconstruction of one image set centered at one time point within the cardiac cycle, thereby dramatically reducing radiation exposure in comparison with retrospective gating (**Fig. 3**).[27] The drawback of this technique is its vulnerability for stair-step artifacts in cases of irregular heart rates. However, with improved temporal resolution of newer scanners, and by shifting the data acquisition to end-systole, artifact-free images can be obtained even at high

and irregular heart rates.[29] ECG-assisted data acquisition of the thorax is usually followed by an ungated CTA of the abdomen and pelvis.

Because CTA of the thoracic aorta constitutes a different examination, scanning parameters should not be adopted from coronary CTA protocols. Tube current-time product can be lowered in comparison with a standard coronary CTA protocol.[27] Adjusting tube voltage and tube current to the body habitus can significantly reduce radiation exposure.[30,31] Based on patients' body habitus, patients of normal weight can be examined with 100 kV and those who

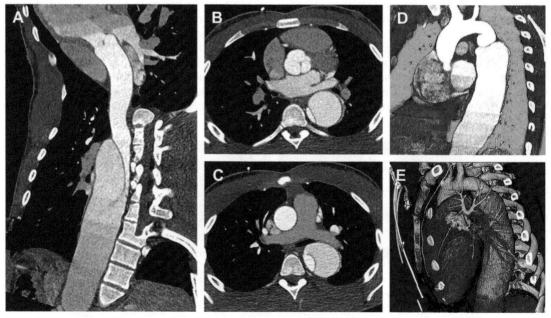

Fig. 3. Prospective ECG-triggered CTA of a 15-year-old male patient with pseudocoarctation and type B dissection. The aneurysmal widening and dissection flap is easily appreciated on the curve-planar reconstruction (*A*) and on axial source images (*B*, *C*). Volume-rendered images with various color settings give an overview of the pseudocoarctation (*D*, *E*).

are overweight and obese with 120 kV.[27] Tube current is usually adjusted by means of automatic exposure control–based tube-current modulation, a common feature of modern scanner generations, usually based on differences in attenuation in the anterior-posterior and, if available, the lateral scout view. This technique also compensates for varying dose requirements between different cross sections of the body such as the shoulder regions and the air-filled chest.

CTA Findings

Frank dissection is characterized by a discernible intimal flap, caused by blood intruding through a tear in the intima into the medial layer, thus creating a true lumen and a false lumen. By definition, an intimal flap is not seen with isolated IMH or PAU, although both entities may evolve into frank dissection. With Stanford type A dissection the primary intimal tear, also referred to as "entry," is usually located within the ascending aorta, predominantly at the great curvature, less commonly at the lesser curvature, anteriorly, or along the posterior aorta.[32] This proximal entry is discernible in approximately 41% of studies with diagnostic quality.[32] Of importance, the proximal tear can be located further distally in the aortic arch or proximal descending aorta with proximal propagation of the intimal flap into the ascending aorta. True lumen can be differentiated from false lumen by following certain characteristics: the beak sign, that is, presence of an acute angle between the dissection flap and the outer wall, and a larger cross-sectional area are indicators of the false lumen.[33] Also, the intimal flap is usually curved toward the false lumen. Features that generally indicate the true lumen are outer wall calcification, eccentric flap calcification, and continuity to a nondissected portion of the aorta.[33] With circumferential dissection, the false lumen wraps around the inner, invariably true lumen.[33] Furthermore, contrast enhancement of the false lumen is usually delayed. Widening of the aorta is seen with frank dissection.

IMH lacks an intimal flap. Instead, aortic wall thickening with hyperdense appearance as compared with the aortic lumen can be noted on unenhanced CT images.

Aortic dissection can be complicated by aortic rupture. Signs of aortic rupture are hemorrhagic pericardial effusion and a mediastinal or pleural fluid collection, which can be appreciated on CT studies. Pericardial tamponade, acute aortic regurgitation, aortic rupture itself, or major aortic branch obstruction will finally lead to death. Other organ involvement depends on the extent of dissection. Extension of dissection membrane into the carotid arteries will compromise cerebral blood flow, resulting in neurologic symptoms in up to 29% and ischemic stroke in up to 16% of patients.[34] This possibility emphasizes the importance of including at least the proximal segments of the major branching vessels of the aortic arch into the scan range, not only for documenting the cause of the neurologic symptoms but also for providing valuable information to the cardiothoracic surgeon regarding optimization of the surgical strategy. Dissection can extend downward and compromise blood flow to the celiac trunk, superior and inferior mesenteric arteries, and their subsequent organs, either by extending into these arteries or by collapse of the true lumen, thereby leading to hepatic or splenic infarction, mesenteric ischemia, and renal ischemia. In particular, compromised renal perfusion can easily be appreciated on CTA as asymmetric attenuation of the renal parenchyma, with hypoattenuation indicating delayed perfusion. Impaired branching vessel perfusion can be caused by two different types of obstruction. Static obstruction occurs when the intimal flap extends into the ostium of the branching vessel without a reentry point, resulting in increased pressure or thrombus formation in the false lumen within the branch vessel, causing focal stenosis and end-organ ischemia.[35] Dynamic obstruction affects vessels arising from the true lumen, when the intimal flap spares the branching vessel but prolapses and covers the branch-vessel ostium like a curtain.[35] Further downwards, dissection can extend beyond the aortic bifurcation into the iliac and even femoral arteries, leading to acute limb ischemia. This process underlines the importance of extending the scan range beyond the level diaphragm to cover the abdomen and pelvis, also providing relevant information for potential endovascular treatment. Proximal propagation of the intimal flap into the aortic root beyond the sinotubular junction can lead to acute aortic regurgitation, either by direct impaired integrity of the valve by the intruding dissection or by acute dilation of the aortic root. Proximal propagation can also compromise myocardial blood supply with subsequent signs and symptoms of myocardial ischemia, by either ostial dissection with formation of a local flap, extension into the coronary artery with a coronary false lumen, or circumferential detachment with an inner-cylinder intussusception.[36]

Pitfalls of CTA

Recent advances in temporal resolution and ECG-assistance technique have greatly diminished artifact burden and thus have increased diagnostic certainty, although this has never been quantified in a formal study.

Nevertheless, especially with nongated CTA studies, one has to be careful not to mistakenly interpret pulsation artifacts of the ascending aorta as a dissection flap. Pulsation artifacts can still be present even with modern MDCT scanners and ECG-assisted data acquisition, especially in the setting of high, irregular heart rates when performing studies on a single-source CT scanner. False-negative results are only conceivable when attributable to inadequate contrast opacification, for example, caused by cardiac failure. However, inadequate contrast opacification should inevitably result in study repetition.

Current Issues and Recent Advances in CTA

Current issues of CTA for AAD mainly involve radiation-dose reduction and improvement of data-acquisition techniques. To perform CTA with the lowest acceptable dose must be the prime concern for each examination, especially when using ECG assistance; this is particularly important for patients who will undergo repeated CT examinations (eg, for postoperative follow-up). Introduction of prospective ECG-triggered data acquisition has cut radiation exposure by approximately 50% compared with retrospective ECG gating. This reduction allows for ECG-assisted CTA of the whole thorax for approximately 2 mSv in normal-weight patients and 4 mSv in overweight and obese patients, when exploiting all dose-reduction strategies including tube-current and tube-voltage adaptation to body habitus.[27] In everyday practice, relative radiation-dose reduction is even higher, as retrospective ECG gating is often used with a wide pulsing window, resulting in radiation doses as high as 14 to 17 mSv.[37,38] One major innovation has been the introduction of the dual-source CT (DSCT) scanner. With two x-ray sources mounted 90° off-set and two corresponding detectors a temporal resolution of 83 milliseconds achieved, allowing for motion-free imaging of the aortic root even in atrial fibrillation.[29] With the introduction of second-generation DSCT scanners in 2009, temporal resolution was improved to 75 milliseconds. Furthermore, different angulation of the x-ray sources allows for high-pitch data acquisition with pitch factors of 3.2 and a table feed of 43 cm/s, avoiding overlapping or redundant data acquisition and resulting in an average radiation exposure of 1.6 and 3.2 mSv for the whole thorax in normal and overweight patients, respectively.[28] Extending high-pitch data acquisition to the entire aorta results in an average radiation exposure of 4.4 mSv when using 100 kV.[39] However, with high-pitch acquisition the axial source images are not acquired during the same time point of the cardiac cycle but are delayed "slice-by-slice" along the craniocaudal z-axis of data acquisition. High-pitch data acquisition can be performed with and without prospective ECG triggering. With prospective ECG triggering, data acquisition is attempted in order to achieve a specific cardiac phase at a specific anatomic location, for example, 60% of the RR-interval at the level of the aortic root, but without an increase in radiation dose, compared with high-pitch data acquisition without prospective ECG triggering.[38] However, with high-pitch data acquisition ECG triggering is only needed for visualization of coronary arteries, because the fast data acquisition itself allows for motion-free imaging of the aortic root.[38]

PULMONARY EMBOLISM

As the third most common cause of cardiovascular death after myocardial ischemia and stroke, PE is a potentially fatal condition associated with significant morbidity and mortality.[40] Evaluating the individual likelihood of PE according to the clinical presentation is of importance in the interpretation of diagnostic test results and selection of the diagnostic strategy. Unfortunately, individual clinical signs and symptoms are neither sensitive nor specific. Pleuritic chest pain is reported in more than half of patients with acute PE, and is due to pleural irritation by pulmonary infarction caused by distal emboli.[41,42] Chest pain may also be retrosternal and angina-like, possibly reflecting right ventricular angina. The pain is either of sudden onset or evolves over a period of days to weeks. The same applies to dyspnea, which is reported in 80% of patients with acute PE,[41] with isolated dyspnea of rapid onset usually attributable to more central PE causing more prominent hemodynamic consequences. Syncope is rare, but indicates a severely reduced hemodynamic reserve.

Common to all symptoms and findings is their nonspecificity. Therefore, imaging plays a pivotal role in establishing the diagnosis of PE,[6,43] but also in determining the subsequent therapy. According to a recently published scientific statement by the American Heart Association (AHA), PE can be classified as massive, submassive, and low-risk PE, in order to tailor medical and interventional therapies.[44] Whereas massive PE is defined by findings of hemodynamic compromise, patients with submassive PE are normotensive but are thought to be at increased risk for adverse short-term outcomes.[44] Of importance, the definition of submassive PE may include CT findings of right ventricular dysfunction,[44] as discussed later.

Imaging Modalities and Diagnostic Accuracies

To discriminate suspected PE patients in categories of clinical or pretest probability of low, intermediate, or high corresponding to an increasing prevalence of PE, prediction rules such as the Wells score or the Geneva score are used, taking predisposing factors, symptoms, and clinical signs into account.[45] In clinically stable, non–high-risk patients, the clinical probability guides further workup.[45]

The value of CTA for decision making in suspected PE has changed, with improvements over the last decade. However, with continuously evolving technology the true accuracy of pulmonary CTA is difficult to estimate. Most of the published data on diagnostic performance of pulmonary CTA has been collected on single detectors with wide variations regarding both the sensitivity (53%–100%) and specificity (73%–100%) of CT.[46,47] With 4-slice and 16-slice CT, the sensitivity and specificity vary between 83% and 100% and 89% and 97%, respectively.[48–51] PIOPED (Prospective Investigation of Pulmonary Embolism Diagnosis) II is the largest study assessing the use of pulmonary CTA (CTPA) in the diagnosis of PE. In PIOPED II the sensitivity and specificity of CTPA was 83% and 96%, respectively. Positive predictive values were 96% with a concordantly high probability of venous thromboembolism on clinical assessment, 92% with an intermediate probability on clinical assessment, and 58% if clinical probability was discordant. Negative predictive values were 96% with a concordantly low probability of venous thromboembolism on clinical assessment, 89% with an intermediate probability on clinical assessment, and 60% if clinical probability was discordant.[51] However, PIOPED II mainly used 4-sclice CT and a few 16-slice CT scanners, and the composite reference standard remains controversial. With modern MDCT scanners of at least 64 slices with submillimeter resolution and shortened data-acquisition times, improved diagnostic accuracy seems conceivable. It has been shown that thinner resolution improves visualization of the subsegmental pulmonary arteries and also improves interobserver agreement regarding the presence or absence of emboli.[52] Prospective, large-scale studies have provided evidence in favor of CTA as a stand-alone test to exclude PE, as occurrence of venous thromboembolism in patients with negative CTA left untreated is

very low.[53,54] Thus a negative CTA with modern scanner technology safely excludes PE. Ventilation/perfusion scintigraphy remains a valid option, especially for patients with contraindications for MSCT, but is limited by a high proportion of inconclusive results.[55] However, because most patients with suspected PE do not have the disease, CT should not be the first-line test. In low-risk patients admitted to the ED, that is, without shock or hypotension, plasma D-dimer measurement combined with clinical probability assessment is the first step and allows PE to be ruled out in approximately 30% of patients.[53,54] However, D-dimer should not be measured in patients with a high clinical probability because of the low negative predictive value in this population.[56] In patients with elevated D-dimer level, MDCT is the second-line test, whereas in patients with high clinical probability MDCT constitutes the first-line modality.[45] In high-risk patients (ie, with shock or hypotension), the direct evidence of PE or indirect signs should be first established with echocardiography before definitive diagnosis is sought by CTA.

CTA Technique

CTA of the pulmonary arteries usually includes the entire chest, starting at the lung apex and going down to the costophrenic angles. Scans are usually performed in inspiratory hold. Caudocranial scanning may be preferred to avoid streak artifacts by contrast material in the superior vena cava.[57] Optimal arterial attenuation remains one of the most crucial determinants of sufficient depiction of the pulmonary arteries, demanding precise timing of the contrast material bolus. The scan duration for CTA ranges from about 20 seconds with 4-slice CT to about 5 seconds with 64-slice CT, and 0.6 to 2 seconds with second-generation DSCT. Thus, contrast injection protocols have to be adapted to the shorter scanning times of the newer scanners. Most often, bolus tracking is used with the region of interest placed in the main pulmonary artery. Deep inspiratory breath-hold may cause a transient interruption of the contrast column in the pulmonary arteries due to pronounced inflow of unopacified blood from the inferior vena cava[58]; this may be prevented by a shallow inspiratory breath-hold. Amounts of contrast media and flow rates vary for different scanner generations. Newer scanner generations with shorter acquisition times should allow for depiction of the entire pulmonary artery with maximum attenuation while simultaneously allowing for reduction of contrast media applied by creating a compact but short bolus. In fact, use of 50 mL contrast media has been reported with high-pitch protocols, yielding sufficient image quality.[59] A saline flush following administration of contrast material avoids pooling of the contrast material in the arm veins and in the injection system, and reduces beam-hardening artifacts in the subclavian veins and the superior vena cava.

For routine CTA of the pulmonary arteries ECG-assisted data acquisition is not needed, as less than 1% of subsegmental pulmonary arteries is subject to cardiac motion.[60] However, for simultaneous assessment of the aorta or coronary arteries ECG assistance is mandatory. With modern CT scanners, collimation is similar to that described for AAD. The pitch used for standard CTA protocols ranges between 0.8 and 1.5, or 3.2 for high-pitch acquisition with second-generation DSCT scanners.

Radiation Dose

Similar to CTA for AAD, CTA for PE should be performed with minimal radiation dose while maintaining diagnostic image quality. Adapting tube voltage and tube current to the individual patient's body habitus should be considered standard. Tube current can be adjusted by means of automatic exposure control as explained earlier, reducing radiation dose by 10% to 50%.[61] Normal-weight patients can be examined with 100-kV tube voltage whereas overweight and obese patients should be examined with 120 kV. Reducing tube voltage from 120 to 100 kV reduces radiation exposure by almost half.[62] In addition, because of the absorption characteristics of iodine the intravascular opacification is increased by approximately 70 HU, compensating for the generally higher image noise.[62] Using a 100-kV protocol usually results in an effective dose of 1.5 to 2 mSv,[62] using high pitch as low as 1.6 mSv.[28]

CTA Findings and Assessment of Right Ventricular Dysfunction

On CTA, acute PE manifests either as arterial occlusion with failure to enhance the entire lumen due to a large filling defect, with the affected artery often being enlarged, or as centrally located partial filling defects. Peripheral wedge-shaped areas of hyperattenuation may be found, representing infarcts.

Besides establishing the diagnosis of PE based on the aforementioned findings, CTA yields further important information. Several studies have evaluated the prognostic value of various pulmonary CTA signs to predict adverse clinical events or early death in patients with acute PE.[57,63–68] These signs include flattening or displacement of the interventricular septum toward the left ventricle (LV), reflux of contrast material into the inferior vena cava, and the ratio of right ventricle (RV) to LV diameter or volume assessed with various measurement techniques using ECG-gated and nongated studies (see **Fig. 3**).[63,67,69,70] Several studies reported that ventricular septal bowing on CTA indicates severe PE[4,71] and right ventricular dysfunction,[72,73] and predicts short-term death. However, this remains controversial.[64,68,73] Reflux of contrast medium into the inferior vana cava is an indirect sign of increased right ventricular pressure. However, reflux of contrast medium is not specific and can be seen in various underlying conditions.[74] Increased RV/LV diameter ratio on axial CTPA has been proposed as a sign of right ventricular dysfunction[72,73,75] and a predictor of short-term death.[76] However, multiple quantitative methods and cutoff points have been described to assess dilatation of the complex-shaped RV, for example, measurements taken at atrioventricular valves[63,72] or maximum minor axis measurements.[68] Furthermore, the cutoff values for RV/LV diameter ratio on axial CTPA to indicate severe PE vary throughout the literature (eg, >1 or >1.5),[68,71–73] while other investigators have been unable to confirm its prognostic capability at all.[66] Instead, RV/LV diameter ratios on reconstructed 4-chamber views were found to be a significant predictor for adverse clinical events.[66] Similarly, Schoepf and colleagues[67] established the prognostic value of reconstructed 4-chamber RV/LV diameter ratio for early death in patients with acute PE, using a cutoff value of 0.9.

Due to the complex anatomy of the ventricles, volumetric analysis may be of advantage to unidimensional diameter measurements. With ECG-gated data acquisition, volumetric RV/LV ratio has been shown to allow for a better discrimination of patients with different embolus location, when compared with the unidimensional diameter ratios.[69] However, because of the additional radiation exposure involved with certain ECG-assistance techniques, this approach is not currently used for routine PE and might not even be necessary. In a recent study on 260 patients with acute PE and nongated CTA, it was shown that abnormal position of the interventricular septum, inferior vena cava contrast reflux, 4-chamber RV/LV diameter ratio greater than 1.0, and volumetric RV/LV ratio greater than 1.2 were predictive of adverse outcomes and 30-day mortality.[77] Of importance, CT findings of right ventricular dysfunction, as an RV/LV diameter ratio greater than 0.9 on a reconstructed 4-chamber view, are incorporated in the definition of submassive PE in the recent AHA scientific statement.[44]

Recent Advances with Dual-Energy CT for Pulmonary Perfusion

In patients with PE, visualization of pulmonary perfusion can help to estimate the hemodynamic significance of clots within the pulmonary arteries. Pulmonary perfusion can be studied with CT. DSCT scanners with two orthogonally mounted x-ray tubes not only allow for increased temporal resolution compared with single-source CT scanners, but also for simultaneous acquisition of data sets acquired at different tube voltages (eg, 80 kVp for one tube and 140 kVp for the other), referred to as dual-energy CT (DECT).[78] Iodine has a higher x-ray attenuation at lower photon energies and thus can be differentiated and quantified in a DECT data set, due to its spectral behavior.[79] This technique provides

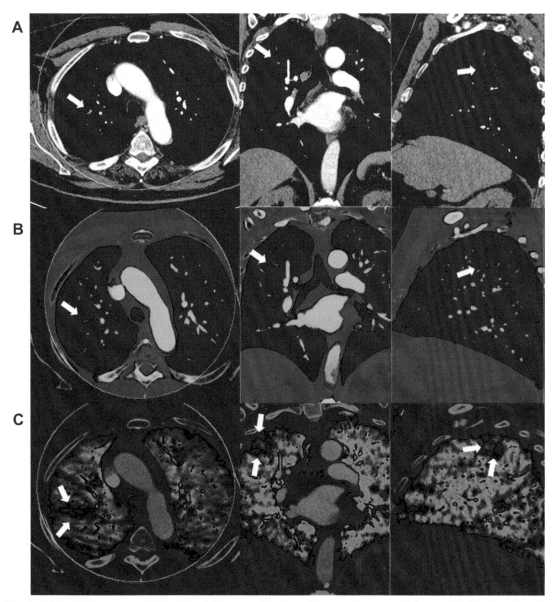

Fig. 4. (*A*) Isolated segmental PE of the right upper lobe in a 41-year-old man, which was initially missed on the axial, coronal, and sagittal maximum-intensity projection gray-scale reformats. Corresponding dual-energy CT displayed the embolism in the dual-energy color-coded images (*B, arrows*) as well as the corresponding color-coded perfusion defect (*C*). The resultant perfusion defect is well visualized on axial, coronal, and sagittal dual-energy perfusion maps (*arrows*).

a comprehensive evaluation of both CTPA for morphologic information and further iodine-based perfusion maps for functional assessment.[80,81] Although DECT actually maps the iodine distribution at a single time point, the term perfusion imaging may be justified, as regional contrast enhancement occurs immediately after arrival of the contrast bolus, providing a reasonably accurate representation of regional blood flow.[82,83] Perfusion defects on DECT show good agreement with perfusion defects observed in ventilation/perfusion scintigraphy, and correspond to embolic vessel occlusion (**Fig. 4**).[83,84] However, circumscribed perfusion defects can be found without visualization of corresponding intravascular clots on pulmonary CTA images.[83,85] This phenomenon is thought to correspond to segments of prior embolism with reperfused segmental vessels and residual peripheral thrombosed vessels that are too small to be visualized on CTA.[85] Thus, DECT lung perfusion images and visualization of vascular iodine distribution may further assist in detecting small pulmonary emboli that are not evident with conventional CTPA (**Fig. 5**).[83] First-generation DSCT scanners were limited by a small field of view for DECT applications, often not covering the entire lung parenchyma.[83] With second-generation DSCT scanners the entire lung parenchyma can be assessed.[86] Use of DECT may be a promising option for adding additional information in the diagnostic workup of acute chest pain;

however, the concrete benefit has still to be determined.

CHEST PAIN CTA

Chest pain or so-called triple rule-out (TRO) CT protocols are aimed at patients with low to intermediate risk for ACS, but with symptoms possibly attributable to PE or AAD. TRO CT comprises tailored ECG-assisted examinations designed to evaluate the aorta, and coronary and pulmonary arteries within one scan. Because of the increase in tube current necessary for evaluation of the coronary arteries and use of retrospective ECG gating, TRO CT is usually associated with effective radiation doses higher than standard CTA examinations tailored to pulmonary arteries or the thoracic aorta alone. The reported effective radiation dose for TRO CT is as high as 19.5 mSv.[87] Use of high-pitch protocols with second-generation DSCT and tube voltage adapted to body mass index results in an estimated radiation exposure of 1.6 to 3.2 mSv.[28] However, high-pitch data acquisition is limited to patients with heart rates lower than 65 beats/min to ensure sufficient image quality of the coronary arteries.[88] Of importance is that TRO usually requires larger amounts of contrast media than pulmonary CTA to achieve sufficient opacification of all vascular structures. Overall, only a minority of patients undergoing TRO CT are found to have PE or AAD.[89]

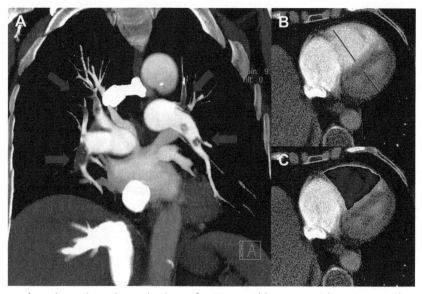

Fig. 5. (*A*) Coronal maximum-intensity projections of a 41-year-old woman with acute central PE and multiple segmental clots (*red arrows*). Elevated RV/LV diameter ratio (*B*) and increased volumetric RV/LV ratio (*C*) indicate right ventricular dysfunction in this patient.

SUMMARY

With advances in CT technology, in particular increased temporal and spatial resolution and decreased examination times, CTA is the accepted standard imaging modality for diagnosis of PE and AAD. Patients may benefit from decreased radiation exposure through the use of modern scanner technology and tailored scan protocols.

REFERENCES

1. McCaig LF, Burt CW. National Hospital Ambulatory Medical Care Survey: 2002 emergency department summary. Adv Data 2004;(340):1–34.

2. Pitts SR, Niska RW, Xu J, et al. National Hospital Ambulatory Medical Care Survey: 2006 emergency department summary. Natl Health Stat Report 2008;(7):1–38.

3. Antman EM, Cohen M, Bernink PJ, et al. The TIMI risk score for unstable angina/non-ST elevation MI: A method for prognostication and therapeutic decision making. JAMA 2000;284(7):835–42.

4. Schoepf UJ, Costello P. CT angiography for diagnosis of pulmonary embolism: state of the art. Radiology 2004;230(2):329–37.

5. Hiratzka LF, Bakris GL, Beckman JA, et al. 2010 ACCF/AHA/AATS/ACR/ASA/SCA/SCAI/SIR/STS/SVM guidelines for the diagnosis and management of patients with Thoracic Aortic Disease: a report of the American College of Cardiology Foundation/ American Heart Association Task Force on Practice Guidelines, American Association for Thoracic Surgery, American College of Radiology, American Stroke Association, Society of Cardiovascular Anesthesiologists, Society for Cardiovascular Angiography and Interventions, Society of Interventional Radiology, Society of Thoracic Surgeons, and Society for Vascular Medicine. Circulation 2010; 121(13):e266–369.

6. Remy-Jardin M, Pistolesi M, Goodman LR, et al. Management of suspected acute pulmonary embolism in the era of CT angiography: a statement from the Fleischner Society. Radiology 2007;245(2):315–29.

7. Clouse WD, Hallett JW Jr, Schaff HV, et al. Acute aortic dissection: population-based incidence compared with degenerative aortic aneurysm rupture. Mayo Clin Proc 2004;79(2):176–80.

8. Meszaros I, Morocz J, Szlavi J, et al. Epidemiology and clinicopathology of aortic dissection. Chest 2000;117(5):1271–8.

9. Sato F, Kitamura T, Kongo M, et al. Newly diagnosed acute aortic dissection: characteristics, treatment modifications, and outcomes. Int Heart J 2005; 46(6):1083–98.

10. Yu HY, Chen YS, Huang SC, et al. Late outcome of patients with aortic dissection: study of a national database. Eur J Cardiothorac Surg 2004;25(5): 683–90.

11. Olsson C, Thelin S, Stahle E, et al. Thoracic aortic aneurysm and dissection: increasing prevalence and improved outcomes reported in a nationwide population-based study of more than 14,000 cases from 1987 to 2002. Circulation 2006;114(24):2611–8. [Epub 2006 Dec 2614].

12. Hagan PG, Nienaber CA, Isselbacher EM, et al. The International Registry of Acute Aortic Dissection (IRAD): new insights into an old disease. JAMA 2000;283(7):897–903.

13. Nienaber CA, Fattori R, Mehta RH, et al. Gender-related differences in acute aortic dissection. Circulation 2004;109(24):3014–21.

14. Parish LM, Gorman JH 3rd, Kahn S, et al. Aortic size in acute type A dissection: implications for preventive ascending aortic replacement. Eur J Cardiothorac Surg 2009;35(6):941–5 [discussion: 945–6].

15. Pape LA, Tsai TT, Isselbacher EM, et al. Aortic diameter > or = 5.5 cm is not a good predictor of type A aortic dissection: observations from the International Registry of Acute Aortic Dissection (IRAD). Circulation 2007;116(10):1120–7.

16. LeMaire SA, Russell L. Epidemiology of thoracic aortic dissection. Nat Rev Cardiol 2011;8(2):103–13.

17. Klompas M. Does this patient have an acute thoracic aortic dissection? JAMA 2002;287(17):2262–72.

18. Slater EE, DeSanctis RW. The clinical recognition of dissecting aortic aneurysm. Am J Med 1976;60(5): 625–33.

19. Hirst AE Jr, Johns VJ Jr, Kime SW Jr. Dissecting aneurysm of the aorta: a review of 505 cases. Medicine 1958;37(3):217–79.

20. Harris KM, Strauss CE, Eagle KA, et al. Correlates of delayed recognition and treatment of acute type A aortic dissection: the International Registry of Acute Aortic Dissection (IRAD). Circulation 2011;124(18): 1911–8.

21. Shiga T, Wajima Z, Apfel CC, et al. Diagnostic accuracy of transesophageal echocardiography, helical computed tomography, and magnetic resonance imaging for suspected thoracic aortic dissection: systematic review and meta-analysis. Arch Intern Med 2006;166(13):1350–6.

22. Sommer T, Fehske W, Holzknecht N, et al. Aortic dissection: a comparative study of diagnosis with spiral CT, multiplanar transesophageal echocardiography, and MR imaging. Radiology 1996;199(2): 347–52.

23. Yoshida S, Akiba H, Tamakawa M, et al. Thoracic involvement of type A aortic dissection and intramural hematoma: diagnostic accuracy–comparison of emergency helical CT and surgical findings. Radiology 2003;228(2):430–5. [Epub 2003 Jun 2020].

24. Zeman RK, Berman PM, Silverman PM, et al. Diagnosis of aortic dissection: value of helical CT with

multiplanar reformation and three-dimensional rendering. AJR Am J Roentgenol 1995;164(6):1375–80.

25. Eggebrecht H, Plicht B, Kahlert P, et al. Intramural hematoma and penetrating ulcers: indications to endovascular treatment. Eur J Vasc Endovasc Surg 2009;38(6):659–65.

26. Roos JE, Willmann JK, Weishaupt D, et al. Thoracic aorta: motion artifact reduction with retrospective and prospective electrocardiography-assisted multi-detector row CT. Radiology 2002;222(1):271–7.

27. Blanke P, Bulla S, Baumann T, et al. Thoracic aorta: prospective electrocardiographically triggered CT angiography with dual-source CT–feasibility, image quality, and dose reduction. Radiology 2010; 255(1):207–17.

28. Lell M, Hinkmann F, Anders K, et al. High-pitch electrocardiogram-triggered computed tomography of the chest: initial results. Invest Radiol 2009;44(11): 728–33.

29. Blanke P, Baumann T, Bulla S, et al. Prospective ECG-triggered CT angiography of the thoracic aorta in patients with atrial fibrillation or accelerated heart rates: feasibility and image quality. AJR Am J Roentgenol 2010;194(1):W111–4.

30. Huda W, Scalzetti EM, Levin G. Technique factors and image quality as functions of patient weight at abdominal CT. Radiology 2000;217(2):430–5.

31. Soderberg M, Gunnarsson M. Automatic exposure control in computed tomography—an evaluation of systems from different manufacturers. Acta Radiol 2010;51(6):625–34.

32. Moon MC, Greenberg RK, Morales JP, et al. Computed tomography-based anatomic characterization of proximal aortic dissection with consideration for endovascular candidacy. J Vasc Surg 2011;53(4):942–9.

33. LePage MA, Quint LE, Sonnad SS, et al. Aortic dissection: CT features that distinguish true lumen from false lumen. AJR Am J Roentgenol 2001;177(1):207–11.

34. Gaul C, Dietrich W, Friedrich I, et al. Neurological symptoms in type A aortic dissections. Stroke 2007;38(2):292–7.

35. Williams DM, Lee DY, Hamilton BH, et al. The dissected aorta: part III. Anatomy and radiologic diagnosis of branch-vessel compromise. Radiology 1997;203(1):37–44.

36. Neri E, Toscano T, Papalia U, et al. Proximal aortic dissection with coronary malperfusion: presentation, management, and outcome. J Thorac Cardiovasc Surg 2001;121(3):552–60.

37. Cornfeld D, Israel G, Detroy E, et al. Impact of Adaptive Statistical Iterative Reconstruction (ASIR) on radiation dose and image quality in aortic dissection studies: a qualitative and quantitative analysis. AJR Am J Roentgenol 2011;196(3):W336–40.

38. Karlo C, Leschka S, Goetti RP, et al. High-pitch dual-source CT angiography of the aortic valve-aortic root complex without ECG-synchronization. Eur Radiol 2011;21(1):205–12.

39. Goetti R, Baumuller S, Feuchtner G, et al. High-pitch dual-source CT angiography of the thoracic and abdominal aorta: is simultaneous coronary artery assessment possible? AJR Am J Roentgenol 2010; 194(4):938–44.

40. Geerts WH, Pineo GF, Heit JA, et al. Prevention of venous thromboembolism: the Seventh ACCP Conference on Antithrombotic and Thrombolytic Therapy. Chest 2004;126(Suppl 3):338S–400S.

41. Stein PD, Saltzman HA, Weg JG. Clinical characteristics of patients with acute pulmonary embolism. Am J Cardiol 1991;68(17):1723–4.

42. Stein PD, Henry JW. Clinical characteristics of patients with acute pulmonary embolism stratified according to their presenting syndromes. Chest 1997;112(4):974–9.

43. Goldhaber SZ. Pulmonary embolism. Lancet 2004; 363(9417):1295–305.

44. Jaff MR, McMurtry MS, Archer SL, et al. Management of massive and submassive pulmonary embolism, iliofemoral deep vein thrombosis, and chronic thromboembolic pulmonary hypertension: a scientific statement from the American Heart Association. Circulation 2011;123(16):1788–830.

45. Torbicki A, Perrier A, Konstantinides S, et al. Guidelines on the diagnosis and management of acute pulmonary embolism: the Task Force for the Diagnosis and Management of Acute Pulmonary Embolism of the European Society of Cardiology (ESC). Eur Heart J 2008;29(18):2276–315.

46. Mullins MD, Becker DM, Hagspiel KD, et al. The role of spiral volumetric computed tomography in the diagnosis of pulmonary embolism. Arch Intern Med 2000;160:293–8.

47. Rathbun SW, Raskob GE, Whitsett TL. Sensitivity and specificity of helical computed tomography in the diagnosis of pulmonary embolism: a systematic review. Ann Intern Med 2000;132:227–32.

48. Safriel Y, Zinn H. CT pulmonary angiography in the detection of pulmonary emboli: a meta-analysis of sensitivities and specificities. Clin Imaging 2002; 26(2):101–5.

49. Qanadli SD, Hajjam ME, Mesurolle B, et al. Pulmonary embolism detection: prospective evaluation of dual-section helical CT versus selective pulmonary arteriography in 157 patients. Radiology 2000; 217(2):447–55.

50. Winer-Muram HT, Rydberg J, Johnson MS, et al. Suspected acute pulmonary embolism: evaluation with multi-detector row CT versus digital subtraction pulmonary arteriography. Radiology 2004;233(3): 806–15.

51. Stein PD, Fowler SE, Goodman LR, et al. Multidetector computed tomography for acute pulmonary embolism. N Engl J Med 2006;354(22):2317–27.

52. Schoepf UJ, Holzknecht N, Helmberger TK, et al. Subsegmental pulmonary emboli: improved detection with thin-collimation multi-detector row spiral CT. Radiology 2002;222(2):483–90.

53. van Belle A, Buller HR, Huisman MV, et al. Effectiveness of managing suspected pulmonary embolism using an algorithm combining clinical probability, D-dimer testing, and computed tomography. JAMA 2006;295(2):172–9.

54. Perrier A, Roy PM, Sanchez O, et al. Multidetector-row computed tomography in suspected pulmonary embolism. N Engl J Med 2005;352(17):1760–8.

55. Value of the ventilation/perfusion scan in acute pulmonary embolism. Results of the Prospective Investigation of Pulmonary Embolism Diagnosis (PIOPED). The PIOPED Investigators. JAMA 1990; 263(20):2753–9.

56. Righini M, Aujesky D, Roy PM, et al. Clinical usefulness of D-dimer depending on clinical probability and cutoff value in outpatients with suspected pulmonary embolism. Arch Intern Med 2004;164(22):2483–7.

57. Ghuysen A, Ghaye B, Willems V, et al. Computed tomographic pulmonary angiography and prognostic significance in patients with acute pulmonary embolism. Thorax 2005;60(11):956–61.

58. Gosselin MV, Rassner UA, Thieszen SL, et al. Contrast dynamics during CT pulmonary angiogram: analysis of an inspiration associated artifact. J Thorac Imaging 2004;19(1):1–7.

59. Kerl JM, Lehnert T, Schell B, et al. Intravenous contrast material administration at high-pitch dual-source CT pulmonary angiography: test bolus versus bolus-tracking technique. Eur J Radiol 2011. [Epub ahead of print].

60. Ghaye B, Szapiro D, Mastora I, et al. Peripheral pulmonary arteries: how far in the lung does multi-detector row spiral CT allow analysis? Radiology 2001;219(3):629–36.

61. Greess H, Wolf H, Baum U, et al. Dose reduction in computed tomography by attenuation-based on-line modulation of tube current: evaluation of six anatomical regions. Eur Radiol 2000;10(2):391–4.

62. Heyer CM, Mohr PS, Lemburg SP, et al. Image quality and radiation exposure at pulmonary CT angiography with 100- or 120-kVp protocol: prospective randomized study. Radiology 2007;245(2):577–83.

63. Araoz PA, Gotway MB, Harrington JR, et al. Pulmonary embolism: prognostic CT findings. Radiology 2007;242(3):889–97.

64. Ghaye B, Ghuysen A, Willems V, et al. Severe pulmonary embolism: pulmonary artery clot load scores and cardiovascular parameters as predictors of mortality. Radiology 2006;239(3):884–91.

65. Mansencal N, Joseph T, Vieillard-Baron A, et al. Diagnosis of right ventricular dysfunction in acute pulmonary embolism using helical computed tomography. Am J Cardiol 2005;95(10):1260–3.

66. Quiroz R, Kucher N, Schoepf UJ, et al. Right ventricular enlargement on chest computed tomography: prognostic role in acute pulmonary embolism. Circulation 2004;109(20):2401–4.

67. Schoepf UJ, Kucher N, Kipfmueller F, et al. Right ventricular enlargement on chest computed tomography: a predictor of early death in acute pulmonary embolism. Circulation 2004;110(20):3276–80.

68. van der Meer RW, Pattynama PM, van Strijen MJ, et al. Right ventricular dysfunction and pulmonary obstruction index at helical CT: prediction of clinical outcome during 3-month follow-up in patients with acute pulmonary embolism. Radiology 2005; 235(3):798–803.

69. Dogan H, Kroft LJ, Huisman MV, et al. Right ventricular function in patients with acute pulmonary embolism: analysis with electrocardiography-synchronized multi-detector row CT. Radiology 2007;242(1):78–84.

70. Henzler T, Krissak R, Reichert M, et al. Volumetric analysis of pulmonary CTA for the assessment of right ventricular dysfunction in patients with acute pulmonary embolism. Acad Radiol 2010;17(3):309–15.

71. Collomb D, Paramelle PJ, Calaque O, et al. Severity assessment of acute pulmonary embolism: evaluation using helical CT. Eur Radiol 2003;13(7):1508–14.

72. Contractor S, Maldjian PD, Sharma VK, et al. Role of helical CT in detecting right ventricular dysfunction secondary to acute pulmonary embolism. J Comput Assist Tomogr 2002;26(4):587–91.

73. Lim KE, Chan CY, Chu PH, et al. Right ventricular dysfunction secondary to acute massive pulmonary embolism detected by helical computed tomography pulmonary angiography. Clin Imaging 2005;29(1):16–21.

74. Gosselin MV, Rubin GD. Altered intravascular contrast material flow dynamics: clues for refining thoracic CT diagnosis. AJR Am J Roentgenol 1997;169(6):1597–603.

75. He H, Stein MW, Zalta B, et al. Computed tomography evaluation of right heart dysfunction in patients with acute pulmonary embolism. J Comput Assist Tomogr 2006;30(2):262–6.

76. Araoz PA, Gotway MB, Trowbridge RL, et al. Helical CT pulmonary angiography predictors of in-hospital morbidity and mortality in patients with acute pulmonary embolism. J Thorac Imaging 2003;18(4):207–16.

77. Kang DK, Thilo C, Schoepf UJ, et al. CT signs of right ventricular dysfunction: prognostic role in acute pulmonary embolism. JACC Cardiovasc Imaging 2011;4(8):841–9.

78. Flohr TG, McCollough CH, Bruder H, et al. First performance evaluation of a dual-source CT (DSCT) system. Eur Radiol 2006;16(2):256–68.

79. Riederer SJ, Kruger RA, Mistretta CA. Limitations to iodine isolation using a dual beam non-K-edge approach. Med Phys 1981;8(1):54–61.

80. Fink C, Johnson TR, Michaely HJ, et al. Dual-energy CT angiography of the lung in patients with

suspected pulmonary embolism: initial results. Rofo 2008;180(10):879–83.

81. Chae EJ, Seo JB, Jang YM, et al. Dual-energy CT for assessment of the severity of acute pulmonary embolism: pulmonary perfusion defect score compared with CT angiographic obstruction score and right ventricular/left ventricular diameter ratio. AJR Am J Roentgenol 2010;194(3):604–10.

82. Schoepf UJ, Bruening R, Konschitzky H, et al. Pulmonary embolism: comprehensive diagnosis by using electron-beam CT for detection of emboli and assessment of pulmonary blood flow. Radiology 2000;217(3):693–700.

83. Thieme SF, Becker CR, Hacker M, et al. Dual energy CT for the assessment of lung perfusion–correlation to scintigraphy. Eur J Radiol 2008; 68(3):369–74.

84. Thieme SF, Johnson TR, Lee C, et al. Dual-energy CT for the assessment of contrast material distribution in the pulmonary parenchyma. AJR Am J Roentgenol 2009;193(1):144–9.

85. Pontana F, Faivre JB, Remy-Jardin M, et al. Lung perfusion with dual-energy multidetector-row CT (MDCT): feasibility for the evaluation of acute pulmonary embolism in 117 consecutive patients. Acad Radiol 2008;15(12):1494–504.

86. Nikolaou K, Thieme S, Sommer W, et al. Diagnosing pulmonary embolism: new computed tomography applications. J Thorac Imaging 2010;25(2):151–60.

87. Johnson TR, Nikolaou K, Becker A, et al. Dual-source CT for chest pain assessment. Eur Radiol 2008;18(4):773–80.

88. Bamberg F, Marcus R, Sommer W, et al. Diagnostic image quality of a comprehensive high-pitch dual-spiral cardiothoracic CT protocol in patients with undifferentiated acute chest pain. Eur J Radiol 2010. [Epub ahead of print].

89. Takakuwa KM, Halpern EJ. Evaluation of a "triple rule-out" coronary CT angiography protocol: use of 64-section CT in low-to-moderate risk emergency department patients suspected of having acute coronary syndrome. Radiology 2008;248(2):438–46.

Cardiac CT in the Emergency Department

Harald Seifarth, MD[a,b], Christopher L. Schlett, MD, MPH[a],
Quynh A. Truong, MD, MPH[a], Udo Hoffmann, MD, MPH[a,*]

KEYWORDS

- Cardiac computed tomography • Emergency department
- Acute coronary syndrome • Triage

Each year more than 6 million patients suffering from chest pain are admitted to the emergency department (ED) in the United States, making it one of the most common causes of ED visits. Of these patients, less than 20% or roughly 1.5 million are diagnosed with a primary or secondary acute coronary syndrome (ACS). On the other hand, the diagnosis is missed in about 2% to 3% of patients.[1–4] It is thus evident that current triage strategies are not optimal in identifying patients suffering from ACS. The diagnostic workup of patients presenting with acute chest pain continues to represent a major challenge for ED personnel. This statement holds especially true for patients with a low to intermediate likelihood for ACS.[5] Taking current concepts for the diagnosis and management of patients presenting with acute chest pain to the ED into account, this article discusses the evidence and potential role of coronary computed tomography (CT) angiography (CCTA) to improve management of patients with possible ACS.

DEFINITION OF ACS

ACS is a clinical syndrome and comprises a spectrum of diagnoses including unstable angina pectoris (UAP), myocardial infarction (MI) without ST-segment elevation (NSTEMI), and MI with ST-segment elevation (STEMI).[6] Although the physiologic substrate for all 3 syndromes is myocardial ischemia, there are important differences. STEMI is defined by increase of markers of myocardial necrosis, in particular troponin T greater than the 99th percentile of a normal population, in conjunction with an ST-segment increase in resting electrocardiography (ECG). In NSTEMI, there is no associated ST increase but biomarkers have the typical "rise and fall" pattern (Table 1). When neither electrocardiographic changes nor biomarkers are increased, but the clinical syndrome is consistent with coronary artery disease (CAD) with documentation of ischemia on noninvasive testing, such as provocative stress testing, or a hemodynamically significant stenotic lesion by cardiac catheterization, then UAP continues the spectrum of ACS.[7] ACS is associated with an increased risk of subsequent MI and cardiac death within 30 days. The individual risk of a patient can be estimated using the TIMI (Thrombolysis in Myocardial Infarction) score.[7]

PATHOPHYSIOLOGY OF ACS

Almost all cases of ACS are related to preexistent atherosclerotic lesions of the coronary arteries and occur when the supply of oxygen to the myocardium is inadequate compared with the demand. The predominant cause of myocardial ischemia is rupture of an atherosclerotic plaque ($\approx 60\%$) followed by plaque erosion ($\approx 40\%$) and rarely a superficial calcified nodule ($\approx 5\%$).[8,9] In STEMI, these events usually lead to the formation of

[a] Cardiac MR PET CT Program, Harvard Medical School, Massachusetts General Hospital, 165 Cambridge Street, Boston, MA 02114, USA
[b] Department of Clinical Radiology, University of Münster, Albert-Schweitzer-Campus 1, 48149 Münster, Germany
* Corresponding author. Cardiac MR PET CT Program, Harvard Medical School, Massachusetts General Hospital, 165 Cambridge Street, Boston, MA 02114.
E-mail address: uhoffmann@partners.org

Cardiol Clin 30 (2012) 117–133
doi:10.1016/j.ccl.2011.12.001
0733-8651/12/$ – see front matter © 2012 Elsevier Inc. All rights reserved.

Table 1
Definition of ACS according to American College of Cardiology/American Heart Association guidelines

	STEMI	NSTEMI	UAP
ECG	New ST elevation >0.2 mV in men or 0.1 mV in women in at least 2 anatomically contiguous leads or T-wave inversion >0.1 mm in at least 2 contiguous precordial leads with prominent R-waves	Prominent ST-segment depression or unspecific changes	
Troponin	Serial levels of cardiac troponins >99 percentile	Serial levels of cardiac troponins increased	Negative cardiac troponins possible
MI	Q-wave MI > Non-Q-wave MI	Non-Q-wave MI > Q-wave MI	No infarction

Data from Wright RS, Anderson JL, Adams CD, et al. 2011 ACCF/AHA Focused Update Incorporated Into the ACC/AHA 2007 Guidelines for the Management of Patients with Unstable Angina/Non–ST-Elevation Myocardial Infarction. J Am Coll Cardiol 2011;57(19):e215–367; and Thygesen K, Alpert JS, White HD. Joint ESC/ACCF/AHA/WHF Task Force for the Redefinition of Myocardial Infarction. Universal definition of myocardial infarction. J Am Coll Cardiol 2007;50(22):2173–95.

a luminal thrombus, reducing or blocking blood flow to the distal coronary segments.[8] Before the event, these lesions do not cause a significant narrowing of the coronary vessel in nearly 60% of patients.[10,11] UAP or NSTEMI is usually caused by a thrombus that does not completely block the lumen. This thrombus can intermittently wax and wane and even become occlusive for a short period, which explains the inconsistent symptoms.[11] Other mechanisms include embolization of thrombus particles distal from the rupture site, vasospasm caused by local vasoconstrictors (eg, thromboxane A_2) released form the rupture site, or a severe coronary stenosis caused by progressive atherosclerosis.[12] In contrast, STEMI is typically caused by an occlusion of an epicardial coronary artery.[6]

Other factors that contribute to the signs and symptoms of ACS are the location of the stenosis, the size of the dependent myocardial territory, the level of myocardial metabolism, coagulatory state of the blood as well as the presence of collateral blood flow because of preexisting CAD.[13–17]

Less common causes of ACS include CAD other than atherosclerosis, vasospasm, embolization to the coronary arteries from other sources than plaque, or hematologic conditions leading to a hypercoagulatory state of the blood.[15] These conditions are believed to cause roughly 3% of ACS, usually in young patients.[18,19]

CURRENT DIAGNOSTIC PATHWAYS AND MANAGEMENT OF PATIENTS PRESENTING TO THE ED WITH SUSPICION OF ACS

Current guidelines recommend the stratification of patients presenting with symptoms suggestive of ACS into 4 categories: (1) noncardiac cause of chest pain, (2) chronic stable angina, (3) possible ACS, and (4) definite ACS.[20] After an initial assessment of the vital signs the likelihood that the patient is suffering from ACS is determined according to the patient's history, physical examination, initial 12-lead electrocardiogram, and presence of increased cardiac biomarkers (**Fig. 1**).[20] However, no single test or risk score exists that allows the reliable stratification of patients and safe discharge of patients without further testing. Risk scores, such as the widely used TIMI score or the Goldman score, can predict the 1-year mortality in patients with ACS; however, sensitivity for prediction of ACS in a low-risk group is poor and even in the lowest-risk group a considerable but short-term mortality has been reported.[21–23] The use of biomarkers of myocardial injury and necrosis such as troponin I, troponin T, or CK-MB to rule out MI provides only delayed assessment because the blood levels of these markers exceed physiologic levels typically within 3 to 8 hours after the event.[15] Serial measurement of cardiac biomarkers significantly improves the sensitivity of this test to 95%.[5] Cardiac biomarkers can be increased because of noncoronary conditions that may lead to myocardial necrosis, such as myocarditis and congestive heart failure, especially in patients with renal disease.[24]

Accordingly the 12-lead electrocardiogram still serves as a hallmark for the decision pathway because it is readily available and offers a relatively high negative predictive value for severe CAD. However, even a normal electrocardiogram does not completely exclude ACS.[7,25–27] Current guidelines suggest the combination of both biomarkers and electrocardiographic testing in patients with symptoms suggestive of ACS.[7] Recently, high sensitive assays for myocardial biomarkers have

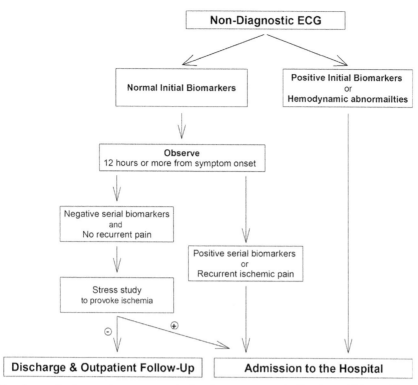

Fig. 1. Algorithm for evaluation and management of patients suspected of having ACS but with a nondiagnostic electrocardiogram according to the current American College of Cardiology/American Heart Association guidelines for unstable angina/NSTEMI. Patients present with possible ACS but are pain free at the time of presentation to the ED. (*Modified from* Wright RS, Anderson JL, Adams CD, et al. 2011 ACCF/AHA Focused Update Incorporated Into the ACC/AHA 2007 Guidelines for the Management of Patients with Unstable Angina/Non–ST-Elevation Myocardial Infarction. J Am Coll Cardiol 2011;57(19):e227; with permission.)

been introduced that offer a high sensitivity at the expense of lower specificity for the detection of MI even at baseline.[7,28,29] However, the clinical role of high-sensitivity troponin assays compared with the standard assays remains unclear. Because of the lack of an effective initial triage tool, dedicated chest pain units have been established in many EDs that accommodate patients until MI is definitely excluded and a provocative stress test can be performed to exclude myocardial ischemia.[30,31] The aim of these units is to define the presence or absence of myocardial ischemia and to further stratify between NSTEMI and unstable angina. Usually, this decision should be reached within 6 to 12 hours. Apart from serial ECG and biomarker measurements, a further diagnostic test is recommended to rule out myocardial ischemia.[7] The use of chest pain units can reduce the number of missed MIs but it also leads to a 10% increase of patients undergoing testing to rule out MI compared with in-hospital testing.[32,33] The current guidelines recommend several provocative testing strategies.[7] Patients with a low to intermediate risk of MI who are capable of exercise and free of

confounding features on the baseline electrocardiogram (eg, bundle branch block, left ventricular (LV) hypertrophy, and paced rhythms) can undergo symptom-limited treadmill testing.

Initial concerns about possible hazards of the treadmill test for potentially unstable patients were proved wrong.[34] A study of 1000 patients with chest pain and a low risk of MI found positive results for ischemia in only 13% and negative results in 64%; however, the test was nondiagnostic in 23% of patients.[35] Because of the high negative predictive value of 89% confirmed by other studies, the test was incorporated into the 2002 guidelines of the American College of Cardiology/American Heart Association for management of patents with non–ST-segment elevation ACS.[36–38] However, the rate of nondiagnostic tests remains problematic. In the study mentioned earlier, further diagnostic testing was required in 34% of patients with a nondiagnostic treadmill test.

For patients unable to exercise or with an uninterpretable baseline electrocardiogram, pharmacologic stress imaging should be considered. For this purpose nuclear perfusion imaging, echocardiography, or magnetic resonance imaging (MRI) can be performed. Among these modalities, single-photon emission tomography (SPECT) is the most commonly used test.

SPECT imaging can be performed at rest, and several studies have shown the ability of rest SPECT to detect significant coronary artery stenosis with a sensitivity exceeding 90% and a specificity between 70% and 80% compared with invasive coronary angiography.[39–41] A large randomized trial of 2475 patients confirmed these results.[42] Patients were randomized to receive usual care with or without an additional rest SPECT. Sensitivity of the 2 approaches was similar (96% and 97%), but patients without acute ischemia in the SPECT arm had a significantly lower hospitalization rate (42% vs 52%). Despite these results, SPECT imaging at rest has limitations, the most important being the inability to differentiate between old and new perfusion defects. Furthermore, SPECT imaging at rest is most sensitive when a patient is experiencing ischemic symptoms and should therefore be performed within 2 hours of symptom resolution.[43] Accordingly current guidelines recommend stress SPECT to exclude CAD if serial ECG and biomarkers are nondiagnostic.[44] This approach has been shown to increase the diagnostic accuracy of the test.[45] In case of nondiagnostic exercise studies (<85% of maximal heart rate achieved) the conversion to a pharmacologic stress test is recommended. The major drawback of SPECT imaging is the radiation exposure of the patients. Using sestamibi, an average effective dose of 10.7 mSv has been reported, with tetrofosmin, the average effective dose is reported to be 8.6 mSv, which is higher than the effective dose resulting from diagnostic invasive coronary angiograms.[46,47] Furthermore, this test is time consuming ($\approx$120 minutes for a complete stress SPECT) and generally not available around the clock.

Similar to SPECT, stress echocardiography provides added information to the evaluation at rest.[48] This technique was reported to have a high negative predictive value (98.8%). While echocardiography at rest is easy to perform, stress echocardiography requires experienced sonographers and physicians and thus it is often not available around the clock.

The third technique available for functional imaging is MRI. Although early studies revealed a high sensitivity and specificity for the detection of NSTEMI and unstable angina, the long examination times and the fact that MRI is not readily available in most centers prevent the technique from being used more frequently.[49] Current guidelines rate perfusion MRI appropriate in patients with suspicion of ACS in whom the electrocardiogram is not interpretable or who are unable to exercise.[50] Recent data show that perfusion MRI is superior to SPECT for detection of CAD in vessels more than 2 mm in diameter.[51] Plein and colleagues[52] found a sensitivity for the detection of significant CAD of 96% with a specificity of 83%. The specificity can be further increased by adding a T2-weighted sequence for assessment of the LV wall.[53]

THE ROLE OF CT IN THE ED

Compared with the imaging modalities mentioned earlier, coronary CT does not routinely provide functional or perfusion data. Recent studies have shown the feasibility of CT perfusion imaging with CT; however, the main focus of CT imaging remains the visualization of the coronary artery tree.[54] Since the introduction of 64-slice CT in 2003, numerous studies on CCTA have been published. A recent meta-analysis reports a very good sensitivity of CCTA for the detection of significant coronary artery stenosis.[55] This finding is also reflected by the fact that CCTA has been added to the European guidelines on diagnosis and management of ACS as a tool for the exclusion of relevant CAD.[7] CCTA has been judged to be useful for evaluation of obstructive CAD in symptomatic patients (class IIa, level of evidence: B) and appropriate for acute chest pain evaluation in patients with a low to intermediate pretest probability of CAD when initial serial ECG and biomarkers are negative.[50,56]

Compared with the imaging methods described earlier, CCTA is generally less time consuming. Modern CT scanners allow for short examination times with the whole imaging process, including patient setup rarely exceeding 20 minutes. The scanners offer a temporal resolution of less than 200 ms, which allows the reliable assessment of the coronary arteries in patients with a heart rate up to 65 bpm.[57,58] Scanners equipped with 2 tube/detector systems offer an even better temporal resolution of less than 90 ms, accommodating for heart rates up to 80 bpm.[59,60] In patients presenting with higher heart rates, a heart rate reduction can be achieved with either oral or intravenous β-blocker. For oral administration either metoprolol or atenolol are recommended 1 hour before the examination; for intravenous administration metoprolol is recommended.[61] Intravenous injection should be performed under electrocardiographic monitoring in 5-mg increments up to a maximum dose of 30 mg.

Diagnostic Accuracy of CCTA in the Diagnosis of ACS

The good performance of CT in detecting coronary artery stenosis and the wide availability of this technology have led to widespread use in the triage of patients with chest pain presenting to the ED.

Several studies comprising more than 1600 patients have been published using dedicated CCTA in the triage of patients presenting to the ED (Table 2).[62–68]

Gallagher and colleagues[63] compared CT with stress myocardial perfusion imaging. Of 92 patients with negative biomarkers and serial ECG in the study, 8% were excluded because of insufficient image quality in CT. In the remaining 85 patients, both CT and stress SPECT were performed. The sensitivity to detect patients with a significant coronary stenosis was 71% for perfusion imaging and 86% for CT. Both techniques had a high negative predictive value (97% for perfusion imaging and 99% for CT).

Goldstein and colleagues[64] published a randomized controlled trial comparing CCTA strategy in assessing patients with chest pain who were deemed low risk after initial ECG and biomarker tests with standard of care (SOC), including serial electrocardiograms and cardiac biomarkers at 4 and 8 hours after the baseline examination as well as a SPECT stress study. The CT-based strategy had a similar diagnostic accuracy compared with the SOC, but reduced diagnostic time compared with SOC (3.4 vs 15.0 hours). On the other hand, the CTA strategy led to a higher number of diagnostic cardiac catheterizations, and 24 of 99 patients had either "stenosis of unclear significance" (25%–70%) or unevaluable segments requiring a stress myocardial perfusion scan, 21 of which showed no perfusion defects. The main reason was likely because of the inclusion of patients with intermediate stenosis, many of whom were found to have nonhemodynamically significant disease. Patients in the CT arm of the study required fewer reevaluations for recurrent chest pain (2% vs 7% in the SOC arm).

The CT-STAT (Coronary Computed Tomographic Angiography for Systematic Triage of Acute Chest Pain Patients to Treatment) trial, a recent multicenter trial by Goldstein and colleagues,[65] studied 699 patients with chest pain, a low to intermediate likelihood of ACS and negative ECG and initial biomarkers. Similar to the study mentioned earlier, patients either received the SOC including a rest-stress SPECT or CCTA. The CT-based strategy reduced the time to diagnosis compared with the SOC by more than 50% (2.9 vs 6.2 hours). Coronary CT was also associated with a smaller radiation exposure compared with SPECT.

Hollander and colleagues[66] studied 568 patients presenting to the ED with chest pain. Patients had a nonischemic initial electrocardiogram and a TIMI risk score of 2 or lower. CTA was negative or showed nonobstructive lesions in 476 (84%) patients, and those patients were discharged from the ED (Fig. 2). None of these patients had a major adverse cardiac event (MACE) within a follow-up period of 30 days. The investigators conclude that patients can be safely discharged home after a negative CCTA.

The ROMICAT (Rule Out Myocardial Infarction using Computer Assisted Tomography) trial published in 2009 studied 368 patients presenting to the ED with chest pain.[67] The study compared the blinded results of CCTA with the standard of care, thus removing the bias of how the results from CCTA could have influenced patient management. Fifty percent of patients were free of CAD and none of these patients had an ACS. Both the extent of coronary plaque and the presence of stenosis predicted ACS independently and incrementally to the TIMI risk score (area under the curve: 0.88, 0.82, vs 0.63, respectively).

Prognosis of CT for MACE During Follow-up

Although these studies show the good performance of CCTA in the acute setting by reliably detecting patients without significant CAD, several studies also report a good prognostic value for CCTA in patients presenting to the ED with chest pain. Two of the trials mentioned earlier also report data on follow-up. In the CT-STAT trial a similarly low rate of MACE was found in both arms for patients with normal results (0.8% for CCTA vs 0.4% for SOC) after a follow-up of 6 months.[65] In the ROMICAT trial, none of the 183 patients with normal CCTA results during index hospitalization developed MACE after a follow-up of 6 months.[67] In the long-term follow-up of this trial Schlett and colleagues[69] report absence of MACE in patients without plaque after a follow-up of 2 years.

Nasis and colleagues[68] studied 203 patients presenting to the ED with chest pain with negative ECG and initial biomarkers. Of these patients, 32% had normal CTA findings and were immediately released from the hospital. After a mean follow-up of 14 months no patient in this group was readmitted to a hospital for recurrent chest pain.

Hollander and colleagues[70] published 1-year outcome data. In 481 patients in whom CTA was negative or showed nonobstructive lesions, there was no MACE and only 1 death of unclear cause (0.2%).

Data from these studies suggest that CCTA can be used to safely rule out significant CAD in patients presenting to the ED with chest pain but in whom initial ECG and biomarkers are negative. This finding is consistent with the results from several studies on the outcome after CCTA in

Table 2
Summary of studies evaluating the diagnostic performance of CCTA in patients presenting with acute chest pain

	Year	Study Type	N	Patients	Outcome of Interest	Prev (%)	CT Criteria	Sens (%)	Spec (%)	NPV (%)	PPV (%)
Gallagher et al[63]	2007	Clinical practice algorithm	85	49 ± 11 y, 53% male	Sig stenosis in ICA or MACE at 30 d	8	Sig stenosis	86	92	99	50
Goldstein et al[64]	2007	Randomized diagnostic trial	99[a]	48 ± 11 y, 43% male	Sig stenosis in ICA or MACE at 6 mo	8	Sig stenosis	100	97	100	73
Rubinshtein et al[62]	2007	Clinical practice algorithm	58	56 ± 10 y, 64% male	ACS during index hospitalization	34	Sig stenosis	100	92	100	87
Hoffmann et al[67]	2009	Observational study	368	53 ± 12 y, 61% male	ACS during index hospitalization	8	Sig stenosis Plaque	77 100	87 54	98 100	35 17

Abbreviations: NPV, negative predictive value; PPV, positive predictive value; Prev, prevalence; Sens, sensitivity; Sig stenosis, stenosis >50%; Spec, specificity.
[a] Number of individuals in the CT arm.

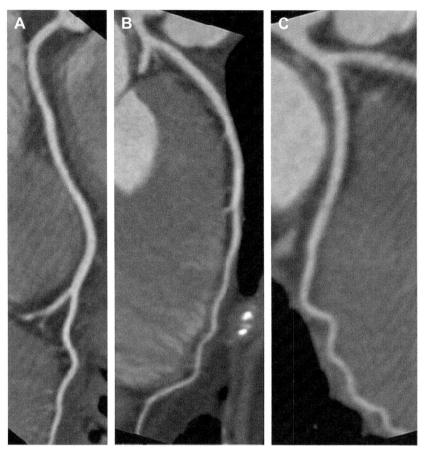

Fig. 2. 52-year-old man presenting to the ED with atypical chest pain. Initial biomarkers and ECG were normal. The CCTA showed no atherosclerotic disease so the patient was dismissed from the hospital. A follow-up telephone call revealed no further episode of chest pain. (*A*) Right coronary artery, (*B*) LAD artery, (*C*) Left circumflex artery.

patients with suspected CAD but without the standardized diagnostic pathway described earlier. A recent meta-analysis of 18 studies with a median follow-up of 20 months found an annualized event rate of only 0.17% in patients with normal CCTA findings.[71] Using CCTA in patients with chest pain and a low risk of having an ACS after initial screening has also been shown to significantly reduce the length of the hospital stay and to reduce costs.[65]

On the other end of the spectrum of CAD, the presence of severe stenosis on CCTA is not necessarily related to ACS. Regarding short-term outcomes, the ROMICAT trial showed that 34 patients had a significant stenosis on CCTA, but only 20 were diagnosed with ACS (**Figs. 3** and **4**).[67] In the trial by Hollander and colleagues[66] only 7 of 54 patients with a stenosis greater than 50% had a stenosis on invasive coronary angiography (ICA) or a MACE within 30 days. Thus, the positive predictive value of CCTA in patients with chest pain remains low; however, it increases significantly when more than 1 stenosis is found.[67] The low

positive predictive value of stenosis has been confirmed by other studies. This finding also holds true for the long-term outcomes. In the meta-analysis mentioned earlier, 2772 patients had obstructive lesions in CT, whereas a MACE was reported in only 381 patients (13.7%), corresponding to an annual event rate of 8.8%.[71] A second meta-analysis confirms these results, reporting an event rate of 6.8% in more than 3600 patients with a follow-up of more than 12 months. Thus, presence of obstructive lesions detected by CT alone should not trigger invasive coronary angiography in patients with acute chest pain.

Data for short-term outcome in patients with intermediate stenosis are scarce. Nasis and colleagues[68] studied 203 patients with chest pain presenting to the ED. Of these patients, 4 had a stenosis between 50% and 70% on CT. All patients had either negative primary or serial troponin and none had ACS. Hollander and colleagues[66] found intermediate stenosis in CT in 41 of 562 patients, of whom only 1 was found to have significant

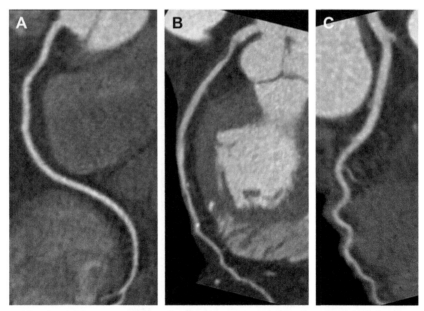

Fig. 3. 78-year-old male patient presenting to the ED after repeated episodes of atypical chest pain. Initial serum biomarkers were normal, but ECG revealed unspecific changes of the T-wave. CCTA showed a large noncalcified plaque in the proximal LAD artery. The right coronary artery and circumflex artery revealed no atherosclerotic plaques. The patient was admitted to the hospital. A SPECT study on the next day revealed no signs of ischemia and normal LV function parameters. Serial biomarkers remained normal. The patient was subsequently discharged with intensified lipid-lowering therapy. (A) Right coronary artery, (B) LAD artery, (C) Left circumflex artery.

disease in ICA. Regarding long-term follow-up, MACE was observed in only 90 of 3185 (2.8%) patients with nonobstructive CAD on CCTA, corresponding to an annualized event rate of 1.4%.[71] Even with a longer follow-up, these numbers remain stable. Sozzi and colleagues[72] followed patients for 5 years after CCTA and reported an annual event rate of 1.2% for patients with nonobstructive disease.

An approach to increase the diagnostic performance of CT in patients with suspected ACS is the integration of cardiac function calculated from the CT examination. This approach is useful both for the diagnosis of ACS as well as for predicting outcomes. In a study including 356 patients with suspected ACS, impaired LV function increased the sensitivity of CCTA to detect ACS by 10%. This approach proved especially valuable in patients with significant stenosis.[73] Data from the CONFIRM registry suggest that a reduced LV ejection fraction (LVEF) of less than 50% incrementally predicts mortality in patients with suspected CAD. Data on LVEF were especially useful in patients with an intermediate risk of having CAD based on clinical variables.[74] These findings were confirmed by other studies.[75,76]

These data suggest that additional studies are needed to make CT an effective tool not only for triage but also to determine appropriate management in patients with CAD. Data from patients

with stable chest pain syndrome suggest that several other factors such as location of CAD and plaque composition may provide incremental value. Similar to the results from older studies using invasive coronary angiography, the strongest predictors of MACE besides the detection of hemodynamically relevant stenosis seem to be obstructive lesions in the left main artery or the proximal left anterior descending (LAD) artery and the number of vessel and segments with disease.[77–80] In contrast to invasive angiography, which can show only the lumen of a coronary artery and offers little information about the morphology of a stenosis, CCTA also allows the evaluation of the vessel wall and to a certain extent the evaluation of the plaque that causes the narrowing of the lumen. This characteristic is of great importance because the processes within the atherosclerotic plaque are responsible for the course of the disease.

POTENTIAL NEW IMAGING TARGETS FOR CT IN PATIENTS PRESENTING WITH ACS

As stated earlier, in most cases the trigger for ACS is rupture of an atherosclerotic plaque. These rupture-prone lesions have been shown to possess distinct features both in histology as well as in invasive imaging techniques. First described by Allen Burke in 1997, the thin fibrous cap fibroatheromas

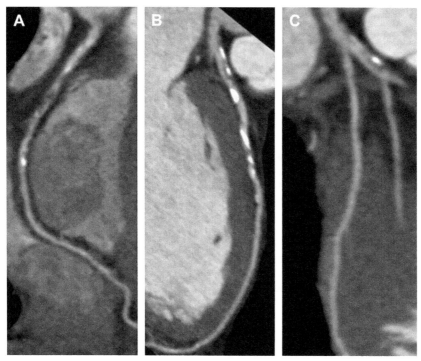

Fig. 4. 47-year-old male patient presenting to the ED with repeated episodes of chest pain after exertion. The initial electrocardiogram was nondiagnostic and initial serum biomarkers were normal. The CCTA revealed a severe stenosis of the mid right coronary artery (RCA) with possible thrombus distal to the stenosis. A second severe stenosis was found in the proximal LAD artery and mild calcified plaques in the mid-LAD artery. The left circumflex artery showed minor wall irregularities. The patient was subsequently transferred to invasive angiography, which confirmed both the severe stenosis and the thrombus in the RCA. The lesion in the LAD artery was rated moderate. After the diagnostic angiography, a stent was placed in the RCA. (*A*) RCA, (*B*) LAD artery, (*C*) Left circumflex artery.

(TCFAs) show a fibrous cap with a thickness of less than 65 μm overlying a large lipid-rich core.[81] The thin fibrous cap can be detected using optical coherence tomography; however, because of the inferior spatial resolution, this feature cannot be detected in intravenous ultrasonography (IVUS) or CCTA.[82–84] In contrast, the lipid core offers a potential target for other imaging modalities. Virmani and colleagues[85] report in a series comprising 400 patients who died of sudden cardiac death that in ruptured plaques, the lipid/necrotic core was larger than 1 mm² and comprised more than 25% of the plaque area in most patients. Although the lipid core is reported to be smaller in TCFAs, it can still be reliably detected using invasive imaging modalities.[84,86] It was recognized early that using CCTA, the spectrum of lesions in patients presenting with ACS is different from patients with stable CAD. Lesions in ACS are predominantly noncalcified, whereas lesions in patients with stable CAD tend to be calcific.[87] Initial reports on CT imaging of coronary atherosclerotic plaques were optimistic about the ability of CT to further differentiate the noncalcified lesions into lipid-rich plaques, potentially at risk of rupture and fibrotic and thus

more stable plaques.[88,89] However, recent studies stated that the reliable differentiation of these plaque types based on the measurement of the mean density is not possible because of significant overlap of the Hounsfield unit (HU) values between the different plaque types.[90] Therefore, researchers have sought to find different approaches to identify high-risk markers of plaques in patients presenting with ACS. One group reported that histogram analysis of the density values can be used to distinguish lipid-rich plaques from fibrous plaques compared with IVUS.[91] Other groups have used multiple, small regions of interest to assess the minimum HU values within the plaque.[92,93] Using this technique a cutoff value of less than 40 HU has been shown to yield sufficient accuracy to distinguish lipid-rich plaques.[91–97]

Over the years several more features have been described that are either commonly found in rupture-prone plaques or are even believed to increase the risk for rupture; the current concept of identifying lesions with a high risk of rupture takes several of these features into account. During progression from early into advanced stages of atherosclerosis most plaques undergo positive remodeling.[98] The diameter of the outer vessel increases, whereas the diameter of the lumen remains nearly unchanged. Several studies using invasive imaging techniques have shown that remodeling is more extensive in plaques at increased risk of rupture.[99–101] This concept has been adapted for CCTA. Hoffmann and colleagues[102] showed that culprit lesions in patients presenting with ACS had increased arterial remodeling compared with nonculprit lesions as defined by invasive angiography. Similar results were reported by Motoyama and colleagues.[96] In a previous study, the same investigators found that the presence of spotty calcifications (ie, calcifications with a maximum size of <3 mm) within a plaque is associated with a higher incidence of ACS.[103] This finding was confirmed by several other invasive and noninvasive studies.[93,104,105] Initial reports state that a direct visualization of the lipid core is possible in some patients using high-resolution CT.[106] These plaques show a hypodense center surrounded by a rim of denser tissue. This ringlike pattern seems to be strongly associated with advanced atherosclerotic plaques and culprit lesions in ACS and is possibly caused by neovascularization of the tissue surrounding the necrotic core of advanced lesions.[95,107,108]

Potential plaque features that can be detected using CCTA in patients with chest pain that might help to identify individuals with a high risk of developing ACS are positive arterial remodeling, the presence of hypodense plaque components, or even the direct visualization of the lipid core and the presence of spotty calcifications.

No data are available on the long-term outcome of patients in whom these features have been detected; however, data do exist on simple plaque characteristics such as noncalcified and mixed plaque. In a study by Min and colleagues,[109] the presence of mixed plaque was associated with the highest likelihood of MACE within a follow-up period of 22 months compared with calcified or purely noncalcified plaque in symptomatic patients. Other studies confirm these results, although the reported odds ratios are smaller.[78,79,110] In all 4 studies, the strongest predictor for MACE was the presence of a significant stenosis in the CCTA scan.

Although further studies are needed to assess the prognostic information of plaque composition detected with CT, data from invasive modalities show that plaque features can predict the outcome in patients with coronary atherosclerosis. The PROSPECT trial published in 2011 included nearly 700 patients undergoing percutaneous coronary intervention. In these patients, nonculprit lesions were assessed using intravascular ultrasound. Plaques responsible for recurrent ACS were associated with a large plaque burden (>70%) at baseline and a small minimal luminal area.[111]

CT Protocols

Most studies using CCTA for the diagnosis of CAD have used an imaging protocol dedicated for imaging the heart and the coronary arteries. Generally, the scan length is tailored to the heart, with the scan starting just above the ostia of the coronary arteries and stretching to the diaphragm. To optimize the spatial resolution in the image, the field of view (FOV) is reduced to the heart.

In contrast, some studies have suggested the use of a so-called triple rule-out protocol that not only allows the assessment of the coronary arteries but also the exclusion of pulmonary embolism and acute aortic syndrome (AAS) as well as other potential causes of chest pain such as pulmonary infiltrates. Although the available data suggest that this approach is feasible, it is consistently associated with a higher radiation exposure because of the longer scan range.[112,113] Furthermore, it has been shown that the use of a triple rule-out protocol compared with a dedicated CCTA scan led to an increased number of additional pulmonary CT angiography scans.[113] Lee and colleagues[114] showed in a retrospective study with 103 patients that most (101 of 103) relevant pulmonary emboli can be identified within the FOV and scan range of the dedicated scan. The same study evaluated 50 patients with AAS. None of the features of AAS such as aortic dissection or intramural hematoma was missed in the FOV or scan range of the dedicated cardiac scan. Madder and colleagues[113] compared the 90-day outcome between dedicated CCTA and the triple rule-out protocol in more than 2000 patients and found no differences between the 2 approaches. Thus it can be concluded that a dedicated CCTA scan can safely be used to assess patients presenting with chest pain and suspicion of ACS.

DOSE ISSUES

Initial reports on CCTA using retrospectively gated 64-slice CT report a high radiation exposure for patients. In individual patients the effective dose sometimes exceeded 20 mSv.[115] Several dose-reduction techniques have been introduced to minimize the exposure. The return to prospectively triggered image acquisition modes (initially used in 4-slice CCTA) has significantly cut the effective dose. In a study comparing prospectively triggered versus retrospectively gated image acquisition, Earls and colleagues[116] reported a reduction of the mean effective dose from 18.4 to 2.8 mSv, preserving the image quality. Herzog and colleagues[47]

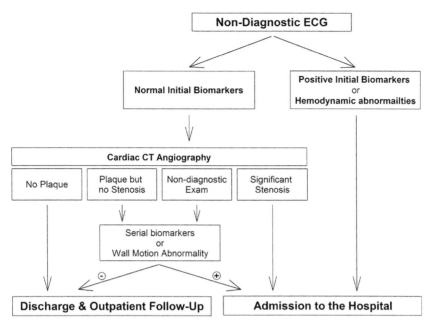

Fig. 5. Proposed algorithm for evaluation and management of patients suspected of having ACS but with a non-diagnostic electrocardiogram. This algorithm is intended for patients with a low to intermediate pretest probability of having CAD. CT stratifies patients into 3 categories: no plaque, plaque but no stenosis, and significant stenosis. A fourth category was created for patients with a nondiagnostic CT examination.

compared CCTA versus invasive coronary angiography and found that the effective dose from CCTA was consistently lower in individual patients (8.5 mSv vs 2.1 mSv). The introduction of even wider detectors and the reduction of the tube voltage to 100 kV in nonobese patients has helped to further reduce the effective dose for CCTA. Several studies report consistent dose values less than 2.5 mSv across different vendors.[117–120] Novel image acquisition techniques use high pitch values for the CCTA scan, allowing extremely short scan times of less than 1 second and low radiation exposure of less than 1 mSv.[118,121,122] The trade-off of both the prospectively triggered and the high-pitch scan protocols is the lack of data for the assessment of cardiac function parameters.

SUMMARY

The impact of CCTA on the management of patients presenting to the ED with chest pain has been proved but only for patients in whom no or minimal plaque is detected (**Fig. 5**). In these patients CCTA can rapidly and safely rule out disease and warrant discharge, thereby saving costs for the care provider.[65] On the other hand, the detection of plaque in CCTA is associated with a certain probability of ACS and MACE. Although some features such as the location of the stenosis in the proximal segments of the left coronary artery and the number of segments with

relevant disease offer incremental value over the detection of stenosis, there is no clear correlation between the findings in CT and the risk of MACE. Recent studies have tried to further integrate CCTA into the workup of patients presenting with chest pain and found the technique useful to more precisely interpret the results from myocardial perfusion studies. In 1 such study, the presence of a perfusion defect on SPECT that matches with the location of a relevant finding in CCTA has been shown to be associated with a rate of MACE twice as high as for unmatched findings.[123] Several trials are under way that include large numbers of patients, such as the RO-MICAT II trial in patients with acute chest pain and the PROMISE trial in patients with stable chest pain, which might be able to provide further clarification on how CT can help to improve management in patients with CAD, guiding medical management or intervention. Possibly, the identification of high-risk plaque features in CCTA may provide incremental value to the detection of hemodynamically relevant atherosclerotic lesions and help to guide the management of patients with chest pain presenting to the ED.

REFERENCES

1. Roger VL, Go AS, Lloyd-Jones DM, et al. Heart disease and stroke statistics–2011 update: a report

from the American Heart Association. Circulation 2011;123(4):e18–209.

2. Pitts SR, Niska R, Xu J, et al. National Hospital Ambulatory Medical Care Survey: 2006 emergency department summary. Natl Health Stat Report 2008;(7):1–39.

3. Pope JH, Aufderheide TP, Ruthazer R, et al. Missed diagnoses of acute cardiac ischemia in the emergency department. N Engl J Med 2000;342(16): 1163–70.

4. Schull M, Vermeulen M, Stukel T. The risk of missed diagnosis of acute myocardial infarction associated with emergency department volume. Ann Emerg Med 2006;48(6):647–55.

5. Sabatine MS, Cannon CP. Approach to the patient with chest pain. 9th edition. Philadelphia: Elsevier; 2010. p. 1076–86. Chapter 53.

6. Antman EM, Anbe DT, Armstrong PW, et al. ACC/ AHA guidelines for the management of patients with ST-elevation myocardial infarction. J Am Coll Cardiol 2004;44(3):E1–211.

7. Wright RS, Anderson JL, Adams CD, et al. 2011 ACCF/AHA focused update incorporated into the ACC/AHA 2007 Guidelines for the Management of Patients with Unstable Angina/Non–ST-Elevation Myocardial Infarction. J Am Coll Cardiol 2011; 57(19):e215–367.

8. Virmani R, Kolodgie FD, Burke AP, et al. Lessons from sudden coronary death: a comprehensive morphological classification scheme for atherosclerotic lesions. Arterioscler Thromb Vasc Biol 2000;20(5):1262–75.

9. Kolodgie FD. Pathologic assessment of the vulnerable human coronary plaque. Heart 2004;90(12): 1385–91.

10. Falk E, Shah PK, Fuster V. Coronary plaque disruption. Circulation 1995;92(3):657–71.

11. Davies MJ. The pathophysiology of acute coronary syndromes. Heart 2000;83(3):361–6.

12. Braunwald E, Angiolillo D, Bates E, et al. The problem of persistent platelet activation in acute coronary syndromes and following percutaneous coronary intervention. Clin Cardiol 2008;31(S1):I17–20.

13. Naghavi M. From vulnerable plaque to vulnerable patient: a call for new definitions and risk assessment strategies: Part II. Circulation 2003;108(15):1772–8.

14. McDaniel M, Galbraith E, Jeroudi A, et al. Localization of culprit lesions in coronary arteries of patients with ST-segment elevation myocardial infarctions: relation to bifurcations and curvatures. Am Heart J 2011;161(3):508–15.

15. Antman EM. ST-segment elevation myocardial infarction: pathology, pathophysiology, and clinical features. 9th edition. Philadelphia: Elsevier; 2010. p. 1087–110. Chapter 54.

16. Ambrose JA. Plaque disruption and the acute coronary syndromes of unstable angina and myocardial infarction: if the substrate is similar, why is the clinical presentation different? J Am Coll Cardiol 1992; 19(7):1653–8.

17. Ambrose JA, Tannenbaum MA, Alexopoulos D, et al. Angiographic progression of coronary artery disease and the development of myocardial infarction. J Am Coll Cardiol 1988;12(1):56–62.

18. Larsen A, Galbraith P, Ghali W, et al. Characteristics and outcomes of patients with acute myocardial infarction and angiographically normal coronary arteries. Am J Cardiol 2005;95(2):261–3.

19. Kardasz I, De Caterina R. Myocardial infarction with normal coronary arteries: a conundrum with multiple aetiologies and variable prognosis: an update. J Intern Med 2007;261(4):330–48.

20. Anderson JL, Adams CD, Antman EM, et al. ACC/ AHA 2007 Guidelines for the Management of Patients with Unstable Angina/non ST-elevation myocardial infarction: a report of the American College of Cardiology/American Heart Association Task Force on Practice Guidelines (Writing Committee to Revise the 2002 Guidelines for the Management of Patients with Unstable Angina/Non ST-Elevation Myocardial Infarction): developed in collaboration with the American College of Emergency Physicians, the Society for Cardiovascular Angiography and Interventions, and the Society of Thoracic Surgeons: endorsed by the American Association of Cardiovascular and Pulmonary Rehabilitation and the Society for Academic Emergency Medicine. Circulation 2007;116(7):e148–304.

21. Antman EM, Cohen M, Bernink PJ, et al. The TIMI risk score for unstable angina/non-ST elevation MI: a method for prognostication and therapeutic decision making. JAMA 2000;284(7):835–42.

22. Morrow DA, Antman EM, Giugliano RP, et al. A simple risk index for rapid initial triage of patients with ST-elevation myocardial infarction: an InTIME II substudy. Lancet 2001;358(9293):1571–5.

23. Manini AF, Dannemann N, Brown DF, et al. Limitations of risk score models in patients with acute chest pain. Am J Emerg Med 2009;27(1):43–8.

24. Jaffe AS, Babuin L, Apple FS. Biomarkers in acute cardiac disease: the present and the future. J Am Coll Cardiol 2006;48(1):1–11.

25. Slater DK, Hlatky MA, Mark DB, et al. Outcome in suspected acute myocardial infarction with normal or minimally abnormal admission electrocardiographic findings. Am J Cardiol 1987;60(10):766–70.

26. Rouan GW, Lee TH, Cook EF, et al. Clinical characteristics and outcome of acute myocardial infarction in patients with initially normal or nonspecific electrocardiograms (a report from the Multicenter Chest Pain Study). Am J Cardiol 1989;64(18): 1087–92.

27. Forest RS, Shofer FS, Sease KL, et al. Assessment of the standardized reporting guidelines ECG

classification system: the presenting ECG predicts 30-day outcomes. Ann Emerg Med 2004;44(3): 206–12.

28. Reichlin T, Hochholzer W, Bassetti S, et al. Early diagnosis of myocardial infarction with sensitive cardiac troponin assays. N Engl J Med 2009; 361(9):858–67.

29. Keller T, Zeller T, Peetz D, et al. Sensitive troponin I assay in early diagnosis of acute myocardial infarction. N Engl J Med 2009;361(9):868–77.

30. Amsterdam EA, Lewis WR, Kirk JD, et al. Acute ischemic syndromes. Chest pain center concept. Cardiol Clin 2002;20(1):117–36.

31. Peacock WF, Fonarow GC, Ander DS, et al. Society of Chest Pain Centers recommendations for the evaluation and management of the observation stay acute heart failure patient-parts 1-6. Acute Card Care 2009;11(1):3–42.

32. Graff LG, Dallara J, Ross MA, et al. Impact on the care of the emergency department chest pain patient from the chest pain evaluation registry (CHEPER) study. Am J Cardiol 1997;80(5):563–8.

33. Roberts RR, Zalenski RJ, Mensah EK, et al. Costs of an emergency department-based accelerated diagnostic protocol vs hospitalization in patients with chest pain: a randomized controlled trial. JAMA 1997;278(20):1670–6.

34. Lewis WR, Amsterdam EA, Turnipseed S, et al. Immediate exercise testing of low risk patients with known coronary artery disease presenting to the emergency department with chest pain. J Am Coll Cardiol 1999;33(7):1843–7.

35. Amsterdam EA, Kirk JD, Diercks DB, et al. Immediate exercise testing to evaluate low-risk patients presenting to the emergency department with chest pain. J Am Coll Cardiol 2002;40(2):251–6.

36. Kirk JD, Turnipseed S, Lewis WR, et al. Evaluation of chest pain in low-risk patients presenting to the emergency department: the role of immediate exercise testing. Ann Emerg Med 1998;32(1):1–7.

37. Ramakrishna G, Milavetz JJ, Zinsmeister AR, et al. Effect of exercise treadmill testing and stress imaging on the triage of patients with chest pain: CHEER substudy. Mayo Clin Proc 2005;80(3): 322–9.

38. Amsterdam EA, Kirk JD, Bluemke DA, et al. Testing of low-risk patients presenting to the emergency department with chest pain: a scientific statement from the American Heart Association. Circulation 2010;122(17):1756–76.

39. Kontos MC, Kurdziel K, McQueen R, et al. Comparison of 2-dimensional echocardiography and myocardial perfusion imaging for diagnosing myocardial infarction in emergency department patients. Am Heart J 2002;143(4):659–67.

40. Heller GV, Stowers SA, Hendel RC, et al. Clinical value of acute rest technetium-99m tetrofosmin tomographic myocardial perfusion imaging in patients with acute chest pain and nondiagnostic electrocardiograms. J Am Coll Cardiol 1998;31(5): 1011–7.

41. Varetto T, Cantalupi D, Altieri A, et al. Emergency room technetium-99m sestamibi imaging to rule out acute myocardial ischemic events in patients with nondiagnostic electrocardiograms. J Am Coll Cardiol 1993;22(7):1804–8.

42. Udelson JE, Beshansky JR, Ballin DS, et al. Myocardial perfusion imaging for evaluation and triage of patients with suspected acute cardiac ischemia: a randomized controlled trial. JAMA 2002;288(21):2693–700.

43. Schaeffer MW, Brennan TD, Hughes JA, et al. Resting radionuclide myocardial perfusion imaging in a chest pain center including an overnight delayed image acquisition protocol. J Nucl Med Technol 2007;35(4):242–5.

44. Klocke FJ, Baird MG, Lorell BH, et al. ACC/AHA/ASNC guidelines for the clinical use of cardiac radionuclide imaging–executive summary: a report of the American College of Cardiology/American Heart Association Task Force on Practice Guidelines (ACC/AHA/ASNC Committee to Revise the 1995 Guidelines for the Clinical Use of Cardiac Radionuclide Imaging). Circulation 2003;108(11):1404–18.

45. Conti A, Gallini C, Costanzo E, et al. Early detection of myocardial ischaemia in the emergency department by rest or exercise (99m)Tc tracer myocardial SPET in patients with chest pain and non-diagnostic ECG. Eur J Nucl Med 2001;28(12):1806–10.

46. Einstein AJ, Moser KW, Thompson RC, et al. Radiation dose to patients from cardiac diagnostic imaging. Circulation 2007;116(11):1290–305.

47. Herzog BA, Wyss CA, Husmann L, et al. First head-to-head comparison of effective radiation dose from low-dose 64-slice CT with prospective ECG-triggering versus invasive coronary angiography. Heart 2009;95(20):1656–61.

48. Bedetti G, Pasanisi E, Tintori G, et al. Stress echo in chest pain unit: the SPEED trial. Int J Cardiol 2005; 102(3):461–7.

49. Kwong RY, Schussheim AE, Rekhraj S, et al. Detecting acute coronary syndrome in the emergency department with cardiac magnetic resonance imaging. Circulation 2003;107(4):531–7.

50. Hendel RC, Patel MR, Kramer CM, et al. ACCF/ACR/SCCT/SCMR/ASNC/NASCI/SCAI/SIR 2006 appropriateness criteria for cardiac computed tomography and cardiac magnetic resonance imaging: a report of the American College of Cardiology Foundation Quality Strategic Directions Committee Appropriateness Criteria Working Group, American College of Radiology, Society of Cardiovascular Computed Tomography, Society for Cardiovascular Magnetic Resonance, American Society of Nuclear Cardiology,

North American Society for Cardiac Imaging, Society for Cardiovascular Angiography and Interventions, and Society of Interventional Radiology. J Am Coll Cardiol 2006;48(7):1475–97.

51. Schwitter J, Wacker CM, van Rossum AC, et al. MR-IMPACT: comparison of perfusion-cardiac magnetic resonance with single-photon emission computed tomography for the detection of coronary artery disease in a multicentre, multivendor, randomized trial. Eur Heart J 2008;29(4):480–9.

52. Plein S, Greenwood JP, Ridgway JP, et al. Assessment of non-ST-segment elevation acute coronary syndromes with cardiac magnetic resonance imaging. J Am Coll Cardiol 2004;44(11):2173–81.

53. Cury RC, Shash K, Nagurney JT, et al. Cardiac magnetic resonance with T2-weighted imaging improves detection of patients with acute coronary syndrome in the emergency department. Circulation 2008;118(8):837–44.

54. Blankstein R, Shturman LD, Rogers IS, et al. Adenosine-induced stress myocardial perfusion imaging using dual-source cardiac computed tomography. J Am Coll Cardiol 2009;54(12):1072–84.

55. Mowatt G, Cook JA, Hillis GS, et al. 64-Slice computed tomography angiography in the diagnosis and assessment of coronary artery disease: systematic review and meta-analysis. Heart 2008; 94(11):1386–93.

56. Budoff MJ, Achenbach S, Blumenthal RS, et al. Assessment of coronary artery disease by cardiac computed tomography: a scientific statement from the American Heart Association Committee on Cardiovascular Imaging and Intervention, Council on Cardiovascular Radiology and Intervention, and Committee on Cardiac Imaging, Council on Clinical Cardiology. Circulation 2006;114(16):1761–91.

57. Dewey M, Vavere AL, Arbab-Zadeh A, et al. Patient characteristics as predictors of image quality and diagnostic accuracy of MDCT compared with conventional coronary angiography for detecting coronary artery stenoses: CORE-64 Multicenter International Trial. AJR Am J Roentgenol 2010;194(1):93–102.

58. Raff GL, Gallagher MJ, O'Neill WW, et al. Diagnostic accuracy of noninvasive coronary angiography using 64-slice spiral computed tomography. J Am Coll Cardiol 2005;46(3):552–7.

59. Seifarth H, Wienbeck S, Püsken M, et al. Optimal systolic and diastolic reconstruction windows for coronary CT angiography using dual-source CT. AJR Am J Roentgenol 2007;189(6):1317–23.

60. Ropers U, Ropers D, Pflederer T, et al. Influence of heart rate on the diagnostic accuracy of dual-source computed tomography coronary angiography. J Am Coll Cardiol 2007;50(25):2393–8.

61. Mahabadi AA, Achenbach S, Burgstahler C, et al. Safety, efficacy, and indications of β-adrenergic receptor blockade to reduce heart rate prior to coronary CT angiography. Radiology 2010;257(3): 614–23.

62. Rubinshtein R, Halon DA, Gaspar T, et al. Usefulness of 64-slice cardiac computed tomographic angiography for diagnosing acute coronary syndromes and predicting clinical outcome in emergency department patients with chest pain of uncertain origin. Circulation 2007;115(13):1762–8.

63. Gallagher MJ, Ross MA, Raff GL, et al. The diagnostic accuracy of 64-slice computed tomography coronary angiography compared with stress nuclear imaging in emergency department low-risk chest pain patients. Ann Emerg Med 2007;49(2):125–36.

64. Goldstein JA, Gallagher MJ, O'Neill WW, et al. A randomized controlled trial of multi-slice coronary computed tomography for evaluation of acute chest pain. J Am Coll Cardiol 2007;49(8):863–71.

65. Goldstein JA, Chinnaiyan KM, Abidov A, et al. The CT-STAT (Coronary Computed Tomographic Angiography for Systematic Triage of Acute Chest Pain Patients to Treatment) trial. J Am Coll Cardiol 2011;58(14):1414–22.

66. Hollander JE, Chang AM, Shofer FS, et al. Coronary computed tomographic angiography for rapid discharge of low-risk patients with potential acute coronary syndromes. Ann Emerg Med 2009;53(3): 295–304.

67. Hoffmann U, Bamberg F, Chae CU, et al. Coronary computed tomography angiography for early triage of patients with acute chest pain: the ROMICAT (Rule Out Myocardial Infarction using Computer Assisted Tomography) trial. J Am Coll Cardiol 2009;53(18):1642–50.

68. Nasis A, Meredith IT, Nerlekar N, et al. Acute chest pain investigation: utility of cardiac CT angiography in guiding troponin measurement. Radiology 2011; 260(2):381–9.

69. Schlett CL, Banerji D, Siegel E, et al. Prognostic value of CT angiography for major adverse cardiac events in patients with acute chest pain from the emergency department. J Am Coll Cardiol Img 2011;4(5):481–91.

70. Hollander JE, Chang AM, Shofer FS, et al. One-year outcomes following coronary computerized tomographic angiography for evaluation of emergency department patients with potential acute coronary syndrome. Acad Emerg Med 2009;16(8):693–8.

71. Hulten EA, Carbonaro S, Petrillo SP, et al. Prognostic value of cardiac computed tomography angiography. J Am Coll Cardiol 2011;57(10):1237–47.

72. Sozzi FB, Civaia F, Rossi P, et al. Long-term follow-up of patients with first-time chest pain having 64-slice computed tomography. Am J Cardiol 2011; 107(4):516–21.

73. Seneviratne SK, Truong QA, Bamberg F, et al. Incremental diagnostic value of regional left ventricular function over coronary assessment by

cardiac computed tomography for the detection of acute coronary syndrome in patients with acute chest pain: from the ROMICAT trial. Circ Cardiovasc Imaging 2010;3(4):375–83.

74. Chow BJ, Small G, Yam Y, et al. Incremental prognostic value of cardiac computed tomography in coronary artery disease using CONFIRM: COroNary computed tomography angiography evaluation for clinical outcomes: an InteRnational Multicenter registry. Circ Cardiovasc Imaging 2011;4(5):463–72.

75. de Graaf FR, van Werkhoven JM, van Velzen JE, et al. Incremental prognostic value of left ventricular function analysis over non-invasive coronary angiography with multidetector computed tomography. J Nucl Cardiol 2010;17(6):1034–40.

76. Min JK, Lin FY, Dunning AM, et al. Incremental prognostic significance of left ventricular dysfunction to coronary artery disease detection by 64-detector row coronary computed tomographic angiography for the prediction of all-cause mortality: results from a two-centre study of 5330 patients. Eur Heart J 2010;31(10):1212–9.

77. Alderman EL, Corley SD, Fisher LD, et al. Five-year angiographic follow-up of factors associated with progression of coronary artery disease in the Coronary Artery Surgery Study (CASS). CASS Participating Investigators and Staff. J Am Coll Cardiol 1993;22(4):1141–54.

78. Pundziute G, Schuijf JD, Jukema JW, et al. Prognostic value of multislice computed tomography coronary angiography in patients with known or suspected coronary artery disease. J Am Coll Cardiol 2007;49(1):62–70.

79. van Werkhoven JM, Schuijf JD, Gaemperli O, et al. Incremental prognostic value of multi-slice computed tomography coronary angiography over coronary artery calcium scoring in patients with suspected coronary artery disease. Eur Heart J 2009;30(21):2622–9.

80. Lin FY, Shaw LJ, Dunning AM, et al. Mortality risk in symptomatic patients with nonobstructive coronary artery disease: a prospective 2-center study of 2,583 patients undergoing 64-detector row coronary computed tomographic angiography. J Am Coll Cardiol 2011;58(5):510–9.

81. Burke AP, Farb A, Malcom GT, et al. Coronary risk factors and plaque morphology in men with coronary disease who died suddenly. N Engl J Med 1997;336(18):1276–82.

82. Jang IK, Bouma BE, Kang DH, et al. Visualization of coronary atherosclerotic plaques in patients using optical coherence tomography: comparison with intravascular ultrasound. J Am Coll Cardiol 2002; 39(4):604–9.

83. Vancraeynest D, Pasquet A, Roelants V, et al. Imaging the vulnerable plaque. J Am Coll Cardiol 2011;57(20):1961–79.

84. Suh WM, Seto AH, Margey RJP, et al. Intravascular detection of the vulnerable plaque. Circ Cardiovasc Imaging 2011;4(2):169–78.

85. Virmani R, Burke AP, Farb A, et al. Pathology of the vulnerable plaque. J Am Coll Cardiol 2006; 47(Suppl 8):C13–8.

86. Nasu K, Tsuchikane E, Katoh O, et al. Accuracy of in vivo coronary plaque morphology assessment: a validation study of in vivo virtual histology compared with in vitro histopathology. J Am Coll Cardiol 2006;47(12):2405–12.

87. Leber A. Composition of coronary atherosclerotic plaques in patients with acute myocardial infarction and stable angina pectoris determined by contrast-enhanced multislice computed tomography. Am J Cardiol 2003;91(6):714–8.

88. Leber A. Accuracy of multidetector spiral computed tomography in identifying and differentiating the composition of coronary atherosclerotic plaques: a comparative study with intracoronary ultrasound. J Am Coll Cardiol 2004;43(7):1241–7.

89. Schroeder S, Kuettner A, Leitritz M, et al. Reliability of differentiating human coronary plaque morphology using contrast-enhanced multislice spiral computed tomography: a comparison with histology. J Comput Assist Tomogr 2004;28(4):449–54.

90. Pohle K, Achenbach S, Macneill B, et al. Characterization of non-calcified coronary atherosclerotic plaque by multi-detector row CT: comparison to IVUS. Atherosclerosis 2007;190(1):174–80.

91. Marwan M, Taher MA, Meniawy El K, et al. In vivo CT detection of lipid-rich coronary artery atherosclerotic plaques using quantitative histogram analysis: a head to head comparison with IVUS. Atherosclerosis 2011;215(1):110–5.

92. Motoyama S, Kondo T, Anno H, et al. Atherosclerotic plaque characterization by 0.5-mm-slice multislice computed tomographic imaging. Circ J 2007;71(3):363–6.

93. Kitagawa T, Yamamoto H, Horiguchi J, et al. Characterization of noncalcified coronary plaques and identification of culprit lesions in patients with acute coronary syndrome by 64-slice computed tomography. J Am Coll Cardiol Img 2009;2(2):153–60.

94. Tanaka A, Shimada K, Yoshida K, et al. Non-invasive assessment of plaque rupture by 64-slice multidetector computed tomography–comparison with intravascular ultrasound. Circ J 2008;72(8):1276–81.

95. Kashiwagi M, Tanaka A, Kitabata H, et al. Feasibility of noninvasive assessment of thin-cap fibroatheroma by multidetector computed tomography. JCMG 2009;2(12):1412–9.

96. Motoyama S, Sarai M, Harigaya H, et al. Computed tomographic angiography characteristics of atherosclerotic plaques subsequently resulting in acute

coronary syndrome. J Am Coll Cardiol 2009;54(1): 49–57.

97. Nishio M, Ueda Y, Matsuo K, et al. Detection of disrupted plaques by coronary CT: comparison with angioscopy. Heart 2011;97(17):1397–402.

98. Glagov S, Weisenberg E, Zarins CK, et al. Compensatory enlargement of human atherosclerotic coronary arteries. N Engl J Med 1987;316(22):1371–5.

99. Schoenhagen P, Ziada KM, Kapadia SR, et al. Extent and direction of arterial remodeling in stable versus unstable coronary syndromes: an intravascular ultrasound study. Circulation 2000;101(6): 598–603.

100. Nakamura M, Nishikawa H, Mukai S, et al. Impact of coronary artery remodeling on clinical presentation of coronary artery disease: an intravascular ultrasound study. J Am Coll Cardiol 2001;37(1): 63–9.

101. Raffel OC, Merchant FM, Tearney GJ, et al. In vivo association between positive coronary artery remodelling and coronary plaque characteristics assessed by intravascular optical coherence tomography. Eur Heart J 2008;29(14):1721–8.

102. Hoffmann U, Moselewski F, Nieman K, et al. Noninvasive assessment of plaque morphology and composition in culprit and stable lesions in acute coronary syndrome and stable lesions in stable angina by multidetector computed tomography. J Am Coll Cardiol 2006;47(8):1655–62.

103. Motoyama S, Kondo T, Sarai M, et al. Multislice computed tomographic characteristics of coronary lesions in acute coronary syndromes. J Am Coll Cardiol 2007;50(4):319–26.

104. Ehara S. Spotty calcification typifies the culprit plaque in patients with acute myocardial infarction: an intravascular ultrasound study. Circulation 2004; 110(22):3424–9.

105. Takaoka H, Ishibashi I, Uehara M, et al. Comparison of image characteristics of plaques in culprit coronary arteries by 64 slice CT and intravascular ultrasound in acute coronary syndromes. Int J Cardiol 2011. DOI:10.1016/j.ijcard.2011.04.014.

106. Maurovich-Horvat P, Hoffmann U, Vorpahl M, et al. The napkin-ring sign: CT signature of high-risk coronary plaques? J Am Coll Cardiol Img 2011; 3(4):440–4.

107. Nakazawa G, Tanabe K, Onuma Y, et al. Efficacy of culprit plaque assessment by 64-slice multidetector computed tomography to predict transient noreflow phenomenon during percutaneous coronary intervention. Am Heart J 2008;155(6):1150–7.

108. Pflederer T, Marwan M, Schepis T, et al. Characterization of culprit lesions in acute coronary syndromes using coronary dual-source CT angiography. Atherosclerosis 2010;211(2):437–44.

109. Min JK, Feignoux J, Treutenaere J, et al. The prognostic value of multidetector coronary CT angiography for the prediction of major adverse cardiovascular events: a multicenter observational cohort study. Int J Cardiovasc Imaging 2010; 26(6):721–8.

110. Gaemperli O, Valenta I, Schepis T, et al. Coronary 64-slice CT angiography predicts outcome in patients with known or suspected coronary artery disease. Eur Radiol 2008;18(6):1162–73.

111. Stone GW, Maehara A, Lansky AJ, et al. A prospective natural-history study of coronary atherosclerosis. N Engl J Med 2011;364(3):226–35.

112. Rogers IS, Banerji D, Siegel EL, et al. Usefulness of comprehensive cardiothoracic computed tomography in the evaluation of acute undifferentiated chest discomfort in the emergency department (CAPTURE). Am J Cardiol 2011;107(5):643–50.

113. Madder RD, Raff GL, Hickman L, et al. Comparative diagnostic yield and 3-month outcomes of "triple rule-out" and standard protocol coronary CT angiography in the evaluation of acute chest pain. J Cardiovasc Comput Tomogr 2011;5(3): 165–71.

114. Lee HY, Song IS, Yoo SM, et al. Rarity of isolated pulmonary embolism and acute aortic syndrome occurring outside of the field of view of dedicated coronary CT angiography. Acta Radiol 2011;52(4): 378–84.

115. Hausleiter J, Meyer T, Hermann F, et al. Estimated radiation dose associated with cardiac CT angiography. JAMA 2009;301(5):500–7.

116. Earls J, Berman E, Urban B, et al. Prospectively gated transverse coronary CT angiography versus retrospectively gated helical technique: improved image quality and reduced radiation dose. Radiology 2008;246(3):742–53.

117. Buechel RR, Pazhenkottil AP, Herzog BA, et al. Prognostic performance of low-dose coronary CT angiography with prospective ECG triggering. Heart 2011;97(17):1385–90.

118. Alkadhi H, Stolzmann P, Desbiolles L, et al. Low-dose, 128-slice, dual-source CT coronary angiography: accuracy and radiation dose of the high-pitch and the step-and-shoot mode. Heart 2010;96(12):933–8.

119. Stolzmann P, Leschka S, Scheffel H, et al. Dual-source CT in step-and-shoot mode: noninvasive coronary angiography with low radiation dose. Radiology 2008;249(1):71–80.

120. Zhang C, Zhang Z, Yan Z, et al. 320-row CT coronary angiography: effect of 100-kV tube voltages on image quality, contrast volume, and radiation dose. Int J Cardiovasc Imaging 2010;27(7): 1059–68.

121. Lell M, Marwan M, Schepis T, et al. Prospectively ECG-triggered high-pitch spiral acquisition for coronary CT angiography using dual source CT: technique and initial experience. Eur Radiol 2009; 19(11):2576–83.

122. Achenbach S, Goroll T, Seltmann M, et al. Detection of coronary artery stenoses by low-dose, prospectively ECG-triggered, high-pitch spiral coronary CT angiography. J Am Coll Cardiol Img 2011;4(4): 328–37.

123. Pazhenkottil AP, Nkoulou RN, Ghadri JR, et al. Prognostic value of cardiac hybrid imaging integrating single-photon emission computed tomography with coronary computed tomography angiography. Eur Heart J 2011;32(12):1465–71.

Myocardial Perfusion by CT Versus Hybrid Imaging

Richard T. George, MD[a],*, Vishal C. Mehra, MD, PhD[b],
Antti Saraste, MD[c,d], Juhani Knuuti, MD[c]

KEYWORDS

- Myocardial perfusion imaging • Ischemia • Atherosclerosis
- Positron emission tomography
- Single-photon emission computed tomography
- Computed tomography

Multislice computed tomography (CT) can visualize the coronary arteries with high resolution and offers an attractive noninvasive alternative to invasive coronary angiography.[1] However, anatomic imaging does not accurately indicate whether the coronary lesions detected cause ischemia, which is the target of revascularization therapy. Thus, before elective invasive coronary angiography, ischemia testing is strongly recommended by clinical practice guidelines.[2] The revascularization procedures performed in patients with documented ischemia have been shown to reduce mortality through reduction of ischemia.[1–4] The nuclear substudy of the COURAGE (Clinical Outcomes Utilizing Revascularization and Aggressive Drug Evaluation) trial showed that coronary interventions were more effective in alleviating myocardial ischemia compared with optimal medical treatment, and the reduction of ischemia was associated with the prognosis of the patient.[2] The FAME (Fractional Flow Reserve vs Angiography for Guiding PCI in Patients with Multivessel Coronary Artery Disease) trial showed that the measurement of fractional flow reserve (FFR), a functional measure of coronary stenosis before coronary intervention, resulted in a 35% reduction in mortality and rate of myocardial infarctions compared with anatomic evaluation of stenoses alone.[4]

Because discrepancies between the apparent anatomic severity of a lesion and its hemodynamic significance are common,[5] functional evaluation of intermediate stenoses is considered essential for therapeutic decisions. The most obvious solution for this problem is to combine anatomic imaging with functional imaging. Software-based coregistration of image datasets

Financial disclosures: Richard T. George, MD: Dr George receives research support from Toshiba Medical Systems Corporation and General Electric. Dr George is a consultant for ICON Medical Imaging. The terms of these arrangements are managed by Johns Hopkins University in accordance with its conflict of interest policies. Dr Knuuti is a consultant for Lantheus Inc.

Funding support: Dr George receives funding support from the National Institutes of Health - National Heart, Lung, and Blood Institute (1R21HL106586-01A1 and RO1 HL095129), Toshiba Medical Systems, and General Electric for research in the areas of computed tomography and radionuclide imaging. Dr Knuuti and Saraste have received support from the Centre of Excellence in Molecular Imaging in Cardiovascular and Metabolic Research, supported by the Academy of Finland, and from the Finnish Cardiovascular Foundation and the Hospital District of Southwest Finland.

[a] Division of Cardiology, Department of Medicine, Johns Hopkins University School of Medicine, 600 North Wolfe Street, 565C Carnegie Building, Baltimore, MD 21287, USA
[b] Division of Cardiology, Department of Medicine, Johns Hopkins University School of Medicine, 600 North Wolfe Street, 568 Carnegie Building, Baltimore, MD 21287, USA
[c] Turku PET Centre, c/o Turku University Hospital, University of Turku, PO Box 52 FI-20521, Turku, Finland
[d] Department of Medicine, Turku University Hospital, University of Turku, PO Box 52 FI-20521, Turku, Finland
* Corresponding author.
E-mail address: rgeorge3@jhmi.edu

from stand-alone scanners is reliable, feasible, and fast. The drawback is that more than 1 image session is needed for each patient, which is not easy in routine clinical work. Hybrid imaging systems combining positron emission tomography (PET) or single-photon emission CT (SPECT) with multidetector CT angiography (CTA) are commercially available and allow direct combination of morphologic and functional information.[6] Coregistration of images is immediate and reliable with integrated scanners because of the capability to perform PET/SPECT and CT image acquisition almost simultaneously with the patient's position fixed. Another alternative is to use functional information that can be derived from CT alone by performing stress myocardial CT perfusion (CTP) imaging in the same session with coronary angiography.[7–10] Because only a single device is needed, this allows broader use of hybrid imaging in routine clinical work. CTP is currently being investigated and more clinical data will be available in the near future.[11]

TECHNOLOGY SUMMARY
SPECT and PET Myocardial Perfusion Imaging

Myocardial perfusion SPECT is the most established noninvasive method for the detection of myocardial ischemia. The reported sensitivity of exercise SPECT for the detection of angiographically significant coronary artery disease (CAD) is high (87%–89%).[12,13] The normalcy rate, which corrects for referral bias that affects specificity, has been found to be 89%.[13] Myocardial perfusion SPECT has also been used to assess the extent of ischemic myocardium and viability. Normal perfusion SPECT in patients with suspected or known CAD predicts a low rate of cardiac death or nonfatal myocardial infarction (<1%/y).[14] In addition, patients with a smaller amount of reversible ischemia on SPECT have a survival advantage with medical therapy rather than revascularization, whereas those with more severe ischemia are more likely to benefit from invasive procedures.[2,3] These characteristics make myocardial perfusion scintigraphy a strong technique to guide therapy for patients with CAD.

PET myocardial perfusion imaging offers certain advantages compared with SPECT. PET has better spatial and contrast resolutions and accurate, well-validated attenuation correction. Therefore, image artifacts caused by soft tissue attenuation are rare. Large numbers of studies have shown PET to be an accurate method for detecting obstructive CAD (sensitivity and specificity ≥90%).[15] A unique feature of PET is that myocardial perfusion can be quantified in absolute terms (mL/min/g).[15–18]

The clinical benefits of quantification of myocardial perfusion have been highlighted in recent studies comparing the diagnostic accuracy of quantitative and relative analysis of PET perfusion imaging in patients with suspected CAD.[19–21] The studies have also shown that quantitative analysis of myocardial perfusion improves the diagnostic accuracy of detecting CAD and is particularly helpful for revealing the true extent of CAD in patients with multivessel disease.[19–21] Particularly in obese patients, SPECT is prone to false-positive results because of nonuniform photon attenuation,[15,16] and PET has been suggested as the method of choice.

The limitation of radionuclide perfusion imaging is that it does not provide information about coronary anatomy. Therefore, nonobstructive CAD or earlier coronary atherosclerosis cannot be detected. Also, differentiation of microvascular dysfunction from epicardial stenosis as a cause of abnormally low perfusion as well as assignment of perfusion defects to certain coronary lesions remain problems in the absence of information on individual coronary anatomy.[22]

The integration of coronary morphology and functional information can also be performed by mental coregistration using standardized allocation of myocardial segments to the main coronary arteries.[23] The standardized vascular territories of coronary arteries varies considerably between individuals, leading to disagreement in up to 72% of patients.[24] This is particularly true in the inferior and inferolateral walls. Thus, the most obvious incremental value of hybrid imaging is based on the accurate spatial colocalization of myocardial perfusion defects and individual coronary arteries and direct correlation of the relationship between anatomic stenosis and perfusion abnormalities.

Myocardial CTP Imaging

Given the aforementioned limitations of coronary CTA, extensive investigation and development is ongoing to extend the capabilities of cardiac CT into myocardial perfusion imaging. Because myocardial CTP imaging is less well known, the technology and methods are summarized briefly.

Multidetector detector CT systems are diverse, each having its own advantages and disadvantages. Although 12-row and 16-row detector systems have been studied for coronary CTA and myocardial CTP imaging,[25,26] the consensus is that systems that are capable of acquiring 64 simultaneous slices or more are required for coronary CTA and myocardial CTP imaging. Several studies have used single-source 64-row detector CT and 64-slice dual-source CT with good results.[7,9,27–29] More recently, studies using 128-slice and 320-row detector systems have been published.[10,30] Dual-source CT systems have the advantage of high temporal resolution for acquiring the myocardium during high heart rates experienced during vasodilator stress, but lack significant cardiac coverage. With the introduction of 320-row CT, the entire cardiac volume can be covered in a single heart beat, thus eliminating issues of temporal nonuniformity of the image.

Although radionuclide myocardial perfusion imaging uses tracers tagged with radioisotopes, myocardial CTP imaging uses iodinated contrast agents to trace myocardial perfusion. Iodinated contrast has similar properties to gadolinium-based contrast agents used for magnetic resonance myocardial perfusion imaging. Iodinated contrast distributes in the extracellular space and is excluded from the intracellular space, as long as cellular membranes remain intact. Unlike gadolinium-based contrast agents, the concentration of iodinated contrast in tissue is directly proportional to the measured attenuation (in Hounsfield units) on a CT image.[27,31] This property allows the quantification of myocardial blood flow and volume.[27,32] In addition, the extraction of iodinated contrast from the intravascular to the extracellular space is not linear. The extraction fraction is higher at low flows and is lower at high flows, and thus needs to be considered when quantifying myocardial blood flow with CT.[33,34]

Rest perfusion and delayed enhanced CT imaging have been established as accurate methods for detecting acute and chronic myocardial infarction and myocardial viability.[35–37] However, the detection of myocardial ischemia requires provocative stress testing. Although exercise and dobutamine stress testing have been used in stress echocardiography and nuclear imaging, these methods rely on an increase in heart rate beyond what is feasible for cardiac CT. As a result, myocardial CTP imaging relies on pharmacologic vasodilator agents such as adenosine, dipyridamole, and regadenoson. Each of these agents has advantages and disadvantages, but they share one thing in common. Each agent must be administered before stress imaging, with contrast-enhanced imaging occurring at the time maximum hyperemia is achieved. Each of these agents causes an increase in heart rate averaging 20 to 25 beats per minute. The most studied agent is adenosine, which has the advantage of a short half-life, but requires an infusion pump and can cause various degrees of atrioventricular block and bronchospasm.[7,9,28] Dipyridamole has similar contraindications as adenosine regarding atrioventricular block and bronchospasm. It also needs to be given using an infusion pump and, because of its long half-life, it often needs reversal with aminophylline. Regadenoson is a specific A_{2A} agonist with a lower incidence of side effects. Regadenoson is attractive for myocardial CTP imaging given its convenient administration, but, of the 3 vasodilator agents, it causes the greatest increase in heart rate.[38,39]

Myocardial CTP images can be acquired using a static or a dynamic acquisition. Static imaging acquires an image of the myocardium over a short period of time during the approximate peak of the contrast bolus. This technique provides perfusion data that is qualitative or semiquantitative. Alternatively, dynamic imaging acquires images of the myocardium over time before and during the first pass of a contrast bolus. Dynamic CTP can provide quantitative data on myocardial perfusion imaging.

Static CTP imaging is triggered to occur during the late upslope, peak, and early downslope of the contrast bolus. Depending on the CT scanning system, this may be done with helical CT with retrospective electrocardiogram (ECG)-gating, dose modulation when available, and prospective ECG-triggered protocols. The first studies of stress CTP imaging used helical CT protocols using single-source CT.[7,28,40] Helical acquisitions allow multicycle reconstruction and the improvement in temporal resolution required with vasodilator stress. Dose modulation was then added to helical protocols with a reduction in overall radiation dose.[9] More recently, using wide-area detector scanning, further reductions in radiation dose have been realized with prospective ECG-triggered protocols.[10,11]

Dynamic CTP imaging refers to serial imaging of the heart as the contrast bolus traverses the coronary arteries and the myocardial microvasculature. This technique allows the construction of time-attenuation curves of the myocardium and a reference artery (aorta) and the calculation of myocardial blood flow and flow reserve.[27,41] Ideally, dynamic imaging should cover the entire myocardium. However 64-row and 64-slice CT systems have limited coverage in the z-axis and therefore do not image the entire myocardium. One strategy to circumvent this limitation is to perform imaging using a shuttle mode.[42] This method images the more cranial and caudal portions of the heart by moving the table every other heart beat. Alternatively, wide-area detector scanners such as a 320-row system are capable of covering the entire myocardium without table movement.

CLINICAL EVIDENCE
Hybrid Imaging

Today, most clinical data on hybrid imaging are based on small diagnostic, single-center studies. Many studies have compared the accuracy of hybrid imaging with the stand-alone techniques (eg, either CTA or SPECT/PET alone). Some studies have focused on the incremental clinical value of hybrid imaging rather than the side-by-side analysis of CTA and perfusion imaging. Despite known limitations of invasive coronary angiography (ICA) in detecting ischemia, it has usually been used as the reference standard. Recently, one study with ICA combined with FFR was published.[43]

The feasibility of clinical noninvasive hybrid imaging was first documented by Namdar and colleagues[44] using fusion of [13]NH$_3$ PET with 4-slice CTA in 25 patients with CAD. In this study, ICA combined with PET was used as the reference standard and the hybrid CTA/PET approach detected obstructive coronary stenoses with a sensitivity, specificity, positive predictive value (PPV), and negative predictive value (NPV) of 90%, 98%, 82%, and 99%, respectively. A subsequent study using SPECT and CTA showed that the hybrid approach results in improvement in PPV from 31% to 77% compared with CTA alone for detection of myocardial ischemia.[45] Sato and colleagues[46] found that adding SPECT information in nonevaluable arteries on CTA improved PPV, in particular, from 69% to 85%. A comparable diagnostic performance was reported by Groves and colleagues[47] using an [82]Rb PET/CT hybrid system. One of the largest studies published in 2007 included 107 patients undergoing hybrid H$_2$[15]O PET/64-slice CTA.[48] In this study, the hemodynamic significance of ICA stenoses was confirmed with FFR when feasible. The use of PET/CTA increased the PPV significantly from 76% to 96% compared with CTA alone and the accuracy was 98%.

Several studies have also shown that hybrid imaging has synergistic clinical value. In one study with positive SPECT perfusion imaging findings, the number of equivocal findings was significantly reduced using SPECT/CTA fusion compared with the side-by-side analysis of stand-alone tests[48] and the hybrid approach added important clinical information in 29% of patients. This effect was most evident in patients with multivessel disease and intermediate severity stenoses. Santana and colleagues[49] detected significantly better diagnostic performance of SPECT/CTA imaging compared with SPECT alone and side-by-side analysis of SPECT and CTA. In a recent study, the improved diagnostic value of hybrid imaging was based on greater accuracy in territories of the left circumflex and right coronary arteries.[50]

Therefore, hybrid imaging may not only improve the diagnostic accuracy of noninvasive detection of CAD but also provide vessel-specific functional information to guide treatment strategies.[4] This possibility is also supported by the finding that the accuracy of vessel-based analysis of hybrid PET/CTA was as high as 98%.[43]

The prognostic value of morphologic and functional coronary information was investigated in a multicenter study in more than 500 patients, which found that both need to be investigated in patients with CAD.[51] A recent prospective follow-up trial assessed the incremental prognostic value of hybrid imaging rather than the side-by-side findings.[52] In this study, 324 consecutive patients undergoing hybrid SPECT/CTA were subdivided into 3 groups based on matching or unmatching the imaging findings. On follow-up of about 2.8 years, abnormal findings in both tests was associated with a significantly higher event rate (death or myocardial infarction [MI]) and proved to be an independent predictor for major cardiovascular events. The annual death/MI rate was 6.0%, 2.8%, and 1.3% for patients with matched, unmatched, and normal findings. The corresponding revascularization rates within 2 months were 41%, 11%, and 0%. Thus, hybrid imaging results may have significant impact on patient management. Larger prospective studies are needed to investigate whether changes in treatment based on hybrid imaging will have an impact on the outcome of the patients.

Myocardial CTP

The development of myocardial CTP imaging began in the 1980s with the introduction of electron beam tomography and a custom multislice CT scanner known as the dynamic spatial reconstructor. Several groups showed the feasibility of performing quantitative CTP imaging of the heart, but these systems had several limitations restricting their widespread use.[53–56]

With the introduction of multidetector CT systems and clinical evidence showing the high sensitivity and NPV of coronary CTA, but limitations in the detection of ischemia-causing lesions, investigators sought again to test the feasibility of performing myocardial CTP imaging. In one of the initial studies, investigators performed adenosine stress helical CTP imaging during the upslope of the contrast bolus in a canine model of myocardial ischemia.[28] This study showed the feasibility of static CTP imaging by showing attenuation differences between ischemic and nonischemic myocardium. In addition, this study was extended to adding arterial input function data to the measurement of myocardial perfusion using a combined dynamic/static approach.[57]

Using dynamic CTP imaging, Daghini and colleagues[32] showed that dynamic imaging and Patlak plot analyses are capable of measuring indices of endothelial and microvascular function in a porcine model. Dynamic CTP imaging has also been validated for the absolute quantification of myocardial blood flow, using upslope, model-based deconvolution and Patlak plot analyses,[27,33] and the calculation of myocardial flow reserve.[41]

The clinical evidence supporting the accuracy and feasibility of myocardial CTP comes from at least 15 published single-center studies, some of which are summarized here. In a pilot study by George and colleagues,[7] 40 patients with a history of an abnormal SPECT study were assessed using either a 64-row or 256-row adenosine stress CTP. They showed a per-patient sensitivity and specificity of 86% and 92%, respectively, of combined coronary CTA and myocardial CTP imaging to detect atherosclerosis causing myocardial ischemia, compared with the gold standard of invasive angiography and SPECT.[7] A similar study of 34 patients undergoing adenosine stress dual-source CTP showed similar accuracy of CTP and SPECT to diagnose a stenosis greater than or equal to 50% on invasive angiography. For CTP and SPECT, the sensitivity was 79% and 67% and the specificity was 80% and 83%, respectively.[9] In addition, this same group showed that the combination of CTP with CTA increased all parameters of accuracy to detect obstructive CAD. Sensitivity increased from 83% to 91%; specificity, from 71% to 91%; PPV, from 66% to 86%; and NPV, from 87% to 93%; and the area under the receiver operating characteristic curve, from 0.77 to 0.90 (P<.005).[58] Using quantitative dynamic CTP imaging, Ho and colleagues[30] showed adenosine stress CTP imaging to have a sensitivity and specificity of 83% and 78% for the detection of segmental perfusion deficits on nuclear myocardial perfusion imaging. Two studies have established the use of dipyridamole for stress CTP imaging. A study of 36 patients, 26 with invasive angiography, showed dipyridamole stress CTP to have a sensitivity and specificity of 88% and 79% for diagnosing anatomic stenosis. A second study showed the added value of dipyridamole stress CTP in the setting of intra-coronary stents.[59] For CTA alone, sensitivity, specificity, PPV, NPV, and accuracy for coronary CTA in stent territories were, respectively, 87%, 75%, 84%, 93%, and 81%. Adding myocardial

CTP to CTA showed improvement in accuracy of 95%, 88%, 81%, 97%, and 91%, respectively (P = .029). More importantly, in vessels/territories with impaired stent evaluation (limited or inadequate), the diagnostic performance of coronary CTA alone was 72%, 83%, 76%, 79%, and 77%, and, combined with myocardial CTP, was 94%, 87%, 85%, 95%, and 91% (P = .036), respectively.[59]

Additional studies have been performed and compared with cardiovascular magnetic resonance (CMR) perfusion imaging. This comparison is attractive because magnetic resonance imaging and CTP imaging share some common principles. One study tested the accuracy of adenosine stress dual-energy CT to detect myocardial perfusion abnormalities on CMR in the presence of clinically significant stenoses on invasive angiography in 50 patients.[60] They showed a per vessel sensitivity, specificity, and accuracy of 89%, 76%, and 83%, respectively. Another study compared stress CTP for the detection of perfusion deficits with CMR perfusion imaging, showing excellent per vessel accuracy with a sensitivity of 96% and specificity of 88%. In addition, CTP was highly accurate for the detection of reversible ischemia, with a sensitivity and specificity of 95% and 96%, respectively, compared with CMR.[61]

FFR is considered the invasive gold standard for defining functionally significant coronary stenoses. Ko and colleagues[10] performed 320-row detector CTP and showed per vessel/territory sensitivity, specificity, PPV, and NPVs of 76%, 84%, 82%, and 79%, respectively, for CTP to identify an FFR less than or equal to 0.8. Furthermore, the combination of a stenosis greater than or equal to 50% on CTA and perfusion defect on CTP was 98% specific for ischemia, whereas the presence of stenosis of less than 50% on CTA and normal perfusion on CTP was 100% specific for exclusion of ischemia.

The most robust validations of any diagnostic test are multicenter diagnostic accuracy studies. Presently, there are 2 multicenter diagnostic accuracy studies for myocardial CTP. CORE320 is a multicenter study performed in 16 centers on 4 continents. CORE320 is testing the hypothesis that the combination of coronary CTA and myocardial CTP can accurately diagnose a stenosis greater than or equal to 50% causing myocardial ischemia compared with the combined gold standard of invasive angiography and SPECT. CORE320 has completed the enrollment of more than 400 patients and data analysis is ongoing.[11] A second multicenter, multivendor study has begun. This study is testing the accuracy of regadenoson CTP compared with SPECT.

LIMITATIONS
Hybrid Imaging

Putting together 2 modalities instead of 1 creates specific challenges. In clinical routine, a sequential approach is often used, with additional scans performed only if the results of the first modality are equivocal (eg, the hemodynamic severity of intermediate stenosis in CTA can be confirmed by perfusion imaging). Conversely, the lesion responsible for perfusion defect can be localized by CTA. When a sequential approach is used, the order of the scans can depend on the pretest likelihood of CAD. In patients with low to intermediate pretest likelihood of CAD, the procedure should start with CTA, and perfusion imaging is performed only in those patients with obstructive CAD in CTA, based on the high NPV of CTA. In contrast, when the pretest likelihood of CAD is higher, a large fraction of patients have obstructive disease and starting with perfusion imaging may be a better approach. CTA is needed only if anatomic information is required rather than a positive perfusion result. Each approach has certain limitations. In the first option, knowledge of coronary function or microvascular disease is missed in patients with nonobstructive atherosclerosis. In the second option, nonobstructive CAD that is not physiologically significant may be missed.

The increased costs and radiation exposure from hybrid imaging procedures have also raised concerns. All efforts should be made to minimize the individual radiation exposure.[62] During recent years, imaging methodology has undergone significant development to comply with this principle. Perfusion SPECT using novel dedicated small-footprint cardiac scanners equipped with solid-state detectors allows further reductions in radiation exposure.[63] Recently, the feasibility and high diagnostic quality of half-dose SPECT perfusion imaging with a total radiation dose of 5.8 mSv was reported.[64] The PET perfusion tracers (ie, $H_2^{15}O$ and $^{13}NH_3$, ^{82}Rb) are associated with low radiation doses (1–2 mSv) and therefore may be particularly suitable for hybrid imaging.[44] The radiation dose from CTA has been revolutionized in the last few years. The image acquisition protocols, ECG-driven tube current modulation, body mass index–adapted tube voltage modulation, prospective ECG-triggered sequential scanning, iterative reconstruction, and high-pitch scanning protocols using dual-source CT scanners have lowered doses even further into the submillisievert range.[65–67] Currently, hybrid stress-only SPECT/CTA or PET/CTA studies can be performed with a radiation dose lower than or similar to invasive diagnostic angiography.[68]

The specific problem in the hybrid approach with PET is the availability of perfusion tracers. Currently, using the most validated perfusion tracers requires an on-site cyclotron. ^{82}Rb is a generator-based tracer but, because of the costs of the generator, the cost-effective delivery requires a large patient flow. Commercial tracer delivery similar to [^{18}F]fluorodeoxyglucose is desirable.

Although the results of clinical trials are promising, the published studies have included a limited number of patients and used a variety of hybrid systems; the uniform reference standard was not used. Thus, larger multicenter trials are needed to confirm these early results. Currently it remains unknown what kind of patients should undergo integrated examinations for clinical effectiveness and minimization of costs and radiation dose.

Combined Coronary CTA and Myocardial CTP

The addition of myocardial CTP imaging adds additional complexity but improved diagnostic opportunities for patients. Similar to hybrid imaging, CTA/CTP imaging shares some of the same issues regarding which study should occur first. For patients with low to intermediate pretest likelihood, a CTA first approach makes similar sense. Myocardial CTP is added in those patients with at least moderate stenoses. One limitation of this sequence is the use of β-blockers. Most CTA protocols use β-blockers as standard of care to improve CTA image quality and reduce radiation doses. However, based on the nuclear perfusion literature, β-blockers may mask myocardial ischemia on subsequent stress CTP imaging.[69,70] Despite this, studies with and without β-blockade have shown similar accuracies.[9,10,29,71]

Adding CTP to a CTA examination increases the contrast and radiation dose to the patient. Studies have shown that between 100 and 150 mL of contrast are required for CTA/CTP imaging.[7,9,11] Therefore, CTA/CTP should be used with caution in patients with renal insufficiency. Technological advances in CTA have markedly reduced the radiation dose in the past several years. These same advances are also benefiting CTP imaging. Studies with dual-source and 320-row CT have shown effective radiation doses between 2.5 and 12.7 mSv for a combined protocol, doses that are less than or similar to SPECT.[9,10,61]

CT imaging artifacts are another limitation. CTP imaging can be affected by 3 primary artifacts: motion, beam-hardening, and reconstruction artifacts.[72,73] Motion artifacts are aggravated by the increase heart rate caused by vasodilator stress agents. Strategies to avoid these artifacts included use of β-blockade and improving temporal resolution using multicycle reconstruction or dual-source CT. Beam-hardening artifacts are analogous to attenuation artifacts in SPECT. In CTP, structures with high attenuation (bone and contrast-filled cavities and vessels) absorb low-energy photons and cause low-attenuation streaks on the myocardium. Reading methods to account for these artifacts and corrections built into reconstruction algorithms can adequately compensate for these artifacts.[72,74]

As with any advanced technology, the financial cost of imaging is of concern. CTP imaging modestly increases imaging time (approximately 15 minutes) and additional contrast and a vasodilator stress agent are required. Although cost-effectiveness data are limited, one study suggests that CTP imaging, used as a first-line imaging test for the workup of patients with CAD, has the potential to provide gains in quality-adjusted life-years at lower cost compared with SPECT.[75]

CLINICAL IMPLICATIONS

There are several situations in which hybrid imaging or CTA/CTP imaging can provide clinically beneficial information.

In moderate stenoses, anatomy alone is not a good determinant of physiologic significance. Perfusion imaging added to CTA can determine whether a moderate stenosis is functionally significant. Patients with multivessel CAD are most likely to benefit from this combination. For example, it is

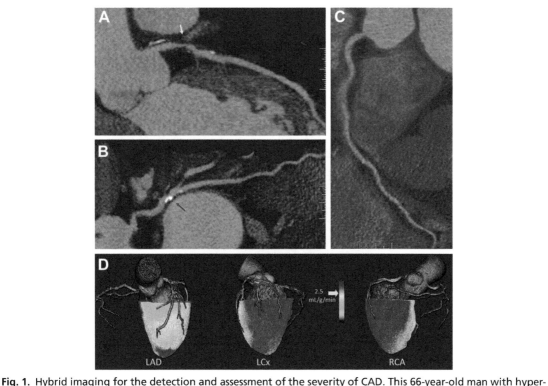

Fig. 1. Hybrid imaging for the detection and assessment of the severity of CAD. This 66-year-old man with hypercholesterolemia and type 2 diabetes mellitus had attacks of anginal pain during the previous weeks. Resting ECG was normal and resting echocardiography showed normal left ventricular and valve function (ejection fraction 65%). An exercise stress test showed good exercise capacity but an ST depression of 1 to 1.5 mm in the lateral leads. CTA showed noncalcified plaque and significant luminal narrowing on proximal left anterior descending artery (LAD) (*arrow, A*). In proximal left circumflex (LCX), a calcified plaque and stenosis was detected (*arrow, B*). The right coronary artery (RCA) was normal, although some motion artifact was seen in the mid-RCA (*C*). In hybrid images (*D*) with stress PET perfusion (absolute scale, 0–3.5 mL/g/min), perfusion was abnormally low in the area supplied by LAD (2.0 mL/g/min) but normal in other vascular regions (LCX 3.4 and RCA 3.2 mL/g/min), which suggests that only the stenosis seen in the LAD was hemodynamically significant. In invasive coronary angiography, similar coronary stenoses were detected but only the LAD stenosis was hemodynamically significant. Scan parameters: CT contrast agent 350 mg I/mL (75 mL), prospective ECG triggering, low radiation protocol (3 mSv); PET perfusion imaging in the same session as CTA using hybrid imaging system, adenosine stress (140 μg/kg/min), O-15-water 900 MBq (0.9 mSv).

possible to identify the culprit flow-limiting lesion. In the setting of balanced 3-vessel disease, imaging of the coronaries does not miss stenoses, but hybrid imaging with quantification of myocardial perfusion allows detection of this phenomenon. Left main stenosis is prognostically important, but is a challenge for perfusion imaging. Left main stenosis noted on CTA with a corresponding large anterior perfusion defect allows accurate detection of these patients. In patients with intermediate or strongly calcified stenosis on CTA, perfusion provides useful information when coronary segments may be limited or uninterpretable. Microvascular disease can be identified based on the presence of reduced perfusion in the absence of obstructive CAD.

One of the major strengths of hybrid imaging is that it powerfully guides the selection of the most appropriate treatment strategy (medical conservative vs percutaneous vs surgical revascularization). However, further studies are warranted to evaluate whether imaging-guided use of interventions will also influence the clinical outcome of patients. It is hoped that the results of ongoing

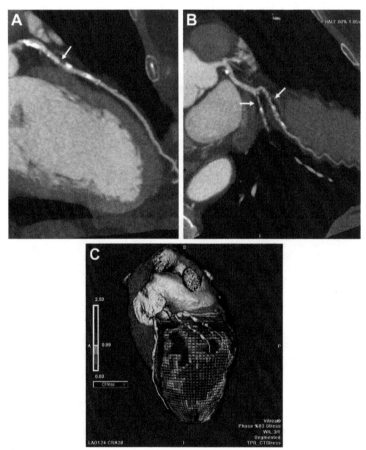

Fig. 2. Combined coronary CTA and myocardial CTP imaging for the detection of physiologically significant CAD. This 64-year-old woman with hypercholesterolemia, hypertension, and tobacco use presented with exertional dyspnea. Resting ECG was normal and resting echocardiography showed normal left ventricular and valve function (ejection fraction 65%). Exercise stress test showed reduced exercise capacity and greater than 1-mm ST depression in the inferolateral leads. CTA showed diffuse calcified and noncalcified plaque and significant luminal narrowing in the proximal LAD (*arrow, A*). In the left circumflex system, there were severe narrowings in the first and second obtuse marginal branches (*arrows, B*). Myocardial CTP imaging showed reduced perfusion in the anterior and anterolateral walls using the transmural perfusion ratio (TPR), a semiquantitative metric of subendocardial ischemia calculated as the ratio of subendocardial and subepicardial attenuation.[7] TPR is color encoded using a scale of 0 to 2.50. Normal perfusion is shown in blue, whereas abnormal perfusion (TPR<0.99) is shown in green, yellow, orange, and red (*C*). ICA showed similar findings and the patient underwent multivessel stenting. Detector CT scan (320 row) parameters: rest coronary CTA-CT contrast agent, 370 mg I/mL (60 mL), prospective ECG triggering, low radiation protocol (5 mSv); stress myocardial CTP-CT contrast agent, 370 mg I/mL (60 mL), prospective ECG triggering (8.7 mSv), adenosine stress (140 μg/kg/min).

prospective multicenter trials such as SPARC, EVINCI, PROMISE, and CORE320 will provide more evidence about the clinical effectiveness of cardiac hybrid imaging.[11,76,77]

Case Histories

Case 1. A 66-year-old man with hypercholesterolemia and type 2 diabetes mellitus had attacks of anginal pain during the previous weeks. His resting ECG was normal and resting echocardiography showed normal left ventricular and valve function (ejection fraction 65%). An exercise stress test showed good exercise capacity but an ST depression of 1 to 1.5 mm in the lateral leads (**Fig. 1**).

Case 2. A 64-year-old woman with hypercholesterolemia, hypertension, and tobacco use presented with exertional dyspnea. Her resting ECG was normal and resting echocardiography showed normal left ventricular and valve function (ejection fraction 65%). An exercise stress test showed reduced exercise capacity and a greater than 1-mm ST depression in the inferolateral leads (**Fig. 2**).

FUTURE PERSPECTIVES

Cardiovascular molecular imaging is designed to visualize and measure biological processes at the molecular and cellular levels.[78,79] Examples of clinical problems that might benefit from molecular imaging include the identification of vulnerable atherosclerotic plaques,[80,81] detection of mechanisms that precede left ventricular remodeling and development of heart failure,[82] and the assessment of risk of ventricular arrhythmias by neuronal imaging.[83] Due to high sensitivity and availability of tracers with low risk of toxicity, PET is the leading imaging technique to proceed with translation of molecular imaging into clinical trials.[78,84] Molecular imaging depends heavily on hybrid imaging approaches, in which the nuclear imaging component is used for molecular targeting and CT imaging is used for localization of the molecular signal. There is preclinical evidence that targeted CT agents can also localize to specific targets. Investigators have shown that the iodine-based contrast agent N1177 localizes to macrophages and can be detected by CT, giving CT the potential to target vulnerable atherosclerotic plaques.[85]

SUMMARY

Cardiac hybrid imaging is entering into routine clinical use. The combination of morphologic imaging of coronary arteries using multidetector CTA and functional imaging of myocardial perfusion using PET, SPECT, and, more recently CT, is a powerful noninvasive imaging method that provides comprehensive information both for diagnosis and decision making for treatment of CAD. Although the performance of hybrid imaging seems to outweigh stand-alone methods, more studies are warranted to demonstrate the cost-effectiveness of this technique.

REFERENCES

1. Wijns W, Kolh P, Danchin N, et al. Guidelines on myocardial revascularization. Eur Heart J 2010;31: 2501–55.
2. Shaw LJ, Berman DS, Maron DJ, et al. Optimal medical therapy with or without percutaneous coronary intervention to reduce ischemic burden: results from the Clinical Outcomes Utilizing Revascularization and Aggressive Drug Evaluation (COURAGE) trial nuclear substudy. Circulation 2008;117:1283–91.
3. Hachamovitch R, Hayes SW, Friedman JD, et al. Comparison of the short-term survival benefit associated with revascularization compared with medical therapy in patients with no prior coronary artery disease undergoing stress myocardial perfusion single photon emission computed tomography. Circulation 2003;107:2900–7.
4. Tonino PA, De Bruyne B, Pijls NH, et al. Fractional flow reserve versus angiography for guiding percutaneous coronary intervention. N Engl J Med 2009; 360:213–24.
5. Gould KL. Identifying and measuring severity of coronary artery stenosis. Quantitative coronary arteriography and positron emission tomography. Circulation 1988;78:237–45.
6. Knuuti J, Kaufmann PA. Hybrid imaging: PET–CT and SPECT–CT. In: Zamorano JL, Bax JJ, Rademakers FE, et al, editors. The ESC textbook of cardiovascular imaging. New York (NY): Springer; 2009. p. 89–101.
7. George RT, Arbab-Zadeh A, Miller JM, et al. Adenosine stress 64- and 256-row detector computed tomography angiography and perfusion imaging: a pilot study evaluating the transmural extent of perfusion abnormalities to predict atherosclerosis causing myocardial ischemia. Circ Cardiovasc Imaging 2009;2:174–82.
8. George RT, Silva C, Ichihara T, et al. Perfusion imaging during first-pass contrast-enhanced helical multi-detector computed tomography. Int J Cardiovasc Imaging 2006;22:S22–3.
9. Blankstein R, Shturman LD, Rogers IS, et al. Adenosine-induced stress myocardial perfusion imaging using dual-source cardiac computed tomography. J Am Coll Cardiol 2009;54:1072–84.
10. Ko BS, Cameron JD, Meredith IT, et al. Computed tomography stress myocardial perfusion imaging in

patients considered for revascularization: a comparison with fractional flow reserve. Eur Heart J 2011. [Epub ahead of print].

11. George RT, Arbab-Zadeh A, Cerci RJ, et al. Diagnostic performance of combined noninvasive coronary angiography and myocardial perfusion imaging using 320-MDCT: the CT angiography and perfusion methods of the CORE320 multicenter multinational diagnostic study. AJR Am J Roentgenol 2011;197:829–37.

12. Klocke FJ, Baird MG, Lorell BH, et al. ACC/AHA/ASNC guidelines for the clinical use of cardiac radionuclide imaging–executive summary: a report of the American College of Cardiology/American Heart Association Task Force on Practice Guidelines (ACC/AHA/ASNC Committee to Revise the 1995 Guidelines for the Clinical Use of Cardiac Radionuclide Imaging). J Am Coll Cardiol 2003;42:1318–33.

13. Underwood SR, Anagnostopoulos C, Cerqueira M, et al. Myocardial perfusion scintigraphy: the evidence. Eur J Nucl Med Mol Imaging 2004;31:261–91.

14. Hachamovitch R, Berman DS, Shaw LJ, et al. Incremental prognostic value of myocardial perfusion single photon emission computed tomography for the prediction of cardiac death: differential stratification for risk of cardiac death and myocardial infarction. Circulation 1998;97:535–43.

15. Di Carli MF, Hachamovitch R. New technology for noninvasive evaluation of coronary artery disease. Circulation 2007;115:1464–80.

16. Knuuti J, Kajander S, Maki M, et al. Quantification of myocardial blood flow will reform the detection of CAD. J Nucl Cardiol 2009;16:497–506.

17. Bergmann SR, Fox KA, Rand AL, et al. Quantification of regional myocardial blood flow in vivo with $H_2{}^{15}O$. Circulation 1984;70:724–33.

18. Hutchins GD, Schwaiger M, Rosenspire KC, et al. Noninvasive quantification of regional blood flow in the human heart using N-13 ammonia and dynamic positron emission tomographic imaging. J Am Coll Cardiol 1990;15:1032–42.

19. Kajander SA, Joutsiniemi E, Saraste M, et al. Clinical value of absolute quantification of myocardial perfusion with 15O-water in coronary artery disease. Circ Cardiovasc Imaging 2011;4:678–84.

20. Parkash R, deKemp RA, Ruddy TD, et al. Potential utility of rubidium 82 PET quantification in patients with 3-vessel coronary artery disease. J Nucl Cardiol 2004;11:440–9.

21. Yoshinaga K, Katoh C, Noriyasu K, et al. Reduction of coronary flow reserve in areas with and without ischemia on stress perfusion imaging in patients with coronary artery disease: a study using oxygen 15-labeled water PET. J Nucl Cardiol 2003;10:275–83.

22. Stone GW, Maehara A, Lansky AJ, et al. A prospective natural-history study of coronary atherosclerosis. N Engl J Med 2011;364:226–35.

23. Cerqueira MD, Weissman NJ, Dilsizian V, et al. Standardized myocardial segmentation and nomenclature for tomographic imaging of the heart: a statement for healthcare professionals from the Cardiac Imaging Committee of the Council on Clinical Cardiology of the American Heart Association. Circulation 2002;105:539–42.

24. Javadi MS, Lautamaki R, Merrill J, et al. Definition of vascular territories on myocardial perfusion images by integration with true coronary anatomy: a hybrid PET/CT analysis. J Nucl Med 2010;51:198–203.

25. Garcia MJ, Lessick J, Hoffmann MH. Accuracy of 16-row multidetector computed tomography for the assessment of coronary artery stenosis. JAMA 2006;296:403–11.

26. Mahnken AH, Bruners P, Katoh M, et al. Dynamic multi-section CT imaging in acute myocardial infarction: preliminary animal experience. Eur Radiol 2006;16:746–52.

27. George RT, Jerosch-Herold M, Silva C, et al. Quantification of myocardial perfusion using dynamic 64-detector computed tomography. Invest Radiol 2007;42:815–22.

28. George RT, Silva C, Cordeiro MA, et al. Multidetector computed tomography myocardial perfusion imaging during adenosine stress. J Am Coll Cardiol 2006;48:153–60.

29. Cury RC, Magalhaes TA, Borges AC, et al. Dipyridamole stress and rest myocardial perfusion by 64-detector row computed tomography in patients with suspected coronary artery disease. Am J Cardiol 2010;106:310–5.

30. Ho KT, Chua KC, Klotz E, et al. Stress and rest dynamic myocardial perfusion imaging by evaluation of complete time-attenuation curves with dual-source CT. JACC Cardiovasc Imaging 2010;3:811–20.

31. George RT, Lardo AC, Lima JA. Computed tomography for the assessment of myocardial perfusion. In: Gerber TC, Kantor B, Williamson EE, editors. Computed tomography of the cardiovascular system. London: Informa Healthcare; 2007.

32. Daghini E, Primak AN, Chade AR, et al. Evaluation of porcine myocardial microvascular permeability and fractional vascular volume using 64-slice helical computed tomography (CT). Invest Radiol 2007;42:274–82.

33. Ichihara T, George RT, Silva C, et al. Quantitative analysis of first-pass contrast-enhanced myocardial perfusion multidetector CT using a Patlak plot method and extraction fraction correction during adenosine stress. IEEE Trans Nucl Sci 2011;58:133–9.

34. Valdiviezo C, Ambrose M, Mehra V, et al. Quantitative and qualitative analysis and interpretation of CT perfusion imaging. J Nucl Cardiol 2010;17:1091–100.

35. Lardo AC, Cordeiro MA, Silva C, et al. Contrast-enhanced multidetector computed tomography

viability imaging after myocardial infarction: characterization of myocyte death, microvascular obstruction, and chronic scar. Circulation 2006;113:394–404.

36. Mahnken AH, Koos R, Katoh M, et al. Assessment of myocardial viability in reperfused acute myocardial infarction using 16-slice computed tomography in comparison to magnetic resonance imaging. J Am Coll Cardiol 2005;45:2042–7.

37. Gerber BL, Belge B, Legros GJ, et al. Characterization of acute and chronic myocardial infarcts by multidetector computed tomography: comparison with contrast-enhanced magnetic resonance. Circulation 2006;113:823–33.

38. Patel AR, Lodato JA, Chandra S, et al. Detection of myocardial perfusion abnormalities using ultra-low radiation dose regadenoson stress multidetector computed tomography. J Cardiovasc Comput Tomogr 2011;5:247–54.

39. Iskandrian AE, Bateman TM, Belardinelli L, et al. Adenosine versus regadenoson comparative evaluation in myocardial perfusion imaging: results of the ADVANCE phase 3 multicenter international trial. J Nucl Cardiol 2007;14:645–58.

40. Kurata A, Mochizuki T, Koyama Y, et al. Myocardial perfusion imaging using adenosine triphosphate stress multi-slice spiral computed tomography: alternative to stress myocardial perfusion scintigraphy. Circ J 2005;69:550–7.

41. Christian TF, Frankish ML, Sisemoore JH, et al. Myocardial perfusion imaging with first-pass computed tomographic imaging: measurement of coronary flow reserve in an animal model of regional hyperemia. J Nucl Cardiol 2010;17:625–30.

42. Bastarrika G, Ramos-Duran L, Schoepf UJ, et al. Adenosine-stress dynamic myocardial volume perfusion imaging with second generation dual-source computed tomography: concepts and first experiences. J Cardiovasc Comput Tomogr 2010;4:127–35.

43. Kajander S, Joutsiniemi E, Saraste M, et al. Cardiac positron emission tomography/computed tomography imaging accurately detects anatomically and functionally significant coronary artery disease. Circulation 2010;122:603–13.

44. Namdar M, Hany TF, Koepfli P, et al. Integrated PET/CT for the assessment of coronary artery disease: a feasibility study. J Nucl Med 2005;46:930–5.

45. Hacker M, Jakobs T, Matthiesen F, et al. Comparison of spiral multidetector CT angiography and myocardial perfusion imaging in the noninvasive detection of functionally relevant coronary artery lesions: first clinical experiences. J Nucl Med 2005;46:1294–300.

46. Sato A, Nozato T, Hikita H, et al. Incremental value of combining 64-slice computed tomography angiography with stress nuclear myocardial perfusion imaging to improve noninvasive detection of coronary artery disease. J Nucl Cardiol 2010;17:19–26.

47. Groves AM, Speechly-Dick ME, Kayani I, et al. First experience of combined cardiac PET/64-detector CT angiography with invasive angiographic validation. Eur J Nucl Med Mol Imaging 2009;36:2027–33.

48. Gaemperli O, Schepis T, Valenta I, et al. Cardiac image fusion from stand-alone SPECT and CT: clinical experience. J Nucl Med 2007;48:696–703.

49. Santana CA, Garcia EV, Faber TL, et al. Diagnostic performance of fusion of myocardial perfusion imaging (MPI) and computed tomography coronary angiography. J Nucl Cardiol 2009;16:201–11.

50. Slomka PJ, Cheng VY, Dey D, et al. Quantitative analysis of myocardial perfusion SPECT anatomically guided by coregistered 64-slice coronary CT angiography. J Nucl Med 2009;50:1621–30.

51. van Werkhoven JM, Schuijf JD, Gaemperli O, et al. Prognostic value of multislice computed tomography and gated single-photon emission computed tomography in patients with suspected coronary artery disease. J Am Coll Cardiol 2009;53:623–32.

52. Pazhenkottil AP, Nkoulou RN, Ghadri JR, et al. Prognostic value of cardiac hybrid imaging integrating single-photon emission computed tomography with coronary computed tomography angiography. Eur Heart J 2011;32:1465–71.

53. Bell MR, Lerman LO, Rumberger JA. Validation of minimally invasive measurement of myocardial perfusion using electron beam computed tomography and application in human volunteers. Heart 1999;81:628–35.

54. Gould RG, Lipton MJ, McNamara MT, et al. Measurement of regional myocardial blood flow in dogs by ultrafast CT. Invest Radiol 1988;23:348–53.

55. Wang T, Wu X, Chung N, et al. Myocardial blood flow estimated by synchronous multislice, high-speed computed tomography. IEEE Trans Med Imaging 1989;8:70–7.

56. Wolfkiel CJ, Ferguson JL, Chomka EV, et al. Measurement of myocardial blood flow by ultrafast computed tomography. Circulation 1987;76:1262–73.

57. George RT, Ichihara T, Lima JA, et al. A method for reconstructing the arterial input function during helical CT: implications for myocardial perfusion distribution imaging. Radiology 2010;255:396–404.

58. Rocha-Filho JA, Blankstein R, Shturman LD, et al. Incremental value of adenosine-induced stress myocardial perfusion imaging with dual-source CT at cardiac CT angiography. Radiology 2010;254:410–9.

59. Magalhães TA, Cury RC, Pereira AC, et al. Additional value of dipyridamole stress myocardial perfusion by 64-row computed tomography in patients with coronary stents. J Cardiovasc Comput Tomogr, in press.

60. Ko SM, Choi JW, Song MG, et al. Myocardial perfusion imaging using adenosine-induced stress

dual-energy computed tomography of the heart: comparison with cardiac magnetic resonance imaging and conventional coronary angiography. Eur Radiol 2011;21:26–35.

61. Feuchtner G, Goetti R, Plass A, et al. Adenosine stress high-pitch 128-slice dual-source myocardial computed tomography perfusion for imaging of reversible myocardial ischemia: comparison with magnetic resonance imaging. Circ Cardiovasc Imaging 2011;4:540–9.

62. Fazel R, Krumholz HM, Wang Y, et al. Exposure to low-dose ionizing radiation from medical imaging procedures. N Engl J Med 2009;361:849–57.

63. Gaemperli O, Kaufmann PA. Lower dose and shorter acquisition: pushing the boundaries of myocardial perfusion SPECT. J Nucl Cardiol 2011;18:830–2.

64. Duvall WL, Croft LB, Ginsberg ES, et al. Reduced isotope dose and imaging time with a high-efficiency CZT SPECT camera. J Nucl Cardiol 2011;18:847–57.

65. Hausleiter J, Martinoff S, Hadamitzky M, et al. Image quality and radiation exposure with a low tube voltage protocol for coronary CT angiography results of the PROTECTION II Trial. JACC Cardiovasc Imaging 2010;3:1113–23.

66. Husmann L, Valenta I, Gaemperli O, et al. Feasibility of low-dose coronary CT angiography: first experience with prospective ECG-gating. Eur Heart J 2008;29:191–7.

67. Achenbach S, Marwan M, Ropers D, et al. Coronary computed tomography angiography with a consistent dose below 1 mSv using prospectively electrocardiogram-triggered high-pitch spiral acquisition. Eur Heart J 2010;31:340–6.

68. Husmann L, Herzog BA, Gaemperli O, et al. Diagnostic accuracy of computed tomography coronary angiography and evaluation of stress-only single-photon emission computed tomography/computed tomography hybrid imaging: comparison of prospective electrocardiogram-triggering vs. retrospective gating. Eur Heart J 2009;30:600–7.

69. Koepfli P, Wyss CA, Namdar M, et al. Beta-adrenergic blockade and myocardial perfusion in coronary artery disease: differential effects in stenotic versus remote myocardial segments. J Nucl Med 2004;45:1626–31.

70. Bottcher M, Czernin J, Sun K, et al. Effect of beta 1 adrenergic receptor blockade on myocardial blood flow and vasodilatory capacity. J Nucl Med 1997;38:442–6.

71. George RT. Computed tomography myocardial perfusion imaging: developmental points of emphasis. Expert Rev Cardiovasc Ther 2009;7:99–101.

72. Mehra V, Valdiviezo C, Arab-Zadeh A, et al. A stepwise approach to the visual interpretation of CT-based myocardial perfusion. J Cardiovasc Comput Tomogr, in press.

73. Mehra VC, Ambrose M, Valdiviezo-Schlomp C, et al. CT-based myocardial perfusion imaging-practical considerations: acquisition, image analysis, interpretation, and challenges. J Cardiovasc Transl Res 2011;4:437–48.

74. Kitagawa K, George RT, Arbab-Zadeh A, et al. Characterization and correction of beam-hardening artifacts during dynamic volume CT assessment of myocardial perfusion. Radiology 2010;256:111–8.

75. Meyer M, Nance JW Jr, Schoepf UJ, et al. Cost-effectiveness of substituting dual-energy CT for SPECT in the assessment of myocardial perfusion for the workup of coronary artery disease. Eur J Radiol 2011. [Epub ahead of print].

76. PROspective Multicenter Imaging Study for Evaluation of Chest Pain (PROMISE). Funded by the National Heart, Lung, and Blood Institute. Available at: http://clinicaltrials.gov/show/NCT01174550. Accessed October 4, 2010.

77. Hachamovitch R, Johnson JR, Hlatky MA, et al. The study of myocardial perfusion and coronary anatomy imaging roles in CAD (SPARC): design, rationale, and baseline patient characteristics of a prospective, multicenter observational registry comparing PET, SPECT, and CTA for resource utilization and clinical outcomes. J Nucl Cardiol 2009;16:935–48.

78. Saraste A, Nekolla SG, Schwaiger M. Cardiovascular molecular imaging: an overview. Cardiovasc Res 2009;83:643–52.

79. Nahrendorf M, Sosnovik DE, French BA, et al. Multimodality cardiovascular molecular imaging, Part II. Circ Cardiovasc Imaging 2009;2:56–70.

80. Rudd JH, Narula J, Strauss HW, et al. Imaging atherosclerotic plaque inflammation by fluorodeoxyglucose with positron emission tomography: ready for prime time? J Am Coll Cardiol 2010;55:2527–35.

81. Gaemperli O, Shalhoub J, Owen DR, et al. Imaging intraplaque inflammation in carotid atherosclerosis with 11C-PK11195 positron emission tomography/computed tomography. Eur Heart J. [Epub ahead of print].

82. Kramer CM, Sinusas AJ, Sosnovik DE, et al. Multimodality imaging of myocardial injury and remodeling. J Nucl Med 2010;51(Suppl 1):107S–21S.

83. Jacobson AF, Senior R, Weiland F, et al. Prognostic significance of 123I-mIBG myocardial scintigraphy in heart failure patients: results from the prospective multicenter international ADMIRE-HF trial. J Am Coll Cardiol 2010;55(20):2212–21.

84. Knuuti J, Bengel FM. Positron emission tomography and molecular imaging. Heart 2008;94:360–7.

85. Hyafil F, Cornily JC, Rudd JH, et al. Quantification of inflammation within rabbit atherosclerotic plaques using the macrophage-specific CT contrast agent N1177: a comparison with 18F-FDG PET/CT and histology. J Nucl Med 2009;50:959–65.

MDCT to Guide Transcatheter Aortic Valve Replacement and Mitral Valve Repair

Jonathon Leipsic, MD, FRCPC, FSCCT[a,b,*],
Cameron J. Hague, MD[b], Ronen Gurvitch, MD[a],
Amr M. Ajlan, MD, FRCPC[b], Troy M. Labounty, MD, FSCCT[c],
James K. Min, MD, FSCCT[c]

KEYWORDS

- Aortic stenosis • Mitral valve repair
- Coronary sinus annuloplasty

TRANSCATHETER AORTIC VALVE REPLACEMENT

Aortic stenosis is becoming increasingly common given our aging population. Estimates suggest that nearly 5% of individuals older than 75 years[1] have aortic stenosis. Historically, the treatment of choice has been aortic valve replacement with conventional surgery for patients with severe aortic stenosis, as the prognosis of untreated patients is poor particularly when symptomatic.[2] Many patients with symptoms related to severe aortic stenosis have numerous comorbidities and are not considered candidates for surgical valve replacement.[3] Transcatheter aortic valve replacement (TAVR) is now available as a minimally invasive option to treat select high-risk patients with severe aortic stenosis.[4–7] At present more than 20,000 procedures have been performed worldwide, mostly confined to patients at high surgical risk. The short- and medium-term outcomes have been promising.[4,6,8]

In September 2010, the landmark PARTNER (Placement of Aortic Transcatheter Valves) B trial was published,[9] in which 358 patients with severe aortic stenosis considered to be at prohibitively high risk for standard surgery were randomized to medical management and balloon aortic valvuloplasty against balloon-expandable transfemoral TAVR. This randomized multicenter trial noted a 20% absolute reduction in 1-year all-cause mortality in the TAVR cohort as compared with the standard of care (30.7% vs 50.7%, $P<.001$), establishing that transfemoral TAVR is superior to conservative therapy for inoperable patients with severe symptomatic aortic stenosis. More recently, the PARTNER A trial results were presented at the American College of Cardiology in 2011, and subsequently published in the *New England Journal of Medicine*.[10] In this study arm, 699 high-risk but operable candidates with severe and symptomatic aortic stenosis were randomized to either TAVR (transfemoral or transapical) or surgical aortic valve replacement (AVR).[10] TAVR

Disclosures: Jonathon Leipsic is on the speaker's bureau and advisory board for Edward Lifesciences. James K. Min is also on the advisory board for Edwards. All other authors report no pertinent disclosures.
[a] Division of Cardiology, St Paul's Hospital, University of British Columbia, Vancouver, BC, Canada
[b] Department of Radiology, St Paul's Hospital, University of British Columbia, Vancouver, BC, Canada
[c] Departments of Medicine, Imaging, and Biomedical Sciences, Cedars-Sinai Heart Institute, Cedars-Sinai Medical Center, Los Angeles, CA, USA
* Corresponding author. Department of Medical Imaging, St Paul's Hospital, 1081 Burrard Street, Vancouver, BC V6S 1Y6, Canada.
E-mail address: jleipsic@providencehealth.bc.ca

Cardiol Clin 30 (2012) 147–160
doi:10.1016/j.ccl.2011.10.003
0733-8651/12/$ – see front matter © 2012 Elsevier Inc. All rights reserved.

was noninferior to AVR for all-cause mortality at 1 year (24.2% vs 26.8%, P = .001), although there was a higher incidence of cerebrovascular events and vascular injury. Many argue that these data are even more impressive given that the transcatheter procedures were performed with first-generation implantable valve technology by operators with limited experience, who were matched against highly experienced surgeons at the premier cardiothoracic centers in the world. Based on current evidence, it is reasonable to suggest that TAVR is an acceptable alternative to surgical AVR in selected patients who are at high risk and operable.

Overview of the TAVR Procedure

Two TAVR systems have seen wide clinical application: the balloon-expandable Edwards SAPIEN and SAPIEN XT valve (Edwards Lifesciences, Irvine, CA, USA) and the self-expandable Core-Valve ReValving system (Medtronic, Minneapolis, MN, USA) (**Fig. 1**). Both systems have been extensively described elsewhere.[9,11,12] Access to the native valve can be achieved using a retrograde transarterial technique typically via the subclavian or femoral arteries, or by using an anterograde transapical technique. In both techniques, balloon aortic valvuloplasty is initially performed to facilitate passage of the valve prosthesis through the stenotic native valve. Subsequently, the unexpanded valve is appropriately positioned within

the native aortic valve. The Edwards SAPIEN valve is expanded by a balloon during burst ventricular pacing to minimize cardiac output and prevent migration of the valve during deployment. The CoreValve is self-expanding and is generally deployed without pacing. Newer routes for transcatheter valve replacement are being developed, such as a transaortic approach via the ascending aorta. Multiple other vendors are also developing new valves for transcatheter implantation.

Achieving optimal positioning of the transcatheter aortic prosthesis is of great importance to the procedural success and patient outcome, as the goal is to displace the native valve leaflets and deploy within the native valve annulus. If the prosthetic valve assumes a low position, there is a risk of heart block, paravalvular regurgitation, and increased risk of mitral valve dysfunction.[13] Alternatively if the valve is implanted too high, there is increased risk of valve embolization into the thoracic aorta, paravalvular regurgitation, and aortic root injury.[14]

Since the inception of this procedure, there has been progressive decrease in size of the delivery catheters required for valve implantation using the transfemoral route. In its first iteration transfemoral access required a large 24F delivery system, and a significant number of vascular complications with resultant morbidity and mortality were encountered. The 22F to 24F sheaths required for the SAPIEN valve and RetroFlex delivery system (Edwards Lifesciences) have been associated

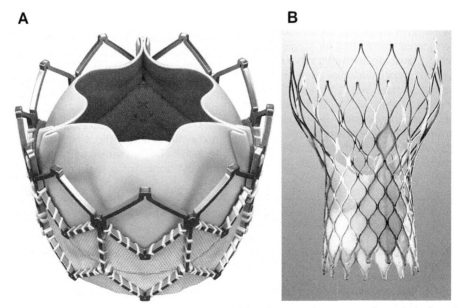

A   **B**

Fig. 1. (*A*) Edwards SAPIEN XT valve. The balloon-expandable valve stent frame comprises cobalt-chromium, with bovine pericardial leaflets (*B*) Medtronic CoreValve. The self-expanding valve stent frame comprises Nitinol, with porcine pericardial leaflets.

with vascular complication rates ranging from 22.9% in the large European SOURCE registry[15] to 30.7% in the North American PARTNER 1B trial.[9] The smaller 18F sheaths required for the third-generation CoreValve delivery system (Medtronic) have been associated with lower vascular complication rates, ranging from 1.9% to 13.3%.[16–18] Similar vascular complication rates with the low-profile, 18F to 19F SAPIEN XT NovaFlex delivery system (Edwards Lifesciences) have not yet been published, but initial experiences suggest similar lower complication rates. Lower profile sheaths and delivery catheters have enabled an improvement in the procedural risk profile through a reduction in the burden of peripheral vascular complications, which has allowed for expanded patient eligibility. In the authors' experience, however, appropriate screening with multidetector computed tomography (MDCT) remains critical. The scope of the problem has been large enough that minor and major vascular access complications have been formally defined by the Valve Academic Research Consortium (VARC)[19] to allow for proper tracking and meaningful comparisons of end points in trials. At the authors' institution, VARC-defined major vascular complications in the last 137 consecutive patients have decreased from 8% in 2009 to 1% in 2010 ($P = .06$), and minor vascular complications have decreased from 24% to 8% ($P<.01$).[20] More importantly, in a subset of 82 patients screened with MDCT, if the diameter of the iliac arteries was less than the external sheath diameter (6.0 mm for 18F sheaths and 6.5 mm for 19F sheaths), vascular complications were found to be much more common (23% vs 5%, $P = .01$).[20] In addition, the presence of moderately or severely calcified iliofemoral arteries, as detected by MDCT, was also a strong predictor of vascular complications (29% vs 9%, $P = .03$).[20]

Iliofemoral Access Assessment

At the authors' institution vascular access evaluation begins with conventional angiography, where all patients undergo fluoroscopic assessment of the descending aorta with fluoroscopic imaging of both iliac and femoral arteries down to the femoral head. A calibrated pigtail catheter (Royal Flush; Cook Inc, Bloomington, IN, USA) is used to facilitate estimation of minimal arterial diameter. Calcification is also graded fluoroscopically as none (0), mild (1), moderate (2), or severe (3). A formal assessment of the abdominal aorta and iliofemoral system is performed in an attempt to detect stenotic, occlusive, and aneurysmal disease. This assessment is done at the time of coronary angiography and provides the operator

a basic assessment of luminal size of the peripheral access, but very limited data regarding vascular atherosclerotic burden and the degree of vessel tortuosity.

MDCT allows a thorough and complete 3-dimensional (3D) assessment of the iliofemoral system, including an evaluation of plaque burden and vessel tortuosity, which provides important data for procedural planning, given the common association of peripheral vascular disease and severe aortic stenosis. Kurra and colleagues[21] recently reported that 33% of patients with severe aortic stenosis had unfavorable iliofemoral arteries for a 24F delivery system; in addition, nearly 80% of the patients evaluated had minimal luminal diameters of less than 8 mm. MDCT provides more accurate luminal assessment than single-plane angiography, due to the additional data afforded by its multiplanar capabilities stemming from the isotropic voxels that are acquired. This potential allows for elaborate 3D reconstructions and accurate assessments of the minimal luminal diameter integrating data from the coronal, sagittal, and transverse axial planes. MDCT can assess vessel tortuosity, burden and pattern of calcification, extent of atherosclerosis, and can identify other high-risk features including dissections and complex atheroma (**Fig. 2**). This additional information is important because successful implants have been completed in patients with arteries of borderline size and mild calcification. However, in the setting of circumferential or horseshoe calcification with small-caliber vessels or stenotic segments of the transfemoral artery, this approach is considered to be contraindicated. Vessels with such anatomy may not allow the artery to expand and accommodate the large-profile delivery catheter, and may increase the risk of arterial dissection or perforation. Early transarterial device delivery failures have been attributed in part to circumferential iliofemoral calcification that was not appreciated on screening angiography.[22]

Another proposed predictor of access complications is a minimal luminal diameter that is less than the sheath diameter. Optimally the minimal lumen diameter should exceed the diameter of the delivery system. In the authors' experience, in the absence of severe calcification, bulky atheromatous burden, or severe tortuosity, short segments of relatively compliant arteries can be up to 1 to 2 mm smaller in diameter than the intended sheath without compromising safety of cannulation.[21,23] As discussed earlier, in a subset of 82 patients screened at the authors' institution with MDCT, a situation whereby the MDCT-determined minimal artery diameter was less

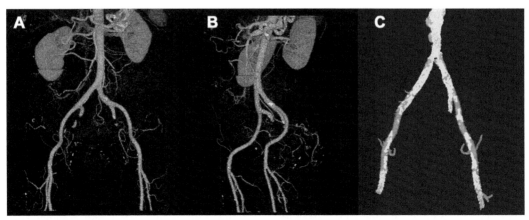

Fig. 2. Iliofemoral assessment of a 79-year-old woman (*A* and *B*) and an 83-year-old man (*C*). Note that when evaluating the iliofemoral system in an anteroposterior fashion (*A*) similar to that done in the catheterization laboratory, one may not appreciate the tortuosity of the iliofemoral system in an anterior posterior dimension, but when obliqued the tortuosity becomes evident (*B*). CT can also provide a valuable assessment of the degree, burden, and distribution of calcification in the iliofemoral system.

than the external sheath diameter was a strong predictor for vascular complications (23% vs 5%, $P = .01$), as was the presence of moderate or severely calcified iliofemoral arteries (29% vs 9%, $P = .03$). Iliofemoral tortuosity of 45° or more did not predict vascular complications ($P = .27$); however, severe tortuosity may become important in the future because lower-profile devices may sacrifice the ability of the delivery system to negotiate tight corners for smaller size.[21] When 2 of the 3 features of vessel diameter less than sheath diameter, circumferential calcification, or severe tortuosity are present, alternative transapical or transaxillary approaches are considered. Recently, Hayashida and colleagues[24] proposed the ratio of sheath and femoral artery size (SFAR) as the most predictive variable in determining those at risk of vascular access injury. These investigators propose an SFAR sliding scale depending on the burden of atherosclerotic calcification with a threshold of 1.05 predicting a higher rate of VARC-defined major complications, with an area under the receiver-operating characteristic curve of 0.727. Hayashida and colleagues suggest that routine application of SFAR improves patient selection, leads to better outcomes, and lowers the morbidity profile for TAVR.

When evaluating the peripheral access with MDCT for TAVR, a standardized approach yields the best results and helps reduce the morbidity and mortality rate from vascular injury.[24] The authors incorporate several reconstructions into their standard iliofemoral evaluation by MDCT, including 3D volume-rendered imaging, curved multiplanar reformats, and maximum-intensity projection images (**Fig. 3**). Multiple measurements are taken along the entire course of the iliofemoral system bilaterally, with the minimum luminal measurement recorded for each side and included in the report. Identifying the specific location of areas with reduced luminal size is important; in some cases, access can be achieved proximal to the site by a cutdown approach. A description of the overall plaque burden and presence of iliofemoral calcification is noted. Attention is given to any region of circumferential or horseshoe

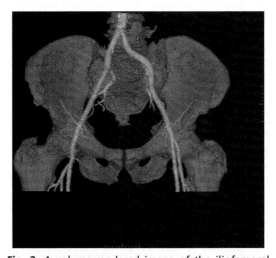

Fig. 3. A volume-rendered image of the iliofemoral system and bony pelvis in an 87-year-old man undergoing workup for TAVR. Note the stenosis in the right common femoral artery at the level of the midfemoral head, suggesting the need for a high puncture on the right and the high bifurcation of the common femoral artery.

calcification. All measurements should be taken in a plane orthogonal to the vessel rather than in the transverse axial plane. To do so, a center-line approach is used to elongate the typically curved and somewhat tortuous iliofemoral vasculature. By elongating the vessel and using an oblique tool, the interpreting physician is able to obtain a true short-axis reformat, allowing reproducible bidimensional measurements.

Coaxial Angle of Deployment Prediction

In addition to access assessment, there is growing evidence that MDCT has potential to assess the aortic root in relation to the body axis.[25] The standard practice has been initially to determine the aortic root orientation using repeated catheter aortograms in 1 or 2 orthogonal planes before commencing the procedure. This process is considered a critical step to ensure a coaxial deployment of the stent along the centerline of the aorta, and thus increase the likelihood that the valve is deployed perpendicular to the aortic root.[25,26] Physicians performing TAVR ideally select an implant projection that is orthogonal to the native valve plane. The need for multiple root angiograms to define this optimal orientation results in longer procedural time, higher effective radiation doses and, perhaps most importantly in this elderly patient population, higher contrast volume. In addition, if accurate orientation is not achieved there is a risk of inappropriate positioning of the device and an increased likelihood of procedural complications, such as stent embolization.[23]

It is now accepted that there are several appropriate angles of stent implantation in any individual. The aortic valve is most commonly directed in a cranial and anterior position with a slight degree of angulation to the right. On this basis, the interventional team typically uses a slight caudal angulation when in a right anterior oblique (RAO) projection and cranial angulation when in the left anterior oblique (LAO) projection. There are, however, significant variations in patient anatomy, and preprocedural assessment of the aortic root geometry has been beneficial in predicting the appropriate angle of implantation.[23,25,26]

Preprocedural computed tomography (CT) examinations provide a data set that can be used to determine the orientation of the aortic root, and thus an opportunity to predict a suitable angle of implantation. At their center the authors use the following method. In a fashion similar to the assessment of the aortic annulus, double oblique transverse projections of the aortic root and

basal ring are created. From this projection, points are deposited on the most inferior aspect of the aortic cusps and the points are then linked to form a triangle. A 3D volume-rendered reconstruction of the aorta is then created with the triangle superimposed on it (**Fig. 4**). The reconstruction can then be rotated through a series of angles. The aim is then to find angiographic projections perpendicular to the native valve plane in 3 axes: (1) cranial-caudal without RAO or LAO angulation, (2) straight RAO to LAO as needed without cranial or caudal angulation, and (3) LAO 30° with cranial or caudal angulation as needed. These axes have been chosen based on past experiences, and they are considered reasonable working angles given the physical constraints of the catheterization laboratory.

Preprocedural angle prediction with MDCT has the potential to decrease the number of aortograms required during the procedure, shortening both procedure time and contrast usage, and to increase the likelihood of coaxial implantation by optimizing the orientation during device placement. This angle prediction may be particularly helpful in patients with unusual anatomy, which often necessitates steep projections that would be difficult to predict at the time of valve implantation. These atypical angles are most commonly observed in patients with musculoskeletal abnormalities, kyphoscoliosis, and tortuous unfolded aortas. There is no single suitable angle for each patient; numerous views are possible. The authors have found that a line of perpendicularity can be generated in each patient (**Fig. 5**),[25] where any point in the RAO to LAO spectrum can be used as long as the correct amount of caudal or cranial angulations is added.

THE ONGOING DEBATE ON HOW TO SIZE THE ANNULUS WITH MDCT

Annular sizing of the aortic valve is essential to TAVR success regardless of the access and approach that is chosen, whether a femoral, subclavian, or transapical approach is used. Reproducible and accurate measurements of the aortic annulus are important in patient selection and proper implantation because current implantable valves are designed for specific annular sizes. During surgical AVR, prosthesis sizing is performed using a sizing probe under direct visualization during open heart surgery. This approach obviously cannot be used in TAVR because there is no opportunity to directly visualize the annulus. As a result, aortic annulus measurements for TAVR rely exclusively on imaging. Annulus measurements are typically performed using 2-dimensional (2D) transthoracic

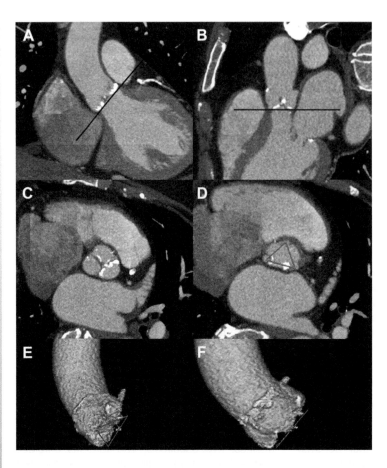

Fig. 4. Coaxial angle prediction with MDCT; an 84-year-old man with critical symptomatic aortic stenosis being evaluated for TAVR. Angle assessment was performed using a stepwise approach. A double oblique transverse image of the aortic root (*C*) is reconstructed from a coronal (*A*) and sagittal oblique reformat (*B*). Points are deposited at inferior aspect of the aortic valve cusps and the points are connected to form a triangle (*D*). The triangle is superimposed on a 3D volume-rendered reconstruction of the aorta to facilitate angle prediction. When the triangle is seen that suggests that the angle is not co-axial (*E*). The triangle was visible with left anterior oblique 14 cranial 8 in this case unlike the predicted coaxial angle of AP Caudal 12 (*F*) where only a line is seen.

echocardiography (TTE), transesophageal echocardiography (TEE), or calibrated aortic angiography, with comparison between methods being limited and controversial.[12]

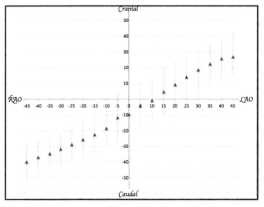

Fig. 5. Graphical display of the line of perpendicularity. The graph is a representation of the typical caudal or cranial angulation needed across varying degrees of RAO to LAO projections (5° intervals) to achieve valve perpendicularity to the x-ray beam. The diamonds denote the mean angles from the last 100 patients, and the bars denote the range.

A unifying limitation of any 2D imaging technique is that diameter measurements are based on a single annular plane, and assume a circular annular orifice. The reality, however, is that the aortic annulus is a complex structure that is often oval.[27–34] There has been significant interest in better defining the shape and size of the annulus by alternative imaging methods. Imaging with 3D TEE has reported larger annular sizes than observed using traditional 2D TEE.[27] Electrocardiographic (ECG)-gated MDCT is typically performed in patients before TAVR implantation, and can also be used to measure the annular size in addition to evaluating vascular access sites.[28,35] The annular size by MDCT is typically larger than when measured with either 2D or 3D TEE,[27,28,30,35] as discussed below.

Current recommendations and clinical practice require patient eligibility for transcatheter valve therapy and prosthesis sizing to be largely based on the aortic annulus measurements on TTE and TEE. Clinical outcomes with TEE-based annulus determination and routine oversizing of the valve by 1 to 2 mm have been good. Although the results with TEE-based sizing have been good, there remains a percentage of patients with paravalvular regurgitation and leak after the procedure,[7] resulting in many investigators pursuing the use of MDCT annular measurements when screening patients for TAVR.[27,28,30,33] At present there are specific annular size limitations for TAVR. For the Edwards SAPIEN valve, the annulus must measure between 18 and 25 mm; for the current generation of CoreValve, the annulus must range between 20 and 27 mm. Recently, both a 20-mm transfemoral and a 29-mm transapical balloon-expandable SAPIEN XT valve have become available. Therefore, accurate annulus determination is becoming increasingly important.

Proposed Annulus Sizing Guide with MDCT

The aortic annulus is not a true ring as the name implies, but is a complex 3D structure. Anatomic studies have established that it is a 3-pronged coronet with 3 anchor points at the inferior aspect of each of the cusps.[27] In addition, the attachment of the aortic cusps is semilunar, extending throughout the aortic root from the left ventricle distally to the sinotubular junction. The annulus is most commonly oval, which was first observed with MDCT[28–34] and then by 3D TEE.[13] Using MDCT the annulus has been reported to have an oval configuration in approximately 50% of patients evaluated for TAVR, with a mean difference between coronal and sagittal measurements of 3.0 ± 1.9 mm.[28] An oval configuration of the annulus was also noted by Delgado and colleagues,[32] who reported a significant difference between mean coronal (25.1 ± 2.4 mm) and sagittal (22.9 ± 2.0 mm) measurements in 53 patients with severe aortic stenosis. This oval geometry of the annulus has been underappreciated on imaging, due to the traditional 2D imaging techniques used for assessment. The elliptical nature of the annulus has been well described in the surgical literature.

The assessment of such a complex structure by a 2D imaging technique is inherently difficult because of the limitations of imaging in specific planes. Previous work has shown that TEE diameters can underestimate the true diameter as measured at surgery by a mean of 1.2 mm, and frequently underestimate it by more than 2 mm.[21] Despite this, operators have become accustomed to echocardiography-guided TAVR, with good results. However, aortic regurgitation, valve embolization, annular rupture, and patient prosthetic mismatch continue to occur, emphasizing the importance of accurate annular evaluation.

Over the past few years, there have been several methods reported in the literature for measurement of the aortic annulus with CT. Regardless of the method used, CT usually yields results of larger size than those from echocardiography, with the differences greater than those between TTE and TEE. These differences could result in clinical implications if simply integrated into echocardiographic-derived sizing criteria, particularly if the annulus is approaching the cutpoints for valve sizing. Messika-Zeitoun and colleagues[30] have shown that MDCT could influence or modify TAVR strategy in 38% of patients using long-axis and short-axis diameters. These differences have resulted in significant confusion among imagers and proceduralists, particularly given that echo-based sizing has yielded good clinical results. Regardless, it is important to consistently report and consider measurements from both TEE and MDCT, and carefully examine both in cases of significant intertest disagreement, as well as to learn from the outcome of the procedure itself. This multimodality approach may reduce the chance for error, and at the very least provides a more comprehensive evaluation of the annulus regarding geometry and size.

More recently, the authors have begun to more formally integrate MDCT annular sizing into their clinical TAVR program. Given the outcome data for recently performed TAVR procedures, it is not reasonable to suggest altering echocardiography-based sizing of the prosthesis in 40% of cases, as may be suggested by MDCT measurements alone.[30–32] Similarly, it is important that a CT-based sizing scale be validated and introduced for annular and prosthesis sizing. The reproducibility and reliability, as well as the knowledge and understanding of how to apply these measurements on CT have been lacking. Because of these limitations, the clinical utility of CT has remained limited in TAVR assessment. The authors therefore sought to first assess the most reproducible measurement of the annulus. Three independent readers reviewed 50 pre-TAVR–MDCT examinations measuring the annulus using 6 previously described methods. The authors evaluated 6 methods: coronal and sagittal oblique, 3-chamber, double oblique transverse short axis of the basal ring,[33] long axis of the basal ring, and an area measurement of the basal ring of the aorta. The results of this assessment confirmed that the most reproducible CT measurements are the mean of the long and short axis of the basal ring and the basal ring area (**Fig. 6**).[33] These measurements are typically 1 to 1.5 mm larger than TEE measurements of the annulus. The authors' proposal is that to develop a CT-based sizing scale for TAVR, one must begin to integrate these differences in the prosthesis selection. The thresholds

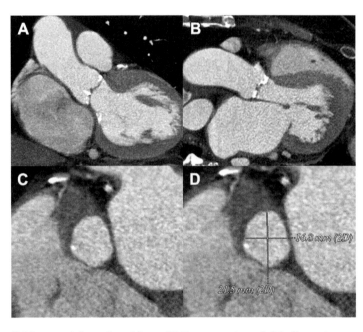

Fig. 6. Stepwise approach to evaluate the aortic annulus and basal ring with MDCT in an 89-year-old woman with severe aortic stenosis. Evaluation begins from a coronal projection of the aorta. A vertically oriented multi-planar tool (*A*) is placed to produce a sagittal oblique reconstruction of the ascending aorta (*B*). A transverse or axial cut-plane is placed on the sagittal reconstruction (*B*) at the level of the commissures. This transverse cut-plane produces a double oblique transverse image of the aortic root. The reviewing physician then scrolls up or down until the caudal attachments of the aortic valve become apparent and then extends approximately 2 mm below (*C*). It is important that the nadir of all 3 cusps must be identified on one transverse image to ensure the appropriate plane for assessment of the aortic annulus. At this point, both short (16.8 mm minimum) and long (21.5 mm maximum) (*D*) dimensions can be obtained, allowing the calculation of the mean diameter of 19.2 mm in this case.

for valve sizing have thus been increased by 1 to 1.5 mm, such that the following sizing guidelines are used when using MDCT: mean basal ring, 23-mm valve for annulus size of more than 19.5 up to 22.5 mm, 26-mm valve for more than 22.5 up to 26.5 mm, and 29-mm valve for more than 26.5 up to 29.5 mm (**Fig. 7, Table 1**).[33] It is important to recognize that this information is now one of many data points that are included in the decision-making process. Future studies, preferably a prospective multicenter trial, are required to gain more understanding of the optimal method for annulus sizing, and although CT remains promising, echocardiographic measurements of annular diameter remain the recommended method for measuring annular dimensions. TAVR outcomes using the conventional anteroposterior (sagittal plane) annular diameter by TEE are excellent.[30]

Reducing Contrast Volume in CT Angiographic Screening for TAVR

One of the limitations of screening TAVR patients with MDCT is the need for additional contrast medium injection. Although CT angiography provides more anatomic detail, it typically requires 50 to 140 mL of intravenous contrast medium, carrying with it the potential risk of contrast-induced nephropathy (CIN). This risk is increased particularly when MDCT is performed in addition to other diagnostic tests, such as coronary

angiography, especially in this elderly cohort with multiple comorbidities. Webb and colleagues[34] documented a prevalence of chronic renal insufficiency approaching 1% in the first 168 patients undergoing transcatheter valve replacement. To help reduce the risk of CIN, several mechanisms for reducing contrast volume have been published. Joshi and colleagues[36] described a new technique for CT angiography of the iliofemoral arterial tree that uses only 10 to 15 mL of iodinated contrast. Their approach was to provide a 15-mL direct aortic injection via pigtail catheter positioned below the renal arteries in the catheterization laboratory. The contrast medium was mixed with normal saline in a 1:3 to 1:4 dilution in a single chamber of the power injector. A total of 40 mL of the contrast/saline mixture was injected at 4 mL/s through the pigtail catheter without a saline chaser. This protocol yielded excellent image quality in more than 90% of cases, and provides an alternative to higher contrast-volume protocols via an intravenous injection.[36]

MDCT FOR MITRAL VALVE REPAIR

After the initial balloon valvuloplasty described for rheumatic mitral stenosis, further technological advancements have made percutaneous mitral valve therapy a reality.[37] Subsequently, percutaneous closure of paravalvular leaks after surgical valve implantation has shown potential, but at present

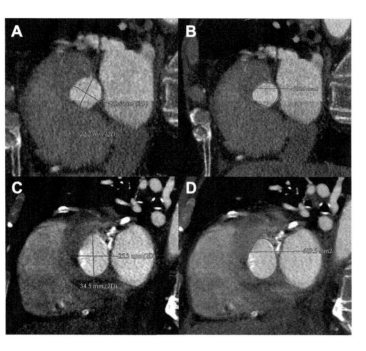

Fig. 7. Basal ring measurements of two patients being evaluated for TAVR. An 88-year-old woman with an annular measurement of 20 mm on TEE underwent an MDCT evaluation and was shown to have a mean basal ring measurement of 21.4 mm (A) (20.6 by 22.2) and an area of 3.80 cm² (B), and was subsequently implanted with a 23-mm Edwards prosthesis. In comparison, a 78-year-old man was shown to have a mean basal ring of 30 mm (25.3 by 34.5) (C) and an area of 6.90 cm² (D), concordant with the TTE measurement of 27 mm. Based on the large annular dimensions, the patient underwent TAVR with a 29-mm prosthesis via a transapical approach.

has a limited role.[37–41] Despite these advances, valvular mitral regurgitation (MR) remains almost exclusively the purview of surgery. Recently, the potential for less invasive percutaneous alternatives replicating these successful surgical procedures without the need for thoracotomy or cardiopulmonary bypass has generated considerable interest. For the most part, these new approaches are modeled after established surgical strategies.

Percutaneous approaches to mitral repair can be broadly divided into procedures that address the various components of the mitral valve. For the purposes of discussion, the mitral valve can be considered to have several component parts: leaflets, subvalvular apparatus (chordae tendinae and papillary muscles), annulus, left atrium, and left ventricle.[39] All are integral to the normal function of the mitral valve and each is a potential avenue for repair. The current status of various percutaneous therapies is presented in **Table 2**.[42,43]

Strategies for transcatheter mitral valve repair include (1) attempting to create a double-orifice mitral valve by using a percutaneous edge-to-edge technique with a clip device or stitch, (2) remodeling of the annulus of the mitral valve by suture-based techniques or application of radiofrequency energy, (3) remodeling of the mitral valvular and annular complex by transventricular and/or transatrial devices, and (4) decreasing mitral insufficiency by attempting to remodel the annulus of the mitral valve by devices implanted in the coronary sinus.

Coronary Sinus Annuloplasty

Mitral annuloplasty using an undersized ring is a routine component of surgical mitral valve repair.[40,41] Many percutaneous devices have attempted to reproduce the beneficial effects of surgical annuloplasty by taking advantage of the proximity of the coronary sinus to the mitral annulus.[42] The coronary sinus and its major tributary, the great cardiac vein, parallel the annulus of the mitral valve along its posterior and lateral aspect. The epicardial coronary venous system is readily accessible via a central venous puncture, as the confluence of the coronary sinus drains

Table 1 Proposed CT sizing			
	Valve Size Chosen		
CT Based	**23 mm**	**26 mm**	**29 mm**
Basal ring mean	≤22.5 mm	≤26.0 mm (short ≤29.5 mm, axis must be ≥18 mm)	—
Basal ring area (cm²)	≤4.3	<5.4	≤6.3

Table 2
Percutaneous MVR and new MVR technological advancements

Anatomic Site	Mechanism	Device	Stage of Development	Limitations
	MVR Technologies			
Leaflets	Edge-to-edge (leaflet plication)	MitraClip	Randomized trial data presented	Results when performed alone may not be durable. Possibility of iatrogenic MS
		MitraFlex	Preclinical development	As for MitraClip
	Space occupier (leaflet coaptation)	Percu-Pro	Phase I trial	Device thrombus formation. Residual MR or iatrogenic MS
Annulus	• CS approach (CS reshaping)	Monarc	Feasibility study ongoing	Position of the CS in relation to the annulus. Risk of compression of the left circumflex
		Carillon	Feasibility study complete	Same risks as above
		Vlacor	First in Man results Feasibility study ongoing	Same risks as above
	• Asymmetrical approach	St. Jude device	Animal models	CS at a distance from MA. Unequal tension on left atrium or MA. Device fracture or erosion, and thrombus formation
	Direct annuloplasty • Percutaneous mechanical cinching • Hybrid	Mitralign Recor Mitral solutions Micardia	First in Man results Preclinical development Preclinical development Preclinical development	Only posterior MA cinching As above Not true percutaneous technique As above
Chordal implants	Transapical • Artificial chord	Neochord, MitraFlex	Preclinical development	Residual leaflet prolapse or restriction with residual MR. Thrombus formation
	Transapical-transseptal • Artificial chord	Babic	Preclinical development	As above
LV	LV (and MA) remodeling	Mardil-BACE	Temporary human implant	Requires mini-thoracotomy. Long-term effects unknown

Abbreviations: CS, coronary sinus; LV, left ventricle; MA, mitral annulus; MR, mitral regurgitation; MS, mitral stenosis; MVR, mitral valve repair.

Data from Chiam PT, Ruiz CE. Technology percutaneous transcatheter mitral valve repair: a classification of the technology. J Am Coll Cardiol Interv 2011;4;1–13.

directly into the right atrium. Percutaneous approaches have generally used internal jugular or subclavian venous access to the right atrium to allow intubation of the coronary sinus. Various remodeling devices can be introduced into the coronary sinus, with the objective being to displace the adjacent posterior mitral annulus toward the anterior aspect of the annulus and thereby improve coaptation of the mitral leaflets.

The coronary sinus approach is an appealing one for many reasons, including the simplicity of the transvenous access and the use of fluoroscopic guidance. This technique is also fraught with significant limitations. Numerous imaging studies have demonstrated that branches of the circumflex artery travel deep to the great cardiac vein in more than one-half of patients.[44–51] Clinical experience has confirmed that coronary artery compression, ischemia, and infarction may occur,[48] and consequently preprocedural screening using noninvasive imaging may be required.

This approach is also limited by other anatomic variants. A nonreliable relationship of the great

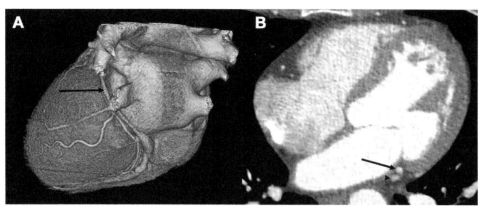

Fig. 8. A 3D volume-rendered image (*A*) and a transaxial image (*B*) of the heart and coronary sinus for evaluation for potential transcatheter mitral annuloplasty. Note that the coronary sinus overlies the atrium rather than the left atrioventricular groove. Also, the circumflex is deep to the great cardiac vein, suggesting a high risk for compromise and compression with a percutaneous coronary sinus device.

cardiac vein and coronary sinus with the annulus, with these venous structures typically lying on the atrial side of the annulus, has also been noted. Given these concerns, MDCT can provide useful information regarding the position and relationship of the coronary sinus, the mitral annulus, and coronary arteries (**Fig. 8**). Careful attention should be given not only to the relationship of the coronary sinus to the circumflex coronary but also to its position in relation to the annulus itself, because the success of the procedure depends on the coronary sinus overlying the annulus.

Mitral Clip Repair

Percutaneous edge-to-edge repair of the mitral valve[52] has gained momentum with recent multicenter trials. The phase I feasibility trial (EVEREST [The Efficacy of Vasopressin Antagonism in Heart Failure Outcome Study With Tolvaptan] I) included 55 patients with functional or degenerative MR grade 3 originating from central malcoaptation. In the 49 patients in whom a clip was implanted, MR grade was reduced to 2 in 42 patients (86%). This benefit seemed durable at 6 months. The ongoing EVEREST registry includes EVEREST I and nonrandomized (roll-in) EVEREST II patients. Clip implantation was successful in 89% of 104 patients, with MR grade reduced to 2 in 79 patients (76%). Success was associated with a sustained clinical benefit (improvement in New York Heart Association class in 73% at 1 year) and a reduction in left ventricular diameter. Therefore, 3D TEE and MDCT may be good complementary imaging modalities to accurately assess mitral valve anatomy, geometry, and function. In particular, 3D TEE permits accurate visualization of the

mitral valve apparatus before, during, and after the procedure and enables accurate selection of the therapeutic strategy, procedural guidance, and evaluation of the immediate results, which may improve the procedural success rate and minimize the number of complications of these novel therapeutic options.[52–57] During the procedure, fluoroscopy remains the mainstay imaging technique to guide the intervention. However, the poor soft-tissue contrast resolution of fluoroscopy does not permit accurate visualization of the mitral valvular apparatus.

Echocardiographic assessment prior to mitral clip repair requires accurate assessment of mitral leaflet morphology, including the presence of flail segments and regurgitant jet location. The regurgitant jet must arise from the central two-thirds of the line of coaptation. The leaflets must coapt over a length of at least 2 mm and over a depth of at least 11 mm. If flail segments are present, the gap must be less than 10 mm and the width less than 15 mm.[52]

Although CT has been explored in evaluation of the mitral valve, no studies that directly evaluate the preprocedural use of MDCT in the placement of the mitral clip device have been published.[52,53] In part, this may be because of the inferior temporal resolution of MDCT in comparison with echocardiography in the assessment of the dynamic nature of mitral valve dysfunction.

SUMMARY

Percutaneous management of valvular heart disease is becoming a reality, with multicenter trials supporting minimally invasive procedures for both aortic and mitral valve disease. Key to the success of percutaneous repair of mitral regurgitation or aortic stenosis is accurate preprocedural assessment of anatomy. MDCT has an established and expanding role in the setting of patient selection and planning of TAVR and percutaneous mitral annuloplasty, with its role in mitral clip placement yet to be defined.

REFERENCES

1. Nkomo VR, Gardin JM, Skelton TN, et al. Burden of valvular heart diseases. Lancet 2006;368:1005–11.
2. Bonow RO, Carabello BA, Kanu C, et al. ACC/AHA 2006 guidelines for the management of patients with valvular heart disease: a report of the American College of Cardiology/American Heart Association Task Force on Practice Guidelines (Writing Committee to Revise the 1998 Guidelines for the Management of Patients With Valvular Heart Disease): developed in collaboration with the Society of Cardiovascular Anesthesiologists: endorsed by the Society for Cardiovascular Angiography and Interventions and the Society of Thoracic Surgeons. J Am Coll Cardiol 2006;48:e1–148.
3. Iung B, Baron G, Butchart EG, et al. Prospective survey of patients with valvular heart disease in Europe. Eur Heart J 2003;24:1231–43.
4. Svensson LG, Dewey T, Kapadia S, et al. United States feasibility study of transcatheter insertion of a stented aortic valve by the left ventricular apex. Ann Thorac Surg 2008;86:46–55.
5. Walther T, Falk V, Kempfert J, et al. Transapical minimally invasive aortic valve implantation; the initial 50 patients. Eur J Cardiothorac Surg 2008; 33:983–8.
6. Grube E, Schuler G, Buellesfeld L, et al. Percutaneous aortic valve replacement for severe aortic stenosis in high-risk patients using the second- and current third-generation self-expanding CoreValve prosthesis: device success and 30-day clinical outcome. J Am Coll Cardiol 2007;50:69–76.
7. Webb JG, Pasupati S, Humphries K, et al. Percutaneous transarterial aortic valve replacement in selected high-risk patients with aortic stenosis. Circulation 2007;116:755–63.
8. Walther T, Simon P, Dewey T, et al. Transapical minimally invasive aortic valve implantation: multicenter experience. Circulation 2007;116:I240–5.
9. Leon MB, Smith CR, Mack M, et al. Transcatheter aortic-valve implantation for aortic stenosis in patients who cannot undergo surgery. N Engl J Med 2010;363(17):1597–607.
10. Smith CR, Leon MB, Mack MJ, et al. Transcatheter versus surgical aortic-valve replacement in high-risk patients. N Engl J Med 2011;364(23):2187–98.
11. Ye J, Cheung A, Lichtenstein SV, et al. Transapical aortic valve implantation in humans. J Thorac Cardiovasc Surg 2006;131:1194–6.
12. Grube E, Laborde JC, Gerckens U, et al. Percutaneous implantation of the CoreValve self-expanding valve prosthesis in high-risk patients with aortic valve disease: the Siegburg First-In-Man study. Circulation 2006;114:1616–24.
13. Al Ali AM, Altwegg L, Horlick EM, et al. Prevention and management of transcatheter balloon-expandable aortic valve malposition. Catheter Cardiovasc Interv 2008;72:573–8.
14. Tuzcu ME. Transcatheter aortic valve replacement malposition and embolization: innovation brings solutions also new challenges. Catheter Cardiovasc Interv 2008;72:579–80.
15. Thomas M, Schymik G, Walther T, et al. Thirty-day results of the SAPIEN aortic Bioprosthesis European Outcome (SOURCE) Registry: a European registry of transcatheter aortic valve implantation using the Edwards SAPIEN valve. Circulation 2010;122(1):62–9.
16. Van Mieghem NM, Nuis RJ, Piazza N, et al. Vascular complications with transcatheter aortic valve implantation using the 18 Fr Medtronic CoreValve System(R): the Rotterdam experience. EuroIntervention 2010;5:673–9.
17. Tchetche D, Dumonteil N, Sauguet A, et al. Thirty-day outcome and vascular complications after transarterial aortic valve implantation using both Edwards Sapien and Medtronic CoreValve bioprostheses in a mixed population. EuroIntervention 2010;5(6): 659–65.
18. Sharp AS, Michev I, Maisano F, et al. A new technique for vascular access management in transcatheter aortic valve implantation. Catheter Cardiovasc Interv 2010;75(5):784–93.
19. Leon M, Piazza N, Nikolsky E, et al. Standardized endpoint definitions for transcatheter aortic valve implantation clinical trials: a consensus report from the Valve Academic Research Consortium. J Am Coll Cardiol 2011;57:253–69.
20. Toggweiler, Leipsic J, Gurvitch R, et al. Improved vascular outcomes with a fully percutaneous procedure. JACC 2011, in press.
21. Kurra V, Schoenhagen P, Roselli EE, et al. Prevalence of significant peripheral artery disease in patients evaluated for percutaneous aortic valve insertion: preprocedural assessment with multidetector computed tomography. J Thorac Cardiovasc Surg 2009;137:1258–64.
22. Descoutures F, Himbert D, Lepage L, et al. Contemporary surgical or percutaneous management of severe aortic stenosis in the elderly. Eur Heart J 2008;29:1410–7.
23. Masson JB, Kovac J, Schuler G, et al. Transcatheter aortic valve implantation: review of the nature, management, and avoidance of procedural complications. JACC Cardiovasc Interv 2009;2:811–20.
24. Hayashida K, Lefevre T, Chevalier B, et al. Transfemoral aortic valve implantation new criteria to

predict vascular complications. JACC Cardiovasc Interv 2011;4:851–8.

25. Gurvitch R, Wood D, Leipsic J, et al. Multislice computed tomography for prediction of optimal angiographic deployment projections during transcatheter aortic valve implantation. JACC Cardiovasc Interv 2010;3(11):1157–65.

26. Kurra V, Kapadia S, Tuzcu M, et al. Pre-procedural imaging of aortic root orientation and dimensions comparison between X-ray angiographic planar imaging and 3-dimensional multidetector row computed tomography. JACC Cardiovasc Interv 2010;3:105–13.

27. Ng A, Delgado V, van der Kley F, et al. Comparison of aortic root dimensions and geometries before and after transcatheter aortic valve implantation by 2- and 3-dimensional transesophageal echocardiography and multislice computed tomography. Circ Cardiovasc Imaging 2010;3:94–102.

28. Tops LF, Wood DA, Delgado V, et al. Noninvasive evaluation of the aortic root with multislice computed tomography. Implications for transcatheter aortic valve replacement. J Am Coll Cardiol Img 2008;1: 321–30.

29. Anderson RH, Lal M, Ho SY. Anatomy of the aortic root with particular emphasis on options for its surgical enlargement. J Heart Valve Dis 1996; 5(Suppl 3):S249–57.

30. Messika-Zeitoun D, Serfaty JM, Brochet E, et al. Multimodal assessment of the aortic annulus diameter. J Am Coll Cardiol 2010;55:186–94.

31. Leipsic J, Gurvitch R, Labounty TM, et al. Multidetector computed tomography in transcatheter aortic valve implantation. JACC Cardiovasc Imaging 2011;4(4):416–29.

32. Delgado V, Ng AC, van de Veire NR, et al. Transcatheter aortic valve implantation: role of multi-detector row computed tomography to evaluate prosthesis positioning and deployment in relation to valve function. Eur Heart J 2010;31:1114–23.

33. Gurvitch R, Webb JG, Yuan R, et al. Aortic annulus diameter determination by multi-detector computed tomography: reproducibility, applicability and implications for transcatheter aortic valve implantation. JACC Interventions, in press.

34. Webb JG, Altwegg L, Boone RH, et al. Transcatheter aortic valve implantation: impact on clinical and valve-related outcomes. Circulation 2009;119(23):3009–16.

35. Wood DA, Tops LF, Webb JG, et al. Role of multislice computed tomography in transcatheter aortic valve replacement. Am J Cardiol 2009;103:1295–301.

36. Joshi S, Mendoza D, Steinberg D, et al. Ultra-low dose intra-arterial contrast injection for iliofemoral computed tomographic angiography. JACC Cardiovasc Imaging 2009;2:1404–11.

37. Inoue K, Owaki T, Nakamura T, et al. Clinical application of transvenous mitral commissurotomy by a new balloon catheter. J Thorac Cardiovasc Surg 1984;87: 394–402.

38. Pate GE, Al Zubaidi A, Chandavimol M, et al. Percutaneous closure of prosthetic paravalvular leaks: case series and review. Catheter Cardiovasc Interv 2006;68:528–33.

39. Pate GE, Thompson CR, Munt BI, et al. Techniques for percutaneous closure of prosthetic paravalvular leaks. Catheter Cardiovasc Interv 2006;67:158–66.

40. Hein R, Wunderlich N, Wilson N, et al. New concepts in transcatheter closure of paravalvular leaks. Future Cardiol 2008;4:373–8.

41. Perloff JK, Rogers WC. The mitral apparatus: functional anatomy of mitral regurgitation. Circulation 1972;46:227–39.

42. Chiam PT, Ruiz CE. Technology percutaneous transcatheter mitral valve repair: a classification of the technology. J Am Coll Cardiol Interv 2011;4:1–13.

43. Savage EB, Ferguson B Jr, DiSesa VJ. Use of mitral valve repair: analysis of contemporary United States experience reported to the Society of Thoracic Surgeons National Cardiac Database. Ann Thorac Surg 2003;75:820–5.

44. Bach DS, Bolling SF. Improvement following correction of secondary mitral regurgitation in end-stage cardiomyopathy with mitral annuloplasty. Am J Cardiol 1996;78:966–9.

45. Webb JG, Harnek J, Munt BI, et al. Percutaneous transvenous mitral annuloplasty: initial human experience with device implantation in the coronary sinus. Circulation 2006;113:851–5.

46. Maselli D, Guarracino F, Chiaramonti F, et al. Percutaneous mitral annuloplasty: an anatomic study of human coronary sinus and its relation with mitral valve annulus and coronary arteries. Circulation 2006;114:377–80.

47. Tops LF, Van de Veire NR, Schuijf JD, et al. Noninvasive evaluation of coronary sinus anatomy and its relation to the mitral valve annulus: implications for percutaneous mitral annuloplasty. Circulation 2007; 115:1426–32.

48. Choure AJ, Garcia MJ, Hesse B, et al. In vivo analysis of the anatomical relationship of coronary sinus to mitral annulus and left circumflex coronary artery using cardiac multidetector computed tomography: implications for percutaneous coronary sinus mitral annuloplasty. J Am Coll Cardiol 2006;48:1938–45.

49. Plass A, Valenta I, Gaemperli O, et al. Assessment of coronary sinus anatomy between normal and insufficient mitral valves by multi-slice computer tomography for mitral annuloplasty device implantation. Eur J Cardiothorac Surg 2008;33:583–9.

50. Sorgente A, Truong QA, Conca C, et al. Influence of left atrial and ventricular volumes on the relation between mitral valve annulus and coronary sinus. Am J Cardiol 2008;102:890–6.

51. Goldberg SL, Van Bibber R, Schofer J, et al. The frequency of coronary artery compression and management using a removable mitral annuloplasty device in the coronary sinus. J Am Coll Cardiol 2008; 51(10 Suppl B):28.

52. Feldman T, Wasserman HS, Herrmann HC, et al. Percutaneous mitral valve repair using the edge-to-edge technique: six-month results of the EVEREST phase I clinical trial. J Am Coll Cardiol 2005;46: 2134–40.

53. Swaans MJ, Van den Branden BJ, Van der Heyden JA, et al. Three-dimensional transoesophageal echocardiography in a patient undergoing percutaneous mitral valve repair using the edge-to-edge clip technique. Eur J Echocardiogr 2009;10:982–3.

54. Feldman T, Glower D. Patient selection for percutaneous mitral valve repair: insight from early clinical trial applications. Nat Clin Pract Cardiovasc Med 2008;5:84–90.

55. Willmann JK, Kobza R, Roos JE, et al. ECG-gated multidetector CT for assessment of mitral valve disease: initial experience. Eur Radiol 2002;12:2662–9.

56. Messika-Zeitoun D, Serfaty JM, Laissy JP, et al. Assessment of mitral valve area in patients with mitral stenosis by multislice computed tomography. J Am Coll Cardiol 2006;48:411–3.

57. Shanks M, Delgado V, Ng AC, et al. Mitral valve morphology assessment: three-dimensional transesophageal echocardiography versus computed tomography. Ann Thorac Surg 2010;90(6):1922–9.

Index

Note: Page numbers of article titles are in **boldface** type.

A

ACS. See Acute coronary syndrome (ACS)
Acute coronary syndrome (ACS)
  coronary CT in, **117–133**
    new imaging targets for, 124–126
    radiation dose in, 126–127
  defined, 117
  diagnosis of
    coronary CTA in
      accuracy of, 120–121
  pathophysiology of, 117–118
  symptoms of
    patients presenting to ED with
      diagnosis and management of, 118–120
Agatston calcium scoring
  prognostic value of coronary CTA in
    comparison with
      in symptomatic patients, 84
Age
  as factor in CAC, 21–23
Angiography
  CAC score as indication for
    contraindications to, 53
  conventional
    CAC on
      vs. fluoroscopy, 27, 31–32
  coronary CT. See Coronary computed
    tomographic angiography (CTA)
  subtraction coronary CT
    for calcified lesions, **147–156**. See also
      Subtraction coronary computed
      tomography angiography (CTA), for
      calcified lesions
Annuloplasty
  coronary sinus
    in mitral valve repair
      MDCT to guide, 155–157
Aortic calcification
  CAC and, 25, 27
Aortic dissection
  clinical presentation of, 103–104
  CT detection of, **103–108**
    CTA
      current issues related to, 108
      findings, 107
      imaging technique, 105–107
      pitfalls, 107–108

    recent advances in, 108
    strategies with, 105
  epidemiology of, 103–104
  imaging of
    modalities for
      diagnostic accuracies of, **103–108**. See also
      Aortic dissection, CT detection of
Aortic valve
  annular sizing of
    MDCT in, 151–154
Artifact(s)
  misregistration
    in subtraction coronary CTA, 100

C

CABG. See Coronary artery bypass graft (CABG)
CAC. See Coronary artery calcium (CAC)
CAC score. See Coronary artery calcium
  (CAC) score
CAD. See Coronary artery disease (CAD)
Calcification
  aortic
    CAC and, 25, 27
    CT-verified vulnerable plaque and, 71
Calcified lesions
  subtraction coronary CTA for, **147–156**. See also
    Subtraction coronary computed tomography
    angiography (CTA), for calcified lesions
Calcium
  coronary artery. See Coronary artery calcium
    (CAC)
Cardiac computed tomography (CT)
  in ED, **117–133**
    role of, 120–124
    for MACE during follow-up
      prognosis of, 121–124
  technical advances in, **1–8**
    future developments, 6–7
    hardware, 1–6
      dual-energy CT, 3, 6
      dual-source CT, 3
      historical development of, 1–2
      wide-detector CT, 2–3
    software, 6
Cardiac gating mode
  in reducing radiation dose in coronary
    CTA, 11–13

Cardiol Clin 30 (2012) 161–165
doi:10.1016/S0733-8651(12)00010-0
0733-8651/12/$ – see front matter © 2012 Elsevier Inc. All rights reserved

Moving?

Make sure your subscription moves with you!

To notify us of your new address, find your **Clinics Account Number** (located on your mailing label above your name), and contact customer service at:

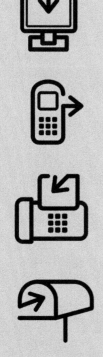

Email: journalscustomerservice-usa@elsevier.com

800-654-2452 (subscribers in the U.S. & Canada)
314-447-8871 (subscribers outside of the U.S. & Canada)

Fax number: 314-447-8029

Elsevier Health Sciences Division
Subscription Customer Service
3251 Riverport Lane
Maryland Heights, MO 63043

Printed and bound by CPI Group (UK) Ltd, Croydon, CR0 4YY

03/10/2024

01040357-0006